Laboratory Test	Normal Value*
albumin	3.5-5.2 g/dl
alkaline phosphatase	38-172 U/L
amylase	27-144 U/L
arterial P_{CO_2}	33-48 mm Hg
arterial pH	7.35-7.45
arterial P_{O_2}	70-100 mm Hg
bicarbonate (HCO_3)	24-31 mEq/L
bilirubin, direct (conjugated)	0.0-0.3 mg/dl
bilirubin, indirect (unconjugated)	0.1-0.7 mg/dl
bilirubin, total	0.1-1.0 mg/dl
blood urea nitrogen (BUN)	8-21 mg/dl
calcium (Ca)	8.9-10.2 mg/dl
chloride (Cl)	98-108 mEq/L
creatine phosphokinase (CPK)	30-285 U/L
creatinine (Cr)	0.3-1.2 mg/dl
erythrocyte sedimentation rate (ESR)	0-15 mm/hr
glucose (Glu)	62-125 mg/dl
hematocrit (HCT)	36-45% female, 38-50% male
lactate dehydrogenase (LDH)	0-190 U/L
lipase	7-51 U/L
mean corpuscular volume (MCV)	81-98 fl
osmolality (Osms)	280-300 mOsm/kg
platelets (PLT)	150,000-400,000/μl
potassium (K)	3.7-5.2 mEq/L
SGOT = AST	10-44 U/L
SGPT = ALT	11-39 U/L
sodium (Na)	136-145 mEq/L
uric acid	2.4-5.7 mg/dl female, 3.4-7.0 mg/dl male
white blood cell count (WBC)	4300-10,000/μl

*Normal values for the University of Washington Medical Center Laboratory

Fractional excretion of sodium:

$$FeNa = \frac{Cr^s \times Na^u}{Cr^u \times Na^s} \times 100$$

Creatinine clearance:

$$CrCl = \frac{(140 - age) \times ideal\ weight\ (kg)}{72 \times (serum\ creatinine)}$$

Osmolal gap:

Osm gap = (measured serum Osms) – (calculated Osms)

Osmolality:

Osm = 2(sodium) + BUN/2.8 + glucose/18

Free water deficit:

Free water deficit = [(serum sodium/140) – 1] × 0.6 × weight (kg)

Alveolar oxygen concentration, P_{AO_2}:

$$P_{AO_2} = F_{IO_2}\ (P_B - 47) - P_{CO_2}/0.8$$
$$= approximately\ 100\ at\ sea\ level\ with\ normal\ P_{CO_2}$$

Where: P_B = atmospheric pressure = 760 mm Hg at sea level
F_{IO_2} = fraction of inspired oxygen = 0.21 at sea level
P_{aO_2} = arterial oxygen concentration = blood gas P_{O_2}
P_{CO_2} = arterial carbon dioxide concentration

Alveolar-arterial oxygen gradient, A-a gradient:

A-a gradient = P_{AO_2} – P_{aO_2}

CLERKSHIP GUIDES

Your Essential Guide to Clinical Clerkships

All you need to succeed:

- Practice Cases
- Frequently Asked Questions
- Key Points
- Practice Exam

Other Titles in the *Clerkship Guides* Series

Manley:
Psychiatry Clerkship Guide

Adams:
Surgery Clerkship Guide

Woodhead:
Pediatrics Clerkship Guide

Forthcoming:
Obstetrics and Gynecology Clerkship Guide

INTERNAL MEDICINE CLERKSHIP GUIDE *Second Edition*

Douglas S. Paauw, MD, FACP

Professor of Medicine
Division of General Internal Medicine
Coordinator for Student Teaching
Rathman Family Foundation
Endowed Chair for Patient-Centered Clinical Education
Department of Medicine
University of Washington School of Medicine
Seattle, Washington

Lisanne R. Burkholder, MD, MPH

Assistant Clinical Professor
Division of General Internal Medicine
Associate Program Director
Primary Care Internal Medicine Residency
University of California, San Francisco, School of Medicine
San Francisco, California

Mary B. Migeon, MD

Assistant Professor
Division of General Internal Medicine
Department of Medicine
University of Washington School of Medicine
Seattle, Washington

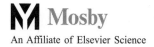

Mosby

An Affiliate of Elsevier Science

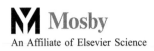
An Affiliate of Elsevier Science

11830 Westline Industrial Drive
St. Louis, Missouri 63146

INTERNAL MEDICINE CLERKSHIP GUIDE   ISBN 0–323–01708–8

Notice

Medicine is an ever-changing field. Standard safety precautions must be followed, but as new research and clinical experience broaden our knowledge, changes in treatment and drug therapy may become necessary or appropriate. Readers are advised to check the most current product information provided by the manufacturer of each drug to be administered to verify the recommended dose, the method and duration of administration, and the contraindications. It is the responsibility of the treating physician, relying on experience and knowledge of the patient, to determine the dosages and the best treatment for each individual patient. Neither the publisher nor the editor assumes any liability for any injury and/or damage to persons or property arising from this publication.

The Publisher

First Edition 1999

Library of Congress Cataloging-in-Publication Data

Internal medicine clerkship guide / [edited by] Douglas S. Paauw, Lisanne R. Burkholder, Mary B. Migeon.–2nd ed.
     p. cm.
  Previously published: Guide to internal medicine. 1st ed. St. Louis: Mosby, 1999.
  ISBN 0-323-01708-8
    1. Internal medicine. 2. Clinical clerkship. I. Paauw, Douglas S. (Douglas Stephen). II. Burkholder, Lisanne R. III. Migeon, Mary B. IV. Guide to internal medicine.
RC46 .G896 2003
616–dc21   2002026456

Acquisitions Editor: William Schmitt
Developmental Editor: Antony Galbraith
Design Coordinator: Gene Harris

KI/QWF

Printed in the United States of America.

Last digit is the print number: 9 8 7 6 5 4 3 2 1

To

Kathy and Carly

Blaine

Jacques, Sophie, and Jonathan

In memory of

George Aagaard and Andrew Epstein

Contributors

Bradley D. Anawalt, MD
Associate Professor
Department of Medicine
University of Washington School of Medicine
Assistant Chief of Medicine
VA Medical Center
Puget Sound
Seattle, Washington

Amy Baernstein, MD
Clinical Instructor
General Internal Medicine
University of Washington School of Medicine
Attending Physician
Emergency Trauma Center
Harborview Medical Center
Seattle, Washington

Robert Baron, MD, MS
Professor
Department of Medicine
Associate Dean for Continuing Medical Education
University of California, San Francisco, School of Medicine
San Francisco, California

Ernie-Paul Barrette, MD, FACP
Assistant Professor
Department of Medicine
Case Western Reserve University School of Medicine
Attending Physician
Metrohealth Medical Center
Cleveland, Ohio

Preetha Basaviah, MD
Assistant Clinical Professor of Medicine
Co-Director, Foundations of Patient Care Course
Moffitt Hospital
Department of Medicine
University of California, San Francisco, School of Medicine
San Francisco, California

Clarence H. Braddock III, MD, MPH
Associate Professor
Associate Chair
Department of Medicine
University of Washington School of Medicine
Seattle, Washington

Janis D. Bridge, MD, MPH
Assistant Professor
Division of General Internal Medicine
Department of Medicine
University of Washington School of Medicine
Seattle, Washington

Sarah L. Clever, MD
Fellow
Robert Wood Johnson Clinical Scholars Program
University of Chicago
Chicago, Illinois

Debra D. Dahlen, MD
Acting Instructor
Department of Medicine
Division of Hematology
University of Washington School of Medicine
Attending Physician
Division of Hematology
Seattle Cancer Care Alliance
Research Fellow
Puget Sound Blood Center and Program
Seattle, Washington

Dawn E. DeWitt, MD, MSC
Associate Professor
Director, WWAMI Regional Community-Based Education in
    Internal Medicine
Attending Physician
Department of Medicine
Adjunct Associate Professor
Department of Medical Education
University of Washington School of Medicine
Seattle, Washington

Keith D. Eaton, MD, PhD
Fellow
Division of Oncology
Department of Medicine
University of Washington School of Medicine
Seattle, Washington

Kelly Fryer-Edwards, PhD
Assistant Professor
Department of Medical History and Ethics
University of Washington School of Medicine
Seattle, Washington

Gregory C. Gardner, MD
Associate Professor
Department of Medicine
Division of Rheumatology
Adjunct Associate Professor of Rehabilitation and Orthopaedics
University of Washington School of Medicine
Seattle, Washington

Barak Gaster, MD
Assistant Professor
Department of Medicine
University of Washington School of Medicine
Seattle, Washington

Karna Gendo, MD
Clinical Instructor
Department of Emergency Services
Harborview Medical Center
Seattle, Washington

Bruce Gilliland, MD, FACP
Professor
Department of Medicine
Professor of Laboratory Medicine
Adjunct Professor of Microbiology
University of Washington School of Medicine
Seattle, Washington

Deborah L. Greenberg, MD
Assistant Professor
Department of Medicine
Division of General Internal Medicine
University of Washington School of Medicine
Seattle, Washington

Karen E. Hauer, MD
Assistant Clinical Professor
Director of Internal Medicine Clerkship
Department of Medicine
University of California, San Francisco, School of Medicine
San Francisco, California

John B. Holroyd, MD
Department of Internal Medicine
Madrona Medical Group
Bellingham, Washington

Robert R. Kempainen, MD
Senior Fellow
Department of Medicine
Division of Pulmonary and Critical Care
University of Washington School of Medicine
Seattle, Washington

Eric E. Kraus, MD
Assistant Professor
Department of Neurology
University of Washington School of Medicine
Seattle, Washington

Uri Ladabaum, MD, MS
Assistant Clinical Professor
Department of Medicine
University of California, San Francisco, School of Medicine
San Francisco, California

Mary B. Laya, MD, MPH
Assistant Professor
Department of Medicine
Division of General Internal Medicine
University of Washington School of Medicine
Seattle, Washington

George Novan, MD
Clinical Associate Professor of Medicine
Department of Medicine
University of Washington School of Medicine
Seattle, Washington
Clerkship Coordinator
Internal Medicine Residency Program
Sacred Heart Medical Center and Deaconess Medical Center
Spokane, Washington

Craig Pepin, MD
Senior Fellow
Department of Medicine
Division of Gastroenterology
University of California, San Francisco, School of Medicine
San Francisco, California

Linda Pinsky, MD
Associate Professor
Department of Medicine
Division of General Internal Medicine
Adjunct Associate Professor of Medical Education
    and Family Medicine
University of Washington School of Medicine
Seattle, Washington

Mark J. Pletcher, MD, MPH
Clinical Research Fellow
Department of Medicine
Division of General Internal Medicine
University of California, San Francisco, School of Medicine
San Francisco, California

Heidi S. Powell, MD
Assistant Professor
Department of Medicine
Division of General Internal Medicine
University of Washington School of Medicine
Seattle, Washington

Caroline S. Rhoads, MD
Assistant Professor of Medicine
Department of Medicine
Division of Infectious Diseases
University of Washington School of Medicine
Associate Director
Adult Medicine Clinic
Harborview Medical Center
Seattle, Washington

Henry Rosen, MD
Professor and Associate Chair
Department of Medicine
Division of Infectious Diseases
University of Washington School of Medicine
Seattle, Washington

Alexander D. Schafir, MD
Clinical Assistant Professor
Oregon Health Sciences University
Providence St. Vincent Medical Center
Portland, Oregon

John V. L. Sheffield, MD
Associate Professor of Medicine
Department of Medicine
University of Washington School of Medicine
Assistant Chief
Harborview Medical Center
Seattle, Washington

C. Scott Smith, MD, FACP
Associate Professor
Department of Medicine and Medical Education
University of Washington School of Medicine
Seattle, Washington
Co-Director
Northwest Regional Faculty Development Center
VA Medical Center
Boise, Idaho

Contributors

Thomas O. Staiger, MD
Associate Professor of Medicine
Department of Medicine
University of Washington School of Medicine
Associate Medical Director for Quality Improvement
   and Risk Management
University of Washington Medical Center
Seattle, Washington

Eliza L. Sutton, MD
Assistant Professor of Medicine
Department of Medicine
University of Washington School of Medicine
Seattle, Washington

Daryl Thornton, MD, MPH
Senior Fellow
Department of Pulmonary and Critical Care
University of Washington School of Medicine
Seattle, Washington

Jeffrey I. Wallace, MD, MPH
Associate Professor and Director of Clinical Geriatrics
University of Colorado School of Medicine
Denver, Colorado

Emily Y. Wong, MD
Assistant Professor
Department of Medicine
Division of General Internal Medicine
University of Washington School of Medicine
Seattle, Washington

Preface

Internal Medicine Clerkship Guide aims to aid and accompany third-year medical students in that all important transition from book learning to the real world practicing of medicine. We present core concepts of internal medicine in a purposefully brief format to allow cover-to-cover reading during the medicine clerkship. Our goal is to help the third-year clerk have a solid foundation of knowledge on which future detailed reading and study may be built. Although targeted for third-year students, as the guide has evolved we have received positive feedback about its utility for learners and educators in other fields including those in Physician's Assistant, Nursing, Nurse Practitioner, and Family Practice residency training programs.

Internal Medicine Clerkship Guide is divided into three sections covering basic skills, common symptoms, and common conditions. The text is structured around basic questions frequently asked by students and instructors to keep the learner engaged and to keep the learning practical. *Key Points* in each chapter help learners focus on core concepts. *Cases* apply new learning to real clinical scenarios. *Learning objectives* accompany answers to each case-based problem and emphasize common internal medicine problems. A *multiple-choice exam* at the end of the guide tests the mastery of the material and prepares learners for clinical and board exams.

We sincerely hope that *Internal Medicine Clerkship Guide* helps students enjoy the process of learning and mastering the basic concepts and skills of internal medicine.

Douglas S. Paauw, MD
Lisanne R. Burkholder, MD
Mary B. Migeon, MD

Acknowledgments

We would like to thank Laura Jewett for invaluable administrative assistance in preparing the manuscript, our contributors for their timely and excellent efforts, D. C. Dugdale and Dawn DeWitt for sage advice about the world of publishing, and Michael Richardson for enthusiastic and generous sharing of his extensive radiologic website resources. We also appreciate the indispensable support of the Divisions of General Medicine at both the University of Washington Medical Center and the University of California, San Francisco. Finally, we would like to thank our students, who inspire us with their enthusiasm and whose thoughtful feedback helped shape this book.

Contents

Contents

Section 3 Patients Presenting with a Known Condition

Abbreviation Terms

A1C	glycosylated hemoglobin	ATN	acute tubular necrosis
ABG	arterial blood gas	AVA	American Urology Association
ABI	ankle/brachial index	AVNRT	AV node reentrant tachycardia
ACEI	angiotensin-converting enzyme inhibitor	AZT	zidovudine (azidothymidine)
ACIP	Advisory Committee on Immunization Practice	BCC	basal cell carcinoma
		β-HCG	beta human chorionic gonadotropin
ACTH	adrenocorticotropic hormone	BMI	body mass index
		BP	blood pressure
AFB	acid-fast bacillus	BPH	benign prostatic hyperplasia
AFP	alpha-fetoprotein		
AIDS	acquired immune deficiency syndrome	BPV	benign positional vertigo
		BUN	blood urea nitrogen
AIN	acute interstitial nephritis	BV	bacterial vaginosis
		CABG	coronary artery bypass graft
ALL	acute lymphocytic leukemia		
		CAD	coronary artery disease
ALT	alanine aminotransaminase (same as SGPT)	cANCA	cytoplasmic antineutrophil cytoplasmic antibody
ANA	antinuclear antibody	CBC	complete blood count
Anti LKM1	antibody to liver, kidney microsome type 1	CCU	cardiac care unit
		CDC	Centers for Disease Control
APAS	antiphospholipid antibody	CEA	carcinoembryonic antigen
AR	aortic regurgitation	CFS	chronic fatigue syndrome
ARF	acute renal failure		
AS	aortic stenosis	CHF	congestive heart failure
ASCUS	atypical cells of undetermined significance	CIE	counter immuno-electrophoresis
		CK	creatine kinase
ASIS	anterior superior iliac spine	CLL	chronic lymphocytic leukemia
AST	aspartate amino-transaminase (same as SGOT)	CML	chronic myelogenous leukemia

Abbreviations

CMV	cytomegalovirus	DXA scan	dual electron x-ray absorptiometry, bone density test
CNS	central nervous system	EBV	Epstein-Barr virus
COPD	chronic obstructive pulmonary disease	ED	emergency department
CP	creatine phosphokinase	EEG	electroencephalogram
CPAP	continuous positive airway pressure	EF	ejection fraction
CPK	creatine phosphokinase	EGD	esophagogastroduodenoscopy
CPR	cardiopulmonary resuscitation	EMG	electromyogram
CR	complete remission	EOMI	extraocular movements intact
CRH	corticotropin-releasing hormone	ERCP	endoscopic retrograde cholangiopancreatogram
CSF	cerebrospinal fluid	ERT	estrogen replacement therapy
CT	computed tomography	ESR	erythrocyte sedimentation rate
CV	cardiovascular	ETT	exercise tolerance test exercise treadmill test
CXR	chest x-ray		
d4T	stavudine		
DCCT	Diabetes Control and Complications Trial	FAP	familial adenomatous polyposis
DDAVP	1-deamino(8-D-arginine) vasopressin	FMP	first menstrual period
ddC	zalcitabine	FNA	fine needle aspiration
ddI	didanosine	FSH	follicle stimulating hormone
DGI	disseminated gonococcal infection	FTA-ABS	fluorescent treponemal antibody absorption (test)
DHT	dihydrotestosterone		
DIC	disseminated intravascular coagulation	GE	gastroesophageal reflux
DKA	diabetic ketoacidosis	GERD	gastroesophageal reflux disease
DLCO	diffusing lung capacity to carbon monoxide	GGT	serum gamma-glutamyltransferase
DM	diabetes mellitus (type 1 or 2)	GI	gastrointestinal
DMARD	disease modifying antirheumatic drug	GYN	gynecologic gynecology
DNR	do not resuscitate	H&P	history and physical
DUB	dysfunctional uterine bleeding	HAART	highly active antiretroviral therapy
DVT	deep venous thrombosis		
Dx	diagnosis		

Abbreviations

HbsAG	hepatitis b surface antigen	IBD	inflammatory bowel disease
HBV	hepatitis B virus	IBS	irritable bowel syndrome
HCM	hypertrophic cardiomyopathy	ICU	intensive care unit
HCT	hematocrit	ID/CC	identification and chief complaint
HCV	hepatitis C virus	IDU	injection drug user
HDV	hepatitis D virus	IL-RA	interleukin/receptor agonist
HEENT	head, eyes, ears, nose, and throat	INH	isoniazid
HEV	hepatitis E virus	INR	international normalized ratio, a standardized prothrombin time
HF	hot flash	ITP	immune thrombocytic purpura
HGSIL	high grade squamous intraepithelial lesion	IVDU	intravenous drug user
HHNC	hyperglycemic hyperosmolar nonketotic (diabetic) coma	IVIG	intravenous immunoglobulin
HIT	heparin-induced thrombocytopenia	JVP	jugular venous pressure
HITT	HIT-associated thrombosis	KOH	potassium hydroxide
HIV	human immunode-ficiency virus	KS	Kaposi's sarcoma
HMG CoA	3-hydroxy-3-methylglutaryl coenzyme A	LCR	ligase chain reaction
		LDH	lactate dehydrogenase
HNPCC	hereditary nonpolyposis colorectal cancer	LE	leukocyte esterase
		LEEP	loop electrical excision procedure
HPI	history of present illness	LFTs	liver function tests
HPV	human papillomavirus	LGSIL	low grade squamous intraep-ithelial lesion
HRT	hormone replacement therapy	LH	luteinizing hormone
		LHRH	luteinizing hormone-releasing factor
HSCT	hematopoietic stem cell transplantation	LLQ	left lower quadrant
		LMW	low molecular weight
		LMWH	low-molecular-weight heparin
HSP	Henoch-Schönlein purpura	LOC	level of consciousness
HSV	herpes simplex virus	LP	lumbar puncture
		LV	left ventricle
HTLV	human T-cell leukemia/lymphoma virus	LVF	left ventricular failure
		LVH	left ventricular hypertrophy

Abbreviations

MAC	*Mycobacterium avium* complex	OSA	obstructive sleep apnea
MCA	middle cerebral artery	PA (view)	posteroanterior
MCP	metacarpophalangeal	PAC	premature atrial contractions
MCV	mean corpuscular volume	PAN	polyarteritis nodosa
MEN-2	multiple endocrine neoplasia syndrome	PANCA	perinuclear antineutrophil cytoplasmic antibody
MI	myocardial infarction		
MMR	measles, mumps, rubella	PCOS	polycystic ovary syndrome
MP	micronized progesterone	PCP	*Pneumocystis carinii* pneumonia
MPAN	microscopic polyarteritis nodosa	PCR	polymerase chain reaction
MR	mitral regurgitation	PE	pulmonary embolus
MRI	magnetic resonance imaging	PEEP	positive end expiratory pressure
MSH	melanocytic stimulating hormone	PERRLA	pupils equal, round, reactive to light and accommodation
MSLT	multiple sleep latency test		
MTP	metatarsophalangeal	PET	positron emission tomography
MVA	motor vehicle accident		
Na	sodium	PHN	postherpetic neuralgia
NCEP	National Cholesterol Education Program	PI	protease inhibitors
NG	nasogastric	PID	pelvic inflammatory disease
NHL	non-Hodgkin's lymphoma	PLMD	periodic leg movement disorder
NIPPV	noninvasive positive pressure ventilation	PMH	past medical history
NNRTI	non-nucleoside reverse transcriptase inhibitors	PMI	point of maximal impulse (of the heart against the chest wall)
NOF	National Osteoporosis Foundation		
NPH	no previous history	PMN	polymorphonuclear, neutrophil (leukocytes)
NPO	nothing by mouth	PMR	polymyalgia rheumatica
NPV	negative predictive value	PN	peripheral neuropathy
NRTI	nucleoside reverse transcriptase inhibitors	PND	postnasal drip or paroxysmal nocturnal dyspnea
NSAID	nonsteroidal anti-inflammatory drug	PPD	packs per day (cigarettes)
NSCLC	non-small cell lung cancer	PPI	proton pump inhibitor
OCP	oral contraceptive pill		

Abbreviations

PPV	positive predictive value	SIADH	syndrome of antidiuretic hormone secretion
PSA	prostate specific antigen		
PSC	primary sclerosing cholangitis	SLE	systemic lupus erythematosus
PSG	polysomnogram	SMBG	self-monitoring blood glucose
PT	prothrombin time		
PTA	prior to admission	SPEP	serum protein electrophoresis
PTH	parathyroid hormone		
PTT	partial thromboplastin time	SS-A	Sjögren's syndrome antigen A
PTU	propylthiouracil	SS-B	Sjögren's syndrome antigen B
PUD	peptic ulcer disease		
PVC	premature ventricular contractions	SSRI	selective serotonin reuptake inhibitor
PVD	peripheral vascular disease	SVT	supraventricular tachycardia
PVR	postvoid residual	T	temperature
RA	radionuclide angiography	TA	temporal arteritis
	rheumatoid arthritis	TB	tuberculosis
		TC	total cholesterol
RAS	reticular activating system	TCA	tricyclic antidepressant
RBC	red blood cells	TEE	transesophageal echocardiography
RF	rheumatoid factor		
RLQ	right lower quadrant	TG	triglycerides
RLS	restless leg syndrome	TIA	transient ischemic attack
RNA	ribonucleic acid		
ROM	range of motion	TIBC	total iron-binding capacity
ROS	review of systems		
RPR	rapid plasma reagin	TIPS	transjugular intrahepatic portosystemic shunt
RR	respiratory rate		
RUQ	right upper quadrant		
SAAG	serum-ascites albumin gradient	TLC	total lung capacity
SAH	subarachnoid hemorrhage	TMP-SMX	trimethoprim sulfamethoxazole
SBE	subacute bacterial endocarditis	tPA	tissue plasminogen activator
SBP	spontaneous bacterial peritonitis	TSH	thryroid-stimulating hormone
SCLC	small cell lung cancer	TTE	transthoracic echocardiography
SERMs	selective estrogen receptor modulators	TURP	transurethral resection of the prostate
SGOT	serum glutamic-oxaloacetic transaminase (AST)	TWAR	Taiwan acute respiratory

Abbreviations

U/S	ultrasound	VS	vital signs
UA	urinalysis	VT	ventricular tachycardia
UBT	urea breath test	Vwd	von Willebrand's
UPEP	urinary protein electrophoresis		disease
		WBC	white blood cell/count
URI	upper respiratory infection	WOB	work of breathing
UTI	urinary tract infection		
VDRL	Venereal Disease Research Laboratory (a test for syphilis)		

Introduction to the Medicine Clerkship

1

Secrets to Being a Successful Medical Student

Medicine is not a trade to be learned but a profession to be entered. It is an ever-widening field that requires continued study and prolonged experience in close contact with the sick. All that the medical school can hope to do is to supply the foundations on which to build.

Francis W. Peabody, 1927

What can I do to be successful in the internal medicine clerkship?

Within the lecture hall, success is often defined by grades. As you enter the clinical years, performance evaluations remain very important, but you must also define personal goals and definitions of success that are more broad than pass/fail. In the medicine clerkship, you may hope to learn how to provide excellent patient care, develop your history-taking and physical examination skills, improve your presentations, acquire time management skills, and become a careful diagnostician. In addition to building these important clinical skills, a vital measure of success is the degree to which you build a foundation of professionalism in your work habits, behavioral attributes, and values as a caretaker and colleague. In these introductory pages, the suggestions made are based on extensive experience in working with students and will hopefully help you excel in the clerkship and enjoy the experience.

Be enthusiastic

Your energy level, desire to learn, and spirit will motivate your residents and attendings to teach and involve you in patient care. With enthusiasm, a student with an average knowledge base can provide fantastic care and be a vital team member. Without enthusiasm, a brilliant student will appear disinterested and be a less effective team member and physician.

Know your patients

An excellent student has complete and timely command of a patient's history, physical exam, and lab test results, strives to understand basic pathophysiological principles underlying patient conditions, is aware of diagnostic and therapeutic options available, and seeks to understand the personal and social factors that may influence his or her patient's response to therapy.

Care about your patients

Assume personal responsibility for the quality of care your patients receive. Monitor their progress closely, and spend time at the bedside to answer questions and discuss matters other than symptoms. Although team hierarchy gives residents and attendings precedence, your patients will view you as their primary physician if you establish a caring rapport.

Communicate with precision

Your chart notes and oral presentations are your opportunity to demonstrate your fund of knowledge, problem solving skills, and ability to think clearly. Legible and precise order writing is essential to good patient care. Careful explanation of the treatment plan to nursing staff will ensure that your intended plan is followed.

Distinguish between major and minor problems

As important as being able to identify all of your patient's problems is the ability to put major and minor problems in perspective. At first, it is natural to consider all problems important, but time constraints make it essential that you prioritize when presenting cases and planning your workday. Attend to all of your patient's issues, but keep a steady focus on the big picture, and you will be able to budget time more efficiently and manage patients more effectively.

Acknowledge your knowledge deficits and seek guidance whenever necessary

At the beginning of the clerkship, you are not expected to know much about taking care of patients. When you encounter uncertainty, take note of it and do not try to hide it from others. Seek guidance from housestaff, nurses, attendings, patients, therapists, and reading. Don't judge yourself harshly. Instead, get excited to learn something new. Your patients will benefit greatly from your honesty about what you don't know.

Develop sound reading habits to use throughout your career

It is impossible to know everything, but it's a good idea to avoid being ignorant about the same thing twice. Each day, keep a list of things you don't understand and read about them later. You may be amazed by how much you retain when the material you read is relevant to your patients.

Behave professionally

It is expected that you will approach patients with empathy and respect their individual dignity and confidentiality. Strive to be cooperative, patient, and attentive at all times, even with difficult persons. It is a privilege to care for fellow human beings. When in doubt treat others as you would have them treat you or your family.

Be a team player

Medical care is provided by professionals from multiple disciplines who share the common goal of serving the patient. To contribute, you must understand the special role of nurses, therapists, and pharmacists and utilize them appropriately. Strong team spirit can motivate you to provide excellent care in spite of fatigue and stress. Earn respect by being respectful.

Work well with nurses

Nurses spend their entire day at your patient's bedside and can provide valuable insight into patient progress. Experienced nurses know a lot about patient assessment and ways to provide comfort. Some students find this intimidating and treat nurses unpleasantly. It is far preferable to acknowledge nursing expertise openly and try to learn from the suggestions made.

Strike a healthy balance between medicine and personal life

Sleep, exercise, good food, and leisure activities with family and friends are vital to your soul. To sustain your energy and focus at the hospital, you must attend to your personal happiness. A healthy balance in your life can help you cope with the anxiety of adapting to your new role and responsibilities and to accept this challenge eagerly. If all goes well on the rotation, you will glimpse the profound satisfaction available to those who care for the sick and gain insight into the kind of doctor you want to become.

2

Day-to-Day Inpatient Skills

What are a student's responsibilities on a ward team?

On the inpatient wards, your primary responsibility is being the team's "expert" on all patients you admit and actively participating in all aspects of their care. In addition to knowing everything about your patients (and always having patient data readily available), you should write all but emergent orders (co-signed by housestaff or attending), represent and speak for your team wherever your patients are discussed, complete chart notes in timely fashion, perform procedures with appropriate supervision, and contribute to all diagnostic and treatment planning. You may also be asked to research interesting aspects of your patients' cases and teach the team during rounds. In addition, you should pay attention on rounds in order to learn from all patients on the team, and you should be ready and willing to help care for any patient as necessary. Finally, students can be a very important source of energy, enthusiasm, curiosity, and fresh humanitarian spirit for their teams. This energy is often crucial to team morale.

Do I need to pre-round?

Yes! The workday officially begins with work rounds at which time the team sets a plan for the day for each patient. Prior to work rounds, you should pre-round, which consists of reviewing chart notes (for new consult recommendations and acute events overnight) and vital signs, doing a directed physical exam, and checking labs. Allow ten to fifteen minutes per patient and be ready to start work rounds on time.

How much information should I gather in the history and physical?

Your H & P should be complete on every patient you admit. Outstanding physicians take excellent histories and possess superior physical examination skills. The history provides information to make most diagnoses, and optimal patient care depends on the accuracy of this information and the strength of the doctor-patient relationship created in the process. With practice and repetition, you will gain confidence in your ability to identify your patients' problems and become more efficient, although the medicine clerkship is not a place to cut corners.

What is a good presentation?

Many students approach case presentations as if their primary purpose was student evaluation. Actually, the main objective of the presentation is to convey the essentials of the patient's illness to team members so that all can learn and participate in subsequent discussions of management. This requires more than a simple recitation of what a patient told you, but rather a critical analysis of the information to produce a clear assessment and plan. At the end of a good presentation, your team should understand a patient's most pressing issues and your plan to address them. Anticipate questions. Attributes of good work rounds presentations include:

- **Brevity:** the goal is three to five minutes for a new patient (less for daily progress reports). At first, you will need to learn from your resident what information is appropriate; you only have time for crucial details. Expect questions and leave time for them.
- **Organization:** practice on your on-call day. Don't freelance. People expect to hear information presented in a certain order. Disorganization creates confusion.
- **Eye contact:** engage your team and they will listen. Presenting from memory greatly enhances your ability to achieve this goal. Never, ever, read from your H & P.

What should I include in my write-ups?

Of all the notes in your patient's chart, yours should be the most complete. Initial write-ups generally average three to six pages and should succinctly review the history, exam, labs, diagnostic reasoning, and plan. To avoid common pitfalls, pay attention to the following:

- **Chronology:** use day of admission as a consistent point of reference ("3 days prior to admission [PTA], she noticed chest pain. One day PTA, she noted shortness of breath")
- **Pertinent negatives:** include at the end of the HPI to reflect the differential diagnosis
- **Abbreviations:** use only familiar abbreviations; write everything else out
- **Organization:** use a bulleted outline for patient medical history (PMH), medications, exam, and plan, so details can be found at a glance
- **Completeness:** describe physical findings completely; be attentive to detail

How do I write a good Assessment and Plan?

The Assessment and Plan section is probably the source of greatest confusion for most students. It's actually quite simple. First, state the problem (diagnosis, symptom, sign, or lab result). Second, give a realistic differential diagnosis for that problem. Third, state which diagnosis is most likely and why others are not, incorporating data from your H&P. Finally, for each problem list the diagnostic and therapeutic plan so that readers can rapidly find and review your plan. By following this formula, you will avoid the two most common mistakes:

- **Don't ramble:** rambling assessments that regurgitate textbook differentials and pathophysiology reflect poor synthesis of information and are not relevant to the case
- **Don't be too brief:** very brief assessments reflect poor understanding of the differential diagnosis and rationale for evaluation and treatment

What should I try to learn when reading about my patients?

In order to monitor your patients effectively and contribute to diagnostic and therapeutic decision-making, begin by reviewing the following information:

- **Differential diagnosis:** for common presenting conditions
- **Pathophysiology:** disease processes of the major diagnoses in your patients
- **Typical signs and symptoms:** for the major conditions in the differential diagnosis
- **Diagnostic algorithm:** rationale for tests, sequence of testing, cost, and potential ramifications of test results on therapeutic options
- **Treatment algorithm:** rationale for choosing treatment options including efficacy, cost
- **Drug therapy:** side effects/toxicities, drug interactions, and convenience

Which reading sources are most useful?

Anything you read in the attempt to provide excellent patient care will be better retained than information reviewed out of context, but different sources have different attributes. *Syllabus/spiral-bound manuals* provide concise reviews with practical management advice. *Texts* are strong on pathophysiology and typical disease signs and symptoms, but can be out of date regarding work-up and therapy. *Online texts* are updated frequently and often contain more practical and timely information. *Medline* is a comprehensive guide to the medical literature. Being able to construct a literature search to answer a clinical question is an essential skill, but be sure that the articles you find are relevant to your patient.

3

Day-to-Day Outpatient Skills

How do I prioritize the outpatient visit?

Whereas inpatients often have a single problem leading to hospitalization, outpatients usually present several issues for you to address in a brief period of time. Often you will not have time to deal with every issue and must determine which to address in a single visit. Each visit should begin with an attempt to set an agenda for that visit. Before entering the room, review the problem list and set some goals. When you see the patient, ask what goals they have: "What are your concerns today?" After you have heard the patient's list, try to cover key management goals, special patient concerns, and avoid overlooking potentially serious new problems. You may respond: "Those are a lot of important issues. Let's cover your blood pressure and sore leg today. We probably won't have time to discuss the chronic shoulder pain, but let's do that carefully next time, okay?"

What is an appropriate exam?

Your exam should address the problems of the day. For a patient with a sore throat, vital signs, a good HEENT, neck, and lung exam should suffice. A complete exam is generally done only with new patients, those with vague or troubling symptoms, and when patients request it specifically.

What should I present to my attending?

In clinic, your presentations should clarify the issues you discussed and your plan for each. Be sure to let your attendings know when you are running behind and how they might help you most. One popular and effective format is as follows:

Identify the patient and frame a question that you want the attending to address

Mr. K is a 45-year-old man with diabetes, hypertension, and depression. He is here for a new lesion on his leg and for a blood pressure check. I'd like you to look at his leg with me, and I need your thoughts on his BP.

Give an efficient, problem-based history, exam, and plan

Leg lesion. He noticed this lesion a few months ago, and it's gradually grown. He doesn't recall injuring himself, and it's non-tender. He has not had fever or chills. On exam, the temperature is 37°C, and on his right anterior shin he has a smooth, shiny, well-demarcated plaque with central atrophy and telangiectasia. The surrounding leg and skin are normal in appearance and sensation is intact. Because he's diabetic, I was originally concerned about infection, but there are no signs or symptoms of that. Could you look at it with me?

Blood pressure. He's had hypertension for 5 years, and it had been well controlled until recently when his medication doses have had to be increased. He's currently taking atenolol 50 mg, hydrochlorothiazide 25 mg, and lisinopril 20 mg. He does not drink and has always been compliant with his medications. Now his pressures at home range from 140s to 150s over 90s. In clinic today, his BP is 152/92 and P is 54. There is no edema. I am uncertain why his hypertension is becoming more difficult to control, and I'd like to review possible explanations and management with you.

Other issues. We didn't talk about his diabetes today. I'd like to schedule an appointment for follow-up in two weeks to go over that and his test results.

Get feedback

Any suggestions for me?

What should I include in my notes?

When reviewing your clinic notes, a reader should be able to rapidly identify your patient's problems, medications, and management plan. With the exception of the Assessment and Plan section, clinic notes are generally much more concise than ward notes. Basic elements include:

- ■ **ID/CC:** briefly frame the patient and purpose of the visit
- ■ **Problem List**
- ■ **Medications**
- ■ **Current Concerns:** concise histories of problems addressed
- ■ **Exam:** detailed descriptions of exam performed that day
- ■ **Labs:** summarize key findings only
- ■ **Assessment and Plan:** for each problem, discuss your rationale and plan

What is my responsibility for follow-up?

It is your responsibility to follow-up on your patient's test results and determine appropriate timing for a return visit. Before a patient leaves clinic, review how they will learn of test results. You may need to devise a system to remind you to look up results. When tests are back, you should either send a letter or make a phone call to the patient. In some clinics, patients can call in for results, but this may not be adequate for abnormal results. You should also discuss when the patient should return to clinic. There are no clear guidelines to follow, so this can be difficult. Ask your attending if you are unclear. From the standpoint of your education, scheduling return visits before you leave the rotation can enhance your experience significantly.

When should I read?

Although clinic rotations generally include more free time than exists on ward rotations, some find it difficult to incorporate reading into diagnostic and therapeutic decision-making in clinic. Several little breaks in the clinic routine exist, however, and you can use each to advantage. Read *before the visit*, especially when you know the chief complaint and are unsure what an appropriate history and exam would entail. Ask your attending for guidance on what to read. A few minutes of advance preparation can save time in the room. Read *before the exam* to look up something during the minute a patient takes to disrobe, but be quick! Read *before your presentation* to clarify questions about diagnosis, elements of the story, exam, or labs before you present to the attending. Read *between visits*, to take advantage of any gaps in your schedule.

4

Communicating with Patients

What do I accomplish with a good patient interview?

A good interview provides key diagnostic information in the majority of cases. Verbal and nonverbal cues help establish a partnership of trust and mutual understanding, setting the stage for compliance with treatment decisions. A good interview elicits patient perceptions about their illness ("what does this illness mean to you?"), about the role they expect their doctor to play in their health care ("what do you hope I can do to help you?"), and sets patient expectations for future interactions.

How should I begin a patient interview?

Say hello using Mr. or Ms. and the patient's last name. You can ask how the patient would like to be addressed if this seems too formal. Never assume you can call someone by their first name because this is offensive to some patients. Next, introduce yourself. Then ask your patient how you can help and listen, listen, listen!

What barriers to communicating with patients will I encounter?

The biggest barrier to good communication is physicians' poor listening skills. Listening is probably the most important skill for any physician. Good listening will transcend many cultural and power differences between patients and their physicians and helps patients feel heard, respected, and understood. Most physicians begin their careers with a good idea of how to listen and with the desire to convey caring and respect. These values, and the listening skills that accompany them, may atrophy during medical training unless specific attention is paid to practicing respectful patient interactions. Listening skills are not just innate features of some personalities—they can be learned (and forgotten). For example, physicians interrupt patients on average within the first seven to eleven seconds of history-taking. Allowing patients to tell their story without interruption sets the visit off to a much better start without actually lengthening the visit time.

After several minutes, if you feel it is necessary, you can gently redirect patients who are rambling: "now let's get back to your chest pain," or "we need to stay focused or I won't be very helpful to you." Patients' stories may unfold in circuitous, unpredictable, and revealing ways. To the physician focused on gathering "the facts," this may seem frustrating. However, there is much to be learned by allowing the patient to tell his or her story. Finding ways to appreciate the breadth of human expression while you are in the midst of gathering data during an interview greatly improves both patient and personal satisfaction with the interaction.

What can I do to be a better listener?

One key listening tool is silence. Use silence to give patients time to answer questions. Use silence, or a simple nod of the head, to encourage patients to share more meaningful information. Another tool is open-ended questions ("tell me more about your pain," "what has this been like for you?") This allows the patient to direct the interview. Closed-ended questions ("is your pain sharp or dull?") are less helpful in creating a good doctor-patient interaction, though they can be useful when used near the end of the interview to flesh out a review of systems. Another tool is reflective statements that summarize what you have heard using the patient's words ("so you have a squeezing feeling around your chest when you walk uphill"). This validates the patient experience and lets the patient know you have been listening. Summary statements also allow you to make transitions from one part of the history to another.

How can my nonverbal cues help communicate caring and respect to patients?

Nonverbal cues may be more important than your words. Sit at eye-level to avoid the power difference implied by looming above a patient. Maintain good eye contact. You can take notes but don't shuffle through the chart while the patient is talking. Practice respectful listening, an exercise in sharing rather than taking control of the conversation. The exam is another powerful venue for nonverbal cues. Don't poke and prod to extract information with your hands. Instead, listen gently, respectfully, and deliberately with your hands. Your patients will feel the difference. Furtive glances at a watch signal you have other more important things to do. Instead, it is better to openly acknowledge time limits and plan with the patient for the best use of time. Stay on schedule, especially in clinic, respecting patients' busy lives.

What can I say during the physical exam?

While silence during the history is a useful tool, silence during the exam can increase patient anxiety as the patient wonders what you are doing, what you are finding and if he or she is going to be OK. During the exam, keep the patient involved as a partner in the experience. Briefly explain what you are doing as you go ("I'll be tapping here to find your liver now"). Reassure patients as you perform the exam when things are normal. Briefly review your findings at the end of the exam. Give patients permission to stop you if the exam becomes uncomfortable.

How do I communicate test results?

Set patient expectations when you order tests for when, how, and with whom you will communicate results. Some patients do not want to hear news directly, but instead prefer that you communicate with a family member. In the clinic, you may mail normal results, and call with abnormal results. In the hospital, you may want to come back in the afternoon with test results—if you promise to return with test results, follow through on your promise! Also explain what you are hoping to learn from the test. In the hospital, significant lab and test results should be shared with patients daily, ideally as soon as they are available. Be brief. Use language the patient can understand to explain the meaning of the test. You may start by asking the patient if he or she remembers your earlier conversation about why the test was obtained. This helps you assess if they have understood prior discussions.

How do I give bad news?

Often, it is effective to start with a screening question to assess patient understanding of why the test was obtained and what they think is likely to be found. This may make it easier to confirm their suspicions with the bad result ("do you understand why we got that CT scan of your abdomen?"). You may also want to establish how much the patient wants to know and if they are ready to hear results. Keep it simple, short, and direct (e.g., "I have bad news. The CT scan shows a growth which could be cancer"). Give people time to absorb bad news—a pause or even a few minutes of silence are often very useful. Some patients will become emotional. This is normal. There is no need to say anything or to try to avoid their emotions. Just being present is often helpful. Some patients will have many questions. If you don't know the answer to a question, say so and offer to find out. Some patients will be quiet.

In general, it is best to keep the message simple and let patient questions guide how much more information you discuss. Offer to answer questions then and later once they have had time to absorb the news. Leave written information letting them know how to reach you if they have questions later. Set a time to return for more discussions and come back at the agreed time. It is often reassuring for patients to hear that you are going to be there to see them through whatever happens next.

How do I do a successful bedside presentation?

Bedside presentation is a tradition that, unfortunately, has fallen out of favor. Bedside presentations work well as the format for daily morning work rounds. The entire team goes to the bedside each day and the intern or student succinctly presents pertinent information regarding hospital course and discusses the plan for the day. Patients prefer hearing bedside presentations on work rounds rather than hearing pieces of conversations about them (or other patients) from the hallway. Teams that do daily bedside rounds often grow to prefer them as well. Bedside presentations provide an efficient way of updating the patient and team simultaneously, including the patient as a partner in plans, making rounds professional and succinct, and allowing quick confirmation of findings. Specific approaches to bedside rounds may vary by team and teaching institution. Basic ground rules include introducing each team member on the first visit, using language the patient can understand, and orienting the patient to the goals of this daily routine ("I'm going to fill the team in on why you came to the hospital and share the information we've gathered about you overnight"). Most patients respond appropriately when encouraged to participate or edit the presentation. Presenters can either speak to the patient, or speak to the team.

Attendings, residents, and students who object to bedside rounds often fear that unanswered questions may arise, or that the patient may see different opinions about how to proceed. However, this is also a strength of bedside rounds since ambiguities and information gathering are a part of medical decision-making. It is fine to say "we don't know" and make a plan for how to find answers and when to get back to the patient with more information. Another fear is that patient questions and concerns may monopolize the conversation and interrupt or prolong rounds. In the rare case that this occurs, the team can acknowledge the need for longer discussion later in the day and plan a time for one team member to return. Most patients appreciate being involved in this patient-centered way of communicating about their care, and benefit greatly from seeing the complex nature of the decision-making process of medicine.

5

Ethics in Medicine

▶ CONFIDENTIALITY

What does the duty of confidentiality require?

Confidentiality is one of the core tenets of medical practice. The obligation of confidentiality prohibits the physician from disclosing information about the patient's case to other parties without permission and encourages the physician to take precautions to ensure only authorized access to information occurs. Discussions about patients with other physicians are often critical for patient care and are an integral part of the learning experience in a teaching hospital. These discussions are justifiable, so long as precautions are taken to limit the ability of others to hear or see confidential information.

What kinds of disclosure are inappropriate?

The realities of communication in medical practice make it difficult to protect patient confidentiality. Inappropriate disclosure of information occurs when cases are discussed in the elevator or hallway, when extra copies of handouts with patient information on them are left out, or when patient family members are informed, even about minor care issues, against the patient's wishes. The patient's right to privacy is not being respected in these situations.

When should confidentiality be breached?

Confidentiality is not an absolute obligation and it may be broken if there is concern for the safety of specific persons or for public welfare. Clinicians have a duty to protect identifiable individuals from any serious threat of harm if they have information that could prevent the harm. In the most clear-cut cases of limited confidentiality, physicians are required by state law to report to public health authorities certain communicable/infectious diseases such as AIDS, hepatitis A and B, measles, and tuberculosis. Suspected cases of child, dependent adult, and elder abuse are reported, as are gunshot wounds. Local municipal code and institutional policies can vary regarding what is reportable and standards of evidence required. It is best to ask about your institution's policy.

▶ INFORMED CONSENT

What is informed consent?

The most important goal of informed consent is to allow the patient to be an informed participant in health care decisions. It originates from the legal and ethical right of the patient to direct what happens to his or her body, and from the ethical duty of the physician to involve the patient in his or her health care. The term "basic consent" entails letting the patient know what you would like to do and asking for their permission. This is appropriate for simple procedures such as drawing blood. Decisions that merit this streamlined approach have a high level of community consensus and a low level of risk. A more formal process of informed consent should occur for more invasive procedures such as lumbar puncture or thoracentesis. The more formal process includes a discussion of several aspects of the procedure (Box 5–1) as well as a consent form signed by the patient and filed in the chart.

What are my responsibilities during the informed consent discussion?

Consent is only valid if given voluntarily by a patient competent to make the decision. Patients often feel powerless and vulnerable and it is easy for coercive situations to arise in this setting. To encourage compliance, the physician must make clear to the patient that he or she is participating in a decision, not merely signing a form. With this understanding, the informed consent process should be seen as an invitation to the patient to participate in decisions. The physician is also generally obligated to share the reasoning process and provide a recommendation to the patient. Comprehension on the part of the patient is equally as important as the information provided. Consequently, the discussion should be carried on in layperson's terms and the patient's understanding should be assessed along the way.

BOX 5–1

Elements to Discuss When Obtaining Formal Patient Consent

▶ nature of the decision/procedure
▶ reasonable alternatives to the proposed intervention
▶ relevant risks, benefits, and uncertainties related to each alternative
▶ assessment of patient understanding
▶ acceptance of the intervention by the patient

What sorts of interventions require informed consent?

For a wide range of decisions, written consent is not required, but some meaningful discussion is needed. For instance, a man contemplating having a prostate-specific antigen (PSA) screen for prostate cancer should know the relevant arguments for and against this screening test, discussed in lay terms. Most health care institutions have policies that state which health interventions require a signed consent form. For example, surgery, anesthesia, and other invasive procedures are usually in this category.

Is there such a thing as implied consent?

Consent can be implied, rather than obtained, in emergency situations when the patient is unconscious or incompetent and no surrogate decision-maker is available. This is based on the principle of beneficence that requires a physician to act on the patient's behalf when the patient's life is at stake. The patient's presence in the hospital ward, ICU, or clinic does not imply consent to undergo treatment or procedures.

▶ DO-NOT-RESUSCITATE ORDERS

What is a Do-Not-Resuscitate order?

A DNR order means the patient will not receive CPR if he or she is found with no pulse or respirations. In some cases, your patient will have a DNR order on the chart. In many cases, the question has never been addressed and you will need to discuss preferences with your patient regarding CPR. Deciding whether to forego future resuscitation involves a careful consideration of potential clinical benefit and the patient's preferences. Real or perceived differences in these two considerations make decisions to forego CPR difficult.

When can CPR be withheld?

If your patient stops breathing or his or her heart stops beating in the hospital, the standard of care is to perform CPR in the absence of a valid physician's order to withhold it. CPR can be withheld when the patient, or the legal surrogate if the patient is not competent, clearly indicates that he or she does not want CPR should the need arise. It can also be withheld when CPR is deemed futile (judged to be of no medical benefit).

When is CPR "futile?"

CPR is deemed futile when it offers the patient no clinical benefit; in such cases, you are ethically justified in withholding it. CPR has been prospectively evaluated in a wide variety of clinical situations. Knowing the probability of success with CPR can help determine futility. For instance, CPR has virtually 0% probability of success in the following clinical circumstances: septic shock, acute stroke, metastatic cancer, and severe pneumonia. Even in other clinical situations, survival after CPR is extremely limited.

How should the patient's quality of life be considered in decisions about CPR?

CPR might also be judged futile when the patient's quality of life is so poor that no meaningful survival is expected even if CPR were successful at restoring circulatory stability. Judging quality of life tempts prejudicial statements about patients with chronic illness or disability. There is substantial evidence that patients with chronic conditions often rate their quality of life much higher than healthy people would. Nevertheless, many would agree that patients in a permanent unconscious state possess a quality of life that virtually no one would accept. Therefore, CPR is usually considered futile for patients in a persistent vegetative state.

Are "slow codes" ever justified?

Slow codes are those in which a half-hearted effort at resuscitation is made. Physicians may be tempted to resort to using a slow code when there is disagreement between the patient and the physician about CPR. Slow codes are not ethically justified.

What if the patient is unable to say what his or her wishes are?

In some cases, the decision about CPR must be made when the patient is unable to participate. There are two general approaches to this dilemma. One is to use an existing Advance Directive, a document that indicates with some specificity the decisions the patient would like made should he or she be unable to participate. The other solution involves identifying a surrogate decision-maker. The law recognizes a hierarchy of family relationships in determining which family member should be the official "spokesperson," (Box 5–2) though ideally all close family members and significant others should be involved in the discussion and reach some consensus.

▶ TERMINATION OF LIFE-SUSTAINING TREATMENTS

When is it justifiable to discontinue life-sustaining treatments?

Occasionally, you will have patients who are receiving treatments or interventions that keep them alive, and you will face the decision of

BOX 5-2

Hierarchy for Choosing a Surrogate Decision-Maker

1. Legal guardian with health care decision-making authority
2. Individual given durable power of attorney for health care decisions
3. Spouse
4. Adult children of patient (all in agreement)
5. Parents of patient
6. Adult siblings of patient (all in agreement)

whether to discontinue these treatments. Examples include dialysis for acute or chronic renal failure and mechanical ventilation for respiratory failure. In some circumstances, these treatments are no longer of benefit, while in others the patient or family no longer wants the treatment. If the patient has the ability to make decisions, fully understands the consequences of the decision, and states that he or she no longer wants a treatment, it is justifiable to withdraw the treatment. Treatment withdrawal is also justifiable if the treatment no longer offers benefit to the patient.

Do different standards apply to withholding and withdrawing care?

Many clinicians feel that it is easier to not start (withhold) a treatment, such as mechanical ventilation, than to stop (withdraw) it. While there is a natural tendency to believe this, there is no ethical or legal distinction between withholding and withdrawing treatment.

What if I'm not sure if the patient is competent?

Patients must be competent to make treatment decisions. A better term is "decision-making capacity" to avoid confusion with legal determinations of competence. For example, an elderly grandfather may be found incompetent to manage a large estate, but may still have intact capacity to make treatment decisions. The capacity to make treatment decisions, including withholding or withdrawing treatment, is considered intact if the patient satisfies all four basic criteria (Box 5-3). If the patient does not meet these criteria, then his or her decision-making capacity should be questioned and the surrogate decision-maker should be consulted. Sometimes the patient is awake, alert, and conversant, but his or her decisions seem questionable or irrational. It is important to distinguish an irrational decision from simple disagreement. In these situations, talk with the patient to clarify their reasoning.

BOX 5-3

Criteria Indicating Patient Competence to Make Treatment Decisions

▶ understands the clinical information presented
▶ appreciates the situation, including the consequences of refusing treatment
▶ displays reason in deliberating about her or his choices
▶ clearly communicates choice

What about the patient whose decision-making capacity varies from day to day?

Patients can move in and out of a coherent state from medication effects or their underlying disease. You should do what you can to catch a patient in a lucid state, lightening up on the medications if necessary, in order to include him or her in the decision-making process.

Does depression or other mental illness impair a patient's decision-making capacity?

Patients with active mental illness, including depression, should have their decision-making capacity evaluated carefully, usually by a psychiatrist. Patients should not be presumed to be unable to make treatment decisions. In several studies, patients voice similar preferences for life-sustaining treatments when depressed as they do after treatment of depression.

K E Y   P O I N T S

▶ With a few exceptions, patient information should be kept in confidence

▶ The ethical principle of respect for persons creates an obligation for physicians to foster patient participation in health care decisions

▶ DNR orders should be written when the patient (or surrogate) states such a preference

▶ Competent, fully informed patients have the right to refuse life-sustaining treatments

CASE 5–1. A 60-year-old man has a heart attack and is admitted to the medical floor with a very poor prognosis. He asks that you not share any of his medical information with his wife as he does not think she will be able to take it. His wife catches you in the hall and asks about her husband's prognosis.

A. Will you tell his wife?
B. What are you required to do legally?

CASE 5–2. A 45-year-old man has a two-week history of chest pain and fainting spells, with a family history of cardiac disease. You feel his symptoms merit cardiac catheterization. After explaining the intervention and the risks of not pursuing treatment, the patient refuses the treatment. He is clear that he understands the implications of letting his symptoms go untreated, but "doesn't want to go there" and gets up to leave.

A. Can the patient refuse to give consent for this intervention?
B. What are your professional obligations in this case?

REFERENCE

Jonsen AR, Siegler M, Winslade WJ: Clinical Ethics. 4th Edition. New York: McGraw Hill, 1998.

USEFUL WEBSITE

University of Washington School of Medicine Ethics in Medicine Website, *http://eduserv.hscer.washington.edu/bioethics*

6

Practical Skills for the Medical Student

▶ HOW TO READ ELECTROCARDIOGRAMS

How do I report ECG findings in my notes?

A normal report covers the six key features of an ECG: rhythm, rate, axis, intervals, chamber sizes, and ischemic changes.

How do I recognize normal sinus rhythm?

Normal sinus rhythm (Figure 6–1) occurs when orderly depolarization begins in the sinus node, progresses through the atria = P wave, traverses the AV node = PR interval, then passes through

Waves: P, Q, R, S, T

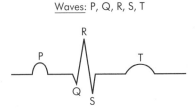

Intervals: PR, QRS, ST, QT

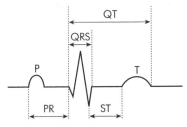

Figure 6–1. Components of a normal ECG tracing.

23

the ventricles = QRS complex, causing a ventricular contraction. After depolarization is finished, there is a brief pause = ST segment, and then the ventricles repolarize = T wave. Thus, in normal sinus rhythm, every QRS complex is preceded by a P wave, every P followed by a QRS, with a constant PR interval for every beat.

How do I calculate the rate?

The heart rate is ventricular contractions per minute. On a standard ECG, a small box passes by in 0.04 seconds, a large box in 0.2 seconds. Estimate rate by counting the large boxes between each QRS complex and memorizing the corresponding rate (Table 6–1). Alternatively, use rate = 300/B, where B is the number of large boxes between each QRS.

Why is it useful to understand vectors?

Understanding vectors in the limb and precordial leads allows you to localize heart muscle injury (Table 6–2). And with vectors you can calculate axis, which helps identify ventricular hypertrophy. You will need to read an ECG text for details about vectors. Normal axis of the QRS reflects the left ventricle's great muscle bulk, which points down and to the left between leads aVF and I. Thus, if QRS is upward in both I and aVF, the axis is normal. Left ventricular hypertrophy shifts the axis to the left and creates a negative QRS in lead aVF. Right ventricular hypertrophy shifts the axis down and to the right with a resultant negative QRS in lead I.

What specific changes will my patient with myocardial damage show on ECG?

In general, ST segment changes and flipped T waves occur with early myocardial damage; significant Q waves appear twenty-four to forty-eight hours later. The spectrum of injury ranges from reversible subendocardial ischemia to irreversible transmural infarction (Figure 6–2). T wave inversions are a nonspecific sign of myocardial ischemia or early infarction. Normal T waves follow the direction of the QRS complex, but flip to the opposite direction with myocardial injury.

TABLE 6–1					
Calculating Rate by the Number of Large Boxes Between QRS Complexes					
Boxes between QRS complexes	1	2	3	4	5
Rate (beats per minute)	300	150	100	75	60

TABLE 6–2

Contiguous Leads that Localize Acute Myocardial Infarction	
Location	Leads Affected (ST, T, Q changes)
Anterior wall of LV	V1–V4
Inferior wall of LV	II, III, aVF
Lateral wall of LV	I, aVL, V5, V6
Posterior wall of LV	V1–V2 (large R waves)
Septal wall	V1–V2
Right ventricle	Right-sided precordial leads

How do I recognize pericarditis on an ECG?

PR segment depression and/or ST elevation in multiple, noncontiguous leads suggests pericarditis. If pericarditis is accompanied by pericardial effusion, the voltages in all leads may be unusually low.

PR >1 large box = MI / meds
QRS > 3 large box = bbb

What are intervals all about?

Prolonged intervals represent delays in conduction. A PR interval greater than 1 large box indicates AV nodal block and can be caused by MI or medications such as digoxin or diltiazem. QRS widening to beyond 3 small boxes (or greater than 0.12 sec) is caused by interventricular conduction delay such as a bundle branch block. Detect left bundle branch block by the "rabbit ears" (RR′) in leads V5-V6. Right bundle branch block causes RR′ in leads V1-V2. QT prolongation is important because it can lead to torsades de pointe, a deadly ventricular arrhythmia. The QT interval depends on the heart rate and is normal if it is less than 1/2 the RR interval. QT prolongation occurs with tricyclic antidepressant overdose, hypomagnesemia, hypocalcemia, some antiarrhythmic drugs, and interactions of some medications (cisapride and erythromycin).

How do I detect chamber wall hypertrophy or enlargement?

LV hypertrophy creates a leftward axis as well as large S waves in leads V1-V2 and large R waves in aVL, V5 and V6 (Table 6-3). RV hypertrophy creates large R waves in leads V1-V2. Left atrial enlargement is best seen in V1 as a late negative deflection in a biphasic P wave. The negative portion of the P wave must be greater than 1 mm deep and 1 box wide. Right atrial enlargement creates a large peaked P wave greater than 2.5 mm high best seen in lead II.

A   Reversible ischemia

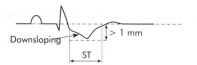

Downsloping

> 1 mm

ST

- Downsloping ST segment depression > 1 mm below baseline

B   Irreversible infarction
Early (minutes/hours)   No longer concave upwards

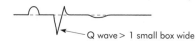

> 1 mm

ST

- ST segment elevation > 1 mm above baseline
- In 2 or more contiguous leads

C   Irreversible infarction
Late (hours/days)

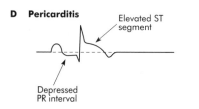

Q wave > 1 small box wide

- T wave inversion
- Q waves > 1 box wide and deep
- In 2 or more contiguous leads

D   Pericarditis
Elevated ST segment

Depressed
PR interval

- Diffuse ST segment elevation
- Diffuse PR segment depression

Figure 6–2. ST segment and Q wave changes with myocardial damage (**A–C**) or pericardial inflammation (**D**).

TABLE 6–3		
Criteria for LVH Using Wave Amplitudes		
R wave in a VL	> 11 mm high	
(S in V1 or V2) + (R in V5 or V6)	> 35 mm high	

USEFUL WEBSITES

http://medstat.med.utah.edu/kw/ecg/
http://www.ecglibrary.com/ecghome.html

HOW TO READ AN ABDOMINAL FILM

When should I obtain abdominal films?

Not all patients with abdominal pain require x-rays, which are often nonspecific. Obtain films when they will aid diagnosis: for perforation, obstruction, or chronic pancreatitis (Figure 6–3).

How do I order abdominal films?

Order an abdominal series, which consists of supine and upright abdominal films as well as a chest x-ray (CXR). The CXR shows the lung fields and diaphragms. This screens for pulmonary pathology such as pneumonia presenting with abdominal symptoms and for free air in the abdomen.

What key findings should I look for in an abdominal series?

Free air, a surgical emergency until proven otherwise, is best seen on CXR as a dark crescent under the right diaphragm in contrast to the radiodense liver. If your patient cannot stand, a cross-table lateral x-ray with the patient's left side down will show free air. Common causes of free air are bowel wall perforation from duodenal ulcer, diverticula, or cancer. Another critical finding is dilated colon from obstruction or ileus. If markedly dilated, toxic megacolon secondary to *Clostridium difficile* should be considered.

What constitutes dilation for large and small bowel?

Roughly 3 cm for small intestine, 6 cm for large intestine, and 9 cm for the cecum constitute dilation. To discern between large and small bowel, consider anatomy. The small bowel valvulae are circumferential and so create lines across the entire bowel; in the large bowel, haustrations only partially embrace the circumference and therefore give a scalloped border. Additionally, the large bowel generally frames the edges of the abdomen whereas the small bowel sits in the center.

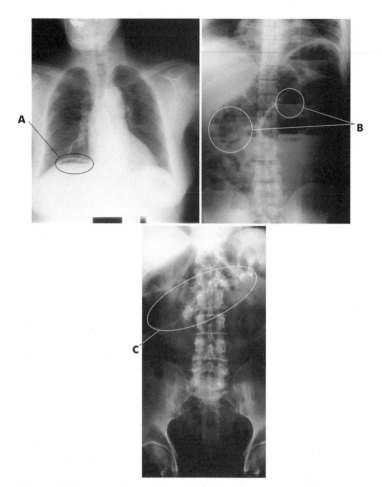

Figure 6–3. Key abdominal series findings. **A,** *Free air* indicates perforation. **B,** *Air fluid levels* of bowel obstruction. **C,** *Pancreatic calcifications* are pathognomonic for chronic pancreatitis.

How can I tell the difference between ileus and bowel obstruction?

In both conditions, air-fluid levels and dilation are seen. Air in the rectum suggests ileus. In true obstruction, no air passes, so the rectum collapses within twenty-four hours. Also, air-fluid levels the same height throughout the gut suggests obstruction, rather than the varying levels seen in ileus.

What other findings can be helpful?

Extensive stool suggests constipation. Arterial calcification raises concern for mesenteric ischemia. Gallstones or kidney stones may be seen. Pneumatosis, air in the bowel wall, is a grim indicator of mesenteric necrosis. Hepatomegaly, splenomegaly, or enlarged kidneys may be suggested. Bowel wall thickening from edema can be seen. Calcifications in the pancreas are diagnostic of chronic pancreatitis.

HOW TO READ CXRs

What should I look for on a CXR?

The key to CXR reading is to proceed systematically through six major steps (Box 6–1). This ensures that you will not overlook anything. Remember, the hardest lesion to see on x-ray is the second one.

Why is technique important?

Technique varies from film to film and must be taken into account. PA (posterior-anterior) and lateral films are preferred, but require the patient to stand. If the patient is unable to stand, anterior-posterior (AP) films are shot with the film behind the patient's back, often in bed. On AP films, divergence of x-ray beams exaggerates heart size. Appropriate *exposure* barely reveals the vertebrae behind the heart. With over-penetration, darkened normal lungs may be mistaken for emphysema. Under-penetration or poor inspiration increases interstitial markings. Adequate *inspiration* is determined by counting at least 10 posterior ribs (appear horizontal) in the lung field. Patient *rotation* artificially widens the mediastinal profile; normally the vertebrae line up between the clavicular heads (Figure 6–4)

BOX 6–1

Key Elements of Reading a CXR

A = Airways and lung fields
B = Bones and soft tissue
C = Cardiac contour and mediastinum
D = Diaphragms and costophrenic angles
E = Examine technique
F = Foreign bodies, tubes, and wires

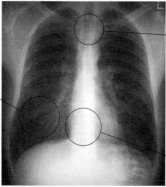

Alignment: Vertebrae aligned between clavicular heads

Inspiration: Count at least10 posterior ribs behind lung fields

Penetration: Vertebrae are just barely visible behind heart

Details: Note patient name, whether PA or AP, and date

Name, Date

Figure 6–4. Elements of techniques important in evaluating a chest x-ray. (© 1997, Mike Richardson)

What can be seen in bones and soft tissue?

Look for bony fractures, dislocations, and lytic lesions from cancer. Severe osteoporosis can be seen as transparent bone or vertebral compression fractures, most clear on the lateral view. Examine soft tissue for swelling, or subcutaneous air suggestive of pneumothorax.

What causes a widened mediastinum?

Patient rotation, thoracic aortic aneurysm, tumor, or lymphadenopathy can widen the mediastinum.

Why should I look at the diaphragms and costophrenic angles?

Free air under the diaphragm occurs with bowel perforation. A blunted costophrenic angle, sometimes the only sign of pleural effusion, should prompt decubitus films (patient lying on his or her side, affected side down) to evaluate the amount of pleural fluid and if it is free flowing or loculated.

What is a silhouette sign?

The silhouette sign occurs when fluid or infection in the lung is adjacent to, and therefore obliterates, the border of the hemidiaphragm or heart. For example, if the right heart border is poorly seen, this is a right middle lobe silhouette sign, indicating a right middle lobe infiltrate (Figure 6–5). Similarly a left lower lobe pneumonia will obliterate the left hemidiaphragm.

What does pneumonia look like?

Pneumonia may have many appearances, including a focal infiltrate, a silhouette sign, diffuse interstitial infiltrates, and unexplained pleural effusions. In a volume-depleted patient, an infiltrate may be very subtle. Apical infiltrates can occur with any form of pneumonia, but are classic for tuberculosis.

What acute catastrophes should I not miss on CXR?

Certain conditions should never be missed (Table 6–4).

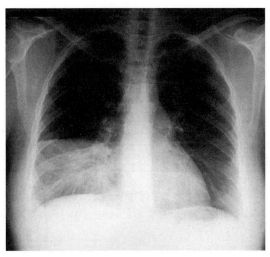

Figure 6–5. Loss of the right heart silhouette with right middle lobe pneumonia. NOTE: Right diaphragm is still clearly seen. (© 1997, Mike Richardson)

TABLE 6–4	
Catastrophes Not to Miss on CXR	
Finding	**Condition**
Subdiaphragmatic "free" air	Intestinal perforation
Widened mediastinum	Aortic aneurysm or dissection
Mediastinal air	Esophageal rupture
Mediastinal shift, air in the pleural space	Pneumothorax

What causes nodules in the lung parenchyma?

Cancer, either primary or metastatic, arteriovenous malformations, focal infection or abscess, hamartomas, or granulomas can all appear as nodules.

What are clues to volume overload or congestive heart failure?

Look for an enlarged cardiac silhouette, greater than half the width of the thorax on PA view, interstitial prominence, Kerley B lines, and cephalization of vessels. *Kerley B lines* are thin horizontal linear densities at the periphery of the lung fields due to edema in the interlobular septa. *Cephalization* is the engorgement of pulmonary vessels in the upper lung fields. Under normal conditions, gravity makes vessels more prominent at the bottom of the lung field. *Blunting of the costophrenic angles* suggests pleural effusion.

USEFUL WEBSITE

http://rad.usuhs.mil/rad/chest_review/

HOW TO PERFORM BASIC PROCEDURES AND BODY FLUID ANALYSIS

What is the first step for all procedures?

All procedures require informed consent. To obtain consent, explain the indication for the procedure, what the procedure involves, the risks (i.e., what a reasonable person would want to know), the alternatives to the procedure, and the consequences of not having the procedure performed. Patient competence is essential in this process. Patients should be able to reiterate the keys points of the procedure and risks. Patients under 18 years of age and those with altered mental status are not considered competent. In these cases, a surrogate decision-maker is sought. In an emergency, informed consent is not necessary if the procedure is considered to be lifesaving. The signed consent should be properly documented in the medical record.

What habits facilitate a successful procedure?

Take time at the outset to review technique, collect and arrange supplies, place a waste receptacle within easy reach, and position the patient. Wash hands before each procedure, observe universal precautions, and always use sterile technique. Out of respect for the hospital staff, clean up following the procedure and dispose of all sharp implements appropriately.

How do I document a procedure?

There is a standard format for procedure notes (Box 6–2).

▶ LUMBAR PUNCTURE

What are the indications for lumbar puncture (LP)?

Any patient with unexplained fever and mental status changes should undergo LP to rule out CNS infection. Patients with new onset "worst headache of their life" and a negative CT scan require LP to rule out subarachnoid hemorrhage, and rare conditions including carcinomatous meningitis and Guillain-Barré. LP's can be used to treat normal pressure hydrocephalus, and to administer intrathecal chemotherapy or epidural anesthesia.

When is LP contraindicated?

Increased intracranial pressure is an absolute contraindication to LP due to the risk of precipitating uncal herniation. Elevated

BOX 6–2

Standard Procedure Note

Date and time _____

Procedure _____

Indication _____

Operators _____

Verbal and written informed consents were obtained following explanation of indications, risks, benefits, and alternative treatments. The area (describe where) was prepped and draped in sterile fashion. ___ of 1 % lidocaine was injected. ___ mL of (type, description) fluid were withdrawn without complication and sent for (name tests). Wound cleansed and dressed. Patient tolerated the procedure well with ___ mL estimated blood loss. Follow-up studies (i.e., CXR following thoracentesis) were negative.

Signature _____

intracranial pressure should be suspected in patients with papilledema or risk factors for space-occupying lesions (HIV, CNS tumor, trauma, focal neurologic exam, or new onset seizure). Under these circumstances, a CT scan prior to LP is mandatory. Coagulopathy is a relative contraindication to LP.

What are the key steps in performing an LP?

Lie the patient on his or her side at the edge of the bed. Position the patient close to you and raise the bed to a comfortable height. The patient's hip bones should be exactly perpendicular to the bed with knees to chest for best access to the intervertebral space. Mark the L4 space at the level of the iliac crests. Prepare and drape the low back in sterile fashion, apply anesthesia to the skin as a wheal, then to the deep tissues, making sure you are not injecting a vessel by pulling back on the syringe plunger prior to injecting. Insert the spinal needle in the same hole used to administer anesthesia, aiming for the umbilicus. Obtain an opening pressure and collect several milliliters of cerebrospinal fluid (CSF) in each of four vials. Replace stylet before removing spinal needle.

What are the complications of LP?

Complications include post-LP headache, infection, hemorrhage, and uncal or tonsillar herniation. LP headache usually resolves with bed rest, nonsteroidal medications, and hydration.

What CSF tests should I order, and how do I interpret them?

Order cell count and differential, glucose, protein, bacterial culture and Gram stain. Glucose should be 50%–60% of the simultaneous blood glucose. If lower, consider bacterial (including tuberculous) meningitis and parameningeal infection. In normal CSF, the WBC count is 0–5 cells per mm^3. A traumatic spinal tap occurs when a blood vessel is nicked on the way into the subarachnoid space. Traumatic taps show a decrease of the RBC count from the first to the fourth vials of CSF. The WBC differential is crucial as predominance of neutrophils suggests bacterial infection. Mononuclear cells are more common with viral, fungal, and tuberculous (TB) meningitis. However, neutrophils may predominate in early viral infection. Protein is usually less than 50 mg/dL. High protein is nonspecific, but is seen in all CNS infections, and is highest with bacterial processes. An isolated increase in protein may be seen in patients with diabetes. Order cytology if malignancy is suspected, and cryptococcal antigen and fungal stain and culture in immunocompromised patients. Specific viral testing is also available.

▶ THORACENTESIS

What are the indications for thoracentesis?

Patients with new or unexplained pleural effusion require thoracentesis for diagnosis. The most common causes of effusions in the U.S. are CHF (500,000 per year), pneumonia (300,000 per year), and malignancy (200,000 per year mostly due to lung, breast cancer, and lymphoma). Thoracentesis in CHF patients is not necessary unless one of the following occurs: 1) asymmetric effusions, 2) pleuritic chest pain, or 3) fever. Effusion associated with pneumonia requires thoracentesis to rule out pleural space infection (empyema) requiring drainage. Thoracentesis can also be used therapeutically to remove large, symptomatic effusions.

When is thoracentesis contraindicated?

Relative contraindications to thoracentesis include coagulopathy, cutaneous infections at the puncture site, and uncooperative patients. Small effusions may be more safely tapped with ultrasound guidance.

What are the key steps to thoracentesis?

Position the patient sitting on the edge of the bed, leaning over a tray-table. Raise the bed to a comfortable height for you. Locate and mark your puncture site two intercostal spaces below where dullness to percussion begins. Be certain your mark is at the upper border of the rib to avoid the neurovascular bundle which lies at the inferior margin of each rib. Prepare with Betadine and drape in sterile fashion. Apply anesthesia generously, especially at the parietal pleura. Advance your 22 gauge, 1.5 inch needle over the top of a rib while pulling back on the plunger until fluid is reached. A diagnostic tap requires about 30 mL of fluid. Therapeutic taps should not exceed 1.5 L to avoid re-expansion pulmonary edema. Fluid collection devices vary. With every device, it is crucial to avoid introducing air into the pleural space. Combat negative intrapleural pressure by having the patient exhale any time you must open the system to change devices. Use a sterile-gloved finger to cover the catheter while changing syringes during fluid collection. Check on the patient several hours after the procedure. If the patient has new shortness of breath or pain, an x-ray should be obtained and promptly reviewed.

What are the complications of thoracentesis?

Pneumothorax, hepatic or splenic puncture, infection, hemothorax, and re-expansion pulmonary edema are complications of thoracentesis.

What pleural fluid tests should I order, and how do I interpret the results?

Use results of pleural fluid and simultaneous blood testing to discern exudates from transudates (Table 6–5). If you suspect a transudate (renal failure, CHF, or cirrhosis), only send fluid for LDH and protein for confirmation and hold extra fluid. This saves almost $200 per patient with very few inaccurate results. Simultaneous serum LDH, protein, and glucose are helpful. If initial results point toward an exudate, send the remaining fluid for cell count and differential, glucose, bacterial cultures, and cytology. Other tests to order as circumstances warrant include amylase and lipids. Cultures for TB, even in the presence of disease, are low yield. pH has fallen out of favor due to difficulty with accuracy but can be helpful in determining if chest tube drainage is needed. Differential diagnosis of exudates includes uninfected parapneumonic effusion, empyema, neoplasm, subdiaphragmatic abscess, pulmonary embolism, pancreatitis, rheumatoid and lupus arthritis, sarcoidosis, and Dressler's syndrome (postpericardiotomy or myocardial infarction). Causes of transudates include congestive heart failure, cirrhosis, and nephrotic syndrome.

▶ PARACENTESIS

What are the indications for paracentesis?

New onset ascites requires paracentesis for diagnosis. Patients with chronic ascites and new abdominal pain, fever, or unexplained increase in ascites should undergo paracentesis to evaluate for spontaneous bacterial peritonitis (SBP). In ascites compromising respiratory status or patient comfort, larger volumes of 2–5 L can be removed therapeutically.

TABLE 6–5		
Interpreting Pleural Fluid		
Test	**Exudate**	**Transudate**
LDH	>200	<200
Pleural LDH/serum LDH	>0.6	<0.6
Protein	>3 gm/dL	<3 gm/dL
Pleural protein/serum protein	>0.5	<0.5
Pleural glucose/serum glucose	<0.5	>0.5
Cell count (per mm^3)	>1000	<1000

When is paracentesis contraindicated?

Paracentesis is hardly ever contraindicated. Although most patients with ascites have coagulopathy, this is not a contraindication because the risk of serious bleeding is low (2%) even with coagulopathy.

What are the key steps to paracentesis?

Have the patient empty his or her bladder and identify your puncture site in the midline below the umbilicus (the bladder is not above the symphysis pubis unless there is significant bladder outlet obstruction). Use either lower quadrant midway between the umbilicus and the anterior superior iliac spine as an alternative site if the patient has a midline scar, because bowel can adhere to scar. The patient can be supine or sitting up slightly. Prepare with Betadine and drape in sterile fashion. Inject 1% lidocaine generously in a skin wheal in the subcutaneous tissues, and especially to the parietal peritoneum. To avoid fluid leakage, advance the needle through a zigzag path in the subcutaneous tissue (Figure 6–6). Pull back on the plunger as you advance. As with thoracentesis, collection devices will vary. After collection, withdraw needle and place a pressure dressing over the site. Check on your patient later to make sure there are no signs of complications.

What are the complications of paracentesis?

Complications include bowel perforation, bladder perforation, abdominal wall hematoma, and infection.

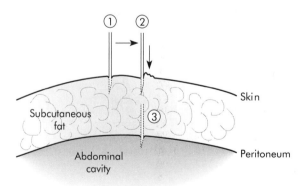

Figure 6–6. Zigzag path through the subcutaneous fat to prevent leakage after paracentesis. *1,* Enter skin; *2,* pull skin 1 to 2 cm away from original entry site with needle perpendicular to skin surface; *3,* advance needle through peritoneum.

What peritoneal fluid tests should I order and how do I interpret them?

Order cell count and differential, protein, bacterial cultures, and cytology. Cell count is the single most important test for deciding presence of infection. Diagnostic criteria for spontaneous bacterial peritonitis are WBC greater than 500 per mm^3 or neutrophils greater than 250 per mm^3. WBC greater than 10,000 indicates peritonitis, such as from perforated duodenal ulcer or colon, and is an indication for immediate CT scan and surgical consult. Calculate the serum-ascites albumin gradient (SAAG): serum albumin minus the ascites albumin. A SAAG greater than 1.1 is consistent with low protein ascitic fluid due to portal hypertension. A SAAG less than 1.1 is consistent with high protein peritoneal fluid due to tuberculosis or peritoneal carcinomatosis. A total ascitic protein greater than 3 gm/dL suggests malignancy or TB. Bacterial cultures are best obtained by inoculating blood culture bottles at the bedside with 10 mL or more per bottle. Cultures for TB in peritoneal fluid are low yield. Yields from cytology are better if several liters are sent.

K E Y P O I N T S

▶ **Proper patient and operator position is key to a comfortable and safe procedure**

▶ **Generous anesthesia, especially at parietal surfaces, is vital to patient comfort and cooperation**

▶ **Use your knowledge of risks, complications, and indications in obtaining patient consent**

ABNORMAL LABORATORY TESTS

My clinic patient has an abnormal lab test. What should I do next?

In the outpatient setting, you have several options for follow-up of abnormal tests: call and ask the patient to return for more history or exam, order follow-up tests, refer for a diagnostic study or consultation, or simply observe over time.

What is the role of screening labs?

Some physicians routinely obtain screening panels of labs; patients may also request these. However, there is no evidence that these "routine" labs are helpful in healthy patients. They generate false positive results and unexpected abnormalities that worry patients, very rarely discover new diseases, and often perplex providers. Since the abnormal range for each test includes normal outliers at the high and low end, a random set of 20 labs will have, on average, one abnormal result just by chance. To avoid this trap, order tests only to pursue your evaluation of symptoms and signs of disease.

Are there any labs that I should order routinely?

In a well adult with no symptoms and a normal exam, reasonable screening tests are total cholesterol, HDL, and glucose. Some physicians also check prostate specific antigen (PSA) in men over age 50, HCT in menstruating women, and thyroid stimulating hormone (TSH) in older women. These screening tests are not uniformly agreed upon.   *Screening- Chol, HDL, Glucose*

♂ PSA   ♀ TSH / HCT

▶ WHITE BLOOD CELL COUNT

What does an elevated white cell count (leukocytosis) mean?   *↑ WBC = infection or steroid.*

The most common causes of leukocytosis are infection and steroids. Bacterial infections usually cause elevation of the neutrophil count with "left shift" (an increase in immature forms of neutrophils). Toxic granulation may also be present with infection, a sign that neutrophils are actively producing digestive enzymes to fight intruding bacteria. Viral infection can cause elevated lymphocytes or atypical lymphocytes. In hospitalized patients, it is not uncommon to see a mild stress-related leukocytosis, a condition that usually rapidly resolves when the patient's condition is more stable, often within 24 hours. Leukemia is an infrequent cause of leukocytosis, usually with immature blast forms in the peripheral circulation.

My patient has elevated eosinophils. What could be causing this?

Eosinophilia may be due to neoplasm, allergy (includes drug reactions), Addison's disease, collagen vascular disease, or parasitic infection (mnemonic NAACP).

▶ ERYTHROCYTE SEDIMENTATION RATE (ESR)

When should I be concerned about an elevated ESR?

The ESR increases with age. In general, an ESR greater than half the age is almost always pathologic and warrants evaluation. More specifically, normal values for men are less than age ÷ 2, and for women are less than (age + 10) ÷ 2. For example, an 80 year old woman should have an ESR less than (80 + 10) ÷ 2, or less than 45. With an ESR greater than 100, the diagnosis is usually obvious during initial evaluation. An elevated ESR is the only hint of disease in 0.06% of cases.

Is the ESR helpful for those with vague symptoms or positive review of systems?

A normal ESR will make the diagnosis of temporal arteritis (TA) and polymyalgia rheumatica (PMR) less likely but is not too help-ful for other disorders. A normal ESR is not strong enough evi-dence to exclude a serious illness. In fact, it is routinely normal in infectious mononucleosis and typhoid fever and in 10% of patients with active tuberculosis.

What causes an ESR greater than 100?

Infection is the most common cause, followed by malignancy and collagen vascular disease. Infections raising the ESR include TB, pulmonary infections, syphilis, chronic bacterial infections (osteomyelitis, endocarditis, septic arthritis, liver/spleen/peri-nephric abscess), urinary tract infections, and AIDS. Malignancy accounts for 15% of ESRs greater than 100, and is almost always metastatic when the ESR is that high. Most likely cancers include multiple myeloma, lymphoma, breast, lung, and colon cancer. Rheumatologic diseases can have a striking elevation in the ESR, especially temporal arteritis, polymyalgia rheumatica, rheumatoid arthritis, and lupus erythematosus.

What evaluation should I pursue when the ESR is greater than 100?

Perform careful history and physical exam including pelvic exam and stool Hemoccult. This should suggest a diagnosis. Blood tests and imaging studies do not substitute for a detailed H & P. Pursue the laboratory tests and studies most likely to confirm the diag-nosis. Consider CBC with differential and urinalysis to look for infection; electrolytes, BUN, and creatinine to check kidney func-tion and acid-base status; and liver function tests to look for hepatic injury. Since myeloma is more common with these extreme elevations in ESR, consider serum and urine electrophoresis (SPEP, UPEP). Obtain CXR to look for lung infection, vasculitis, or tumor. In 5% to 10% of cases with an ESR of greater than 100, no cause will be found.

What about less extreme values, ESR = 35 to 75?

Many of these will be normal when rechecked in several weeks. This should be the extent of the work-up in an asymptomatic patient. Another option is to check a C-reactive protein, or CRP. If the CRP is less than 0.2 mg/dL, the ESR elevation is likely a false positive. For persistently elevated values, a careful history, examination, and careful use of the above tests will lead to the answer. In the asymptomatic patient with a benign examination, almost all elevated ESR results will go unexplained.

▶ LIVER FUNCTION TESTS

How do I interpret liver function tests (ALT, AST, and alkaline phosphatase)?

Elevations of the hepatic transaminases, ALT and AST, suggest parenchymal injury to the liver, with the highest values seen in severe viral hepatitis, toxin or drug injury, and severe hypotension. Most common causes of ALT and AST elevation include medications, alcohol, hepatitis B and C, fatty liver, and hemochromatosis. Increases in alkaline phosphatase and conjugated bilirubin suggest obstructive biliary pathology, either extrahepatic or intrahepatic cholestasis. ALT and AST may be normal or mildly elevated with cholestasis. ALT increases are more specific to liver injury, since AST is found in many other tissues. ALT and AST tend to rise equally except in alcohol ingestion where the AST/ALT ratio is usually greater than 2. ↑ Alk phosc ⊕ Bili = obstruction

ALT more specific to liver

How should I evaluate an elevated alkaline phosphatase (alk phos)?

Biliary obstruction and bone diseases are the main causes of an elevated alk phos. To sort out which is present, obtain a gamma-glutamyl transferase (GGT) or 5'-nucleotidase; either of which will be elevated with biliary tree pathology but not with bone disease. Alk phos isoenzymes also distinguish the source but take several weeks. If biliary pathology is suggested, look for gallstones or tumor compressing the biliary tree (pancreatic, cholangiocarcinoma) by abdominal CT scan. Also consider autoimmune disease such as primary biliary cirrhosis, which is diagnosed by a positive antimitochondrial antibody test in greater than 90% of cases.

↑ Alk phose can be fr. Biliary obstruction or bone, use GGT to distinguish. (or 5'nucleotidase.

Alk phos can also be elevated in hepatitis, cirrhosis, or late in pregnancy, although is rarely more than one to two times the upper limits of normal and not usually greater than the ALT. When bone disease is likely, consider fractures, Paget's disease, bone metastases, or infection.

Bone disease
Pagets
Mets
Infection

▶ TUMOR MARKERS

What are tumor markers?

These are substances produced in excess by particular tumors and found in the blood (Table 6–6). Tumor markers are too nonspecific to use for diagnosis or general screening. They can be used to assess completeness of resection or recurrence after treatment. Occasionally, they can suggest a diagnosis when findings are nonspecific. For example, in the case of a liver mass, elevated α-fetoprotein (AFP) suggests primary liver tumor, while an elevated carcinoembryonic antigen (CEA) suggests colon cancer metastatic to the liver. Patients with cirrhosis at high risk for hepatocellular carcinoma may undergo annual AFP screening, though outcome data are lacking to support this practice. Germ cell tumors are classified based on HCG and AFP production.

HOW TO INTERPRET SENSITIVITY AND SPECIFICITY

What are sensitivity and specificity?

When diagnosing or treating a condition, we need to know "how accurate is this test?" For example, in a screening test for cancer, we want a balance between a big net that catches all cancers (sensitivity) and yet still omits those cases that are not cancer

TABLE 6–6

Common Tumor Markers and Their Clinical Use

Tumor Marker	Associated Tumor	Clinical Use
α-Fetoprotein	Germ cell cancer, liver cancer	Classify tumor type, follow for recurrence; suggest source of liver mass; screen high-risk cirrhosis patients
β-HCG	Germ cell tumor	Classify tumor type
CEA	Colon cancer	Follow for recurrence; suggest source of liver mass
CA-125	Ovarian cancer	Follow for recurrence

(specificity). Put another way, sensitivity is the proportion of people with the condition who test positive; specificity is the proportion of persons without the condition who test negative. You can calculate a test's sensitivity and specificity by using a 2 × 2 table (Table 6–7).

How do levels of sensitivity and specificity impact how I interpret a test?

Some people find the mnemonics **SpPIN** and **SnNOUT** helpful. If a test has high **Sp**ecificity, a **P**ositive test rules the condition **IN**. If a test has high **Sen**sitivity, a **N**egative result rules **OUT** the condition. For example, a peritoneal fluid wave on physical exam is 92% specific for ascites. Therefore, if a fluid wave is present, you can rule ascites in (a highly **sp**ecific test, **p**ositive finding, rule it **in**.) In a study of patients at a VA hospital, a history of ankle edema was 93% sensitive for the presence of ascites. Therefore, if the patient has no history of ankle edema, you can rule ascites out (**sen**sitive test, **n**egative finding, rule it **out**).

If my patient has a positive test, what is the likelihood that she or he actually has the condition?

Sensitivity and specificity relate to characteristics of the test itself. The question of likelihood turns the focus to the characteristics of the patient being tested. We ask, "given a positive test, what is the probability that this patient actually has the condition?" or "given a negative test, what is the probability that the patient doesn't have this condition?" The statistical terms for these concepts are positive and negative predictive value (PPV and NPV), respectively. The predictive value is dependent on the estimated prevalence of a disease, or "pretest probability." In order to determine

TABLE 6–7

Calculating Sensitivity and Specificity

TEST	DISEASE	
	Present	*Absent*
Positive	A (true positive)	B (false positive)
Negative	C (false negative)	D (true negative)

Sensitivity: $\frac{A}{(A + C)}$ or $\frac{\text{(true positive test results)}}{\text{(all patients with disease)}}$ people c̄ disease

Specificity: $\frac{D}{(D + B)}$ or $\frac{\text{(true negative test results)}}{\text{(all patients without disease)}}$ people s̄ disease

how likely it is that a positive test indicates disease, you must have this estimate of the patient's risk, as well as the sensitivity and specificity of the test being applied.

What are the steps to calculating the predictive values?

Calculate predictive values using the same 2 × 2 table (Table 6–8). Pick an arbitrary number of patients, such as 1000, and multiply the pretest probability to get the "disease present" and "disease absent" totals. Then multiply the total "disease present" by the sensitivity to get A = true positives. For D = true negatives, multiply the "disease absent" by the specificity. To get C and B, subtract A from total "disease present" and D from the total "disease absent," respectively. For PPV, divide the true positives, A, by the total positive tests, A plus B. For NPV, divide D by total negative tests, D plus C.

How are predictive values and these calculations applied to a real clinical scenario?

For example, the renal artery duplex is a highly sensitive (92%) and specific (94%) test for renal artery stenosis as a cause of hypertension. But because the incidence of the disease is so low (2%) in the general population, the PPV is 23% while the NPV is 99.8% (Table 6–9). So back to the question, "My patient has a positive renal artery duplex. Does she really have renal artery stenosis?" The answer is "This patient, despite the positive test result, only has a 23% chance of truly having renal artery stenosis."

TABLE 6–8

Calculating Predictive Value*

TEST	DISEASE	
	Present	*Absent*
Positive	A (true positive)	B (false positive)
Negative	C (false negative)	D (true negative)

Positive Predictive Value:

$$\frac{A}{(A + B)} \quad or \quad \frac{\text{(true positive test results)}}{\text{(all positive test results)}}$$

Positive Predictive Value:

$$\frac{D}{(D + C)} \quad or \quad \frac{\text{(true negative test results)}}{\text{(all negative test results)}}$$

*Requires prior knowledge of sensitivity, specificity, and pretest probability, i.e., prevalence of disease.

TABLE 6-9

Predictive Values of Renal Artery Duplex in Renal Artery Stenosis*

| DUPLEX | RENAL ARTERY STENOSIS | |
	Present in 20	Absent in 980
Positive	A = 18†	B = 60
Negative	C = 2	D = 920‡

$$\text{PPV: } \frac{18}{(18 + 60)} = 23\% \qquad \text{NPV: } \frac{920}{(2 + 920)} = 99.8\%$$

*Pretest probability = 2% prevalence of renal artery stenosis in general population. Assume 1000 patients, therefore 20 have disease, 980 do not have disease.
Sensitivity = 92%, specificity = 94% for renal artery duplex.
†Calculated from known sensitivity of 92%; 92% of 20 = 18 true positives.
‡Calculated from known specificity of 94%; 94% of 980 = 920 true negatives.

Case 6-1. A 24-year-old woman desires an HIV test. She is an IV drug user and obtains drugs through prostitution. Assume a pre-test probability of 25%. Sensitivity and specificity are 98%.

  A. Using a 2 × 2 table, calculate the predictive value of a positive test.
  B. Calculate the positive predictive value in monogamous woman with no risk factors (assume a pretest probability of 1/1000).

Case 6-2. When using renal artery duplex for renal artery stenosis, how can you increase the PPV of the test?

HOW TO USE ANTIBIOTICS

How do I approach the task of choosing and dosing antibiotics?

Learning about all antibiotics is almost impossible given the large number of choices available. To complicate matters, many antibiotics sound alike, especially cephalosporins. Your decision to use an individual antibiotic will be based on several factors: coverage of the likely or cultured organisms, drug allergy history, formulary availability, and cost. Once you decide which drug to use, consult a pocket pharmacopoeia, or palm pilot program such as *Epocrates* for dosing, and remember to adjust for renal function.

What is empirical therapy?

Empirical therapy is best guess therapy when a specific pathogen is not yet known. Patients present with signs of infection but definitive culture of blood, urine, or body fluid takes several days. In the interim before the pathogen is known we frequently begin antibiotics. In many cases, especially with pneumonia or skin infections, we never isolate a specific pathogen, and our whole treatment course is based on the most likely pathogen in a given setting.

What is a good starting point for picking antibiotic therapy?

Learn a few antibiotics appropriate for use with common bacterial pathogens: *Staphylococcus aureus*, gram-negative rods, anaerobes, *Enterococcus*, and atypical organisms such as *Chlamydia*, *Legionella*, *Mycoplasma* (Table 6–10)

When do I worry about *S. aureus* infections?

S. aureus is a very common pathogen and its drug resistance makes it particularly troublesome. Typical situations for *S. aureus* infections include endocarditis in injection drug users, skin and wound infections (especially in patients with diabetes), and nosocomial pneumonia.

What are good drugs for treating *S. aureus* infections?

S. aureus infections are divided into methicillin-sensitive and methicillin-resistant (MRSA) infections. In otherwise healthy patients when MRSA is unlikely, the best initial intravenous drugs for *S. aureus* infections are nafcillin or first generation cephalosporins such as cefazolin (Box 6–3). Oral options are dicloxacillin and cephalexin. If the patient has a life-threatening penicillin allergy then vancomycin is the best option. When MRSA is likely, as in frequently hospitalized or institutionalized patients, vancomycin is

BOX 6–3

Best Drugs for Methicillin-Sensitive *S. aureus*
- Nafcillin
- First generation cephalosporin
- Vancomycin

TABLE 6-10

Antibacterial Spectrum of Commonly Used Antibiotics

Antibiotic	Excellent Activity (>85% isolates sensitive)	Fair activity (70%–85% isolates sensitive)	Poor activity
Penicillin	*Streptococcus spp* except enterococci Oral anaerobes		Aerobic gram-negative rods *Staphylococcus aureus* Atypical organisms
Ampicillin	*Streptococcus spp* Oral anaerobes	*Haemophilus influenzae* Enterococci	Most aerobic gram-negative rods *S. aureus* Atypical organisms
Trimethoprim/Sulfa	*Streptococcus spp* except enterococci *Escherichia coli*[*]	*S. aureus*	Anaerobes
Clindamycin	*Streptococcus spp* except enterococci Anaerobes *S. aureus*		Hospital acquired gram-negative rods Aerobic gram-negative rods Atypical organisms
Quinolones Ciprofloxacin Ofloxacin	Aerobic gram-negative rods *S. aureus*	*Streptococcus spp*	Anaerobes *Enterococcus*
Levofloxacin Moxifloxacin* Gatifloxacin*	Aerobic gram-negative rods *S. aureus*/*Streptococcus*	Anaerobes	*Enterococcus*
Azithromycin Clarithromycin	*Streptococcus spp* except enterococci *H. influenzae* *Chlamydia* *Helicobacter pylori* *Mycobacterium avium* complex *Mycoplasma pneumoniae*		Most GNR

*Increasing resistance of *E. coli* approaching 15%. See UTI chapter.

47

used for empirical coverage until sensitivities are available. Oral vancomycin is not absorbed and should only be used for topical therapy of *C. difficile* colitis. Other drugs with good *S. aureus* activity include clindamycin, quinolones, second and third generation cephalosporins, or combination penicillin products with β-lactamase inhibitors such as ampicillin-clavulanate (Unasyn), piperacillin-tazobactam (Zosyn), or ticarcillin-clavulanate (Timentin).

How does anyone keep the cephalosporins straight?

The cephalosporins are confusing because they have similar names. Classify them by generation, with first generation drugs having better gram-positive coverage and third generation drugs having better negative coverage.

gram positives: first generation greater than second generation greater than third generation.

gram negatives: third generation greater than second generation greater than first generation.

Other special features of cephalosporins include: 1) cefotetan and cefoxitin are the only cephalosporins with good anaerobe activity (both are second generation); 2) Ceftazidime and cefoperazone are the only third generation cephalosporins with activity against *Pseudomonas aeruginosa*. Cefepime is a "fourth" generation cephalosporin which has antipseudomonal activity; 3) Ceftriaxone is a third generation cephalosporin that can be given once a day; and 4) no cephalosporin covers *Enterococcus* (group D strep).

When do I worry about gram-negative or anaerobic infections?

Gram-negative bacteria are generally seen with genitourinary tract infections (pyelonephritis, UTI) or infection from a bowel source (biliary tract disease, or peritonitis from bowel wall perforation). In addition to gram-negative rods, the bowels can also be the source of anaerobes and/or gram-positive cocci like *Enterococcus*. The oral gingiva is another common source of anaerobic infections (tooth abscess, aspiration pneumonia). A subcategory of less common gram-negative rods includes nosocomial, or hospital-acquired, gram-negative rods such as *Klebsiella* and *Pseudomonas*.

What are the best antibiotics for treating gram-negative infections?

Aminoglycosides and the monobactam, aztreonam, provide narrow coverage of aerobic gram-negative rods only. They are useful for almost all gram-negative infections, though are usually not used alone as empirical therapy due to their narrow spectrum. For situations where multiple types of organisms are possible, choose broader spectrum empirical therapy such as quinolones (superb gram-negative coverage), extended spectrum penicillins (mezlocillin, piperacillin and ticarcillin), third or fourth generation cephalosporins, imipenem, or meropenem. Of this group, imipenem and meropenem have the broadest spectrum of activity including gram-positive organisms as well as aerobic and anaerobic gram-negative rods. Although it is tempting to always use the broadest antibiotics, in fact this wipes out normal colonizing gut and vaginal flora. Choose the narrowest spectrum possible and narrow therapy promptly when culture results are available.

What antibiotics provide excellent coverage for anaerobic infections?

Anaerobes can be either gram-negative or -positive, and are distinguished by their inability to grow well in the presence of oxygen (Box 6–4). Their response to antibiotics is unique. Anaerobic infections of the mouth are generally sensitive to penicillin or ampicillin. By contrast, anaerobes of the gastrointestinal tract (especially *Bacteroides fragilis*) manufacture β-lactamase, therefore these "below the diaphragm" anaerobes are frequently resistant to penicillin. The best anaerobe drugs in this situation are clindamycin, metronidazole, a penicillin derivative/β-lactamase inhibitor combination, cefotetan, cefoxitin, imipenem, or meropenem.

How do you treat enterococcal infections?

These are difficult to treat. Penicillin, ampicillin, vancomycin, and linezolid are options. Ampicillin has the most activity but resistance is growing. For enterococcal bacteremia, aminoglycosides are frequently combined with ampicillin or vancomycin for synergy. Only about one third of enterococcal strains are sensitive to aminoglycosides.

What drugs are best for the atypical organisms *Legionella, Chlamydia, Mycoplasma*?

Erythromycin and tetracycline are the traditional drugs for these infections. Azithromycin and clarithromycin are newer medications

---

BOX 6–4

Best Drugs for Anaerobes
- Clindamycin
- Metronidazole
- Penicillin derivative with β-lactamase
- Cefotetan/cefoxitin
- Meropenem/imipenem

in the same class as erythromycin and are just as effective against atypical organisms with the benefit of less frequent dosing and fewer side effects, but the drawback of higher cost.

How do I know the cost of antibiotics?

In general, the drug cost of new antibiotics is greater than older antibiotics. For intravenous antibiotics the number of doses is the biggest determining factor in cost. The administration cost of an IV antibiotic is $18 to $24 per dose. As a result an expensive once daily IV antibiotic will have a lower daily cost than a cheaper IV antibiotic that needs to be given several times a day. Example: ceftriaxone 2 gm IV q twenty- four hours = $50 (cost of 2 gm of ceftriaxone) + $20 for one IV administration = $70 per day is cheaper than ampicillin 1 gm IV q six hours = $6 (cost of four doses of 1 gm of ampicillin) + $80 for four IV administrations = $86.

K E Y   P O I N T S

▶ Nafcillin and first generation cephalosporins are the most potent antibiotics for methicillin-sensitive *S. aureus*

▶ In general, for gram-positive coverage by the cephalosporins, first generation greater than second generation greater than third generation; gram-negative coverage is third greater than second greater than first generation

▶ The best antibiotics for anaerobe coverage are clindamycin, metronidazole, penicillin derivatives plus β-lactamase inhibitor, and cefotetan/cefoxitin

---

USEFUL WEBSITE

http://hopkins-abxguide.org/

Patients Presenting with a Symptom, Sign, or Abnormal Lab Value

7

Abdominal Pain

▶ ETIOLOGY

How do I begin to categorize the many causes of abdominal pain?

The acuity, duration, and location of abdominal pain can be helpful clues in narrowing the differential diagnosis early in your history-taking. The list of likely causes of acute abdominal pain, seen usually in hospitalized patients, is different than for chronic abdominal pain, occurring over weeks in outpatients (Tables 7–1 and 7–2). Diffuse abdominal pain is characteristic of a number of common conditions (Box 7–1). Focal pain should be approached geographically, with a differential diagnosis that includes pathology in organs located in the area involved (Figure 7–1). This chapter will not address the issue of functional abdominal pain, a common source of chronic abdominal pain without identifiable physical pathology.

What are some abdominal catastrophes I shouldn't miss?

Some causes of abdominal pain can lead to rapid clinical decline and death, especially if diagnosis is delayed (Box 7–2). Bowel perforation and ischemic bowel can cause gram-negative sepsis. Aortic aneurysm rupture and ectopic pregnancy cause rapid volume depletion and shock.

What important extra-abdominal problems masquerade as abdominal pain?

Angina may present atypically as epigastric pain. The other more typical characteristics of angina may still be present (e.g., pain worsened by exercise, relieved by resting, associated dyspnea, diaphoresis or nausea). Lower lobe pneumonia or pulmonary embolus can irritate the diaphragm and cause upper quadrant abdominal pain, usually worsened by breathing. Abdominal wall pain from muscle strain, hernia, nerve entrapment, rectus sheath

TABLE 7-1

Causes of Acute Abdominal Pain, Associated Risk Factors, and Key Features

Common Causes	Risk Factors	Key Features
Cholecystitis	"Fat, forty, female", prior biliary colic or gallstone	RUQ postprandial pain Fever, nausea, vomiting, anorexia May radiate to the right shoulder
Acute mesenteric infarction	Elderly, atherosclerotic risk factors, atrial fibrillation or other embolic risk	Soft abdominal exam ("pain out of proportion to exam") Acidosis
Appendicitis	Generally young but not always	Diffuse or periumbilical pain progresses over hours to RLQ pain Lying still with peritoneal signs if adjacent peritoneum inflamed Anorexia (severe) Steadily worsening fever, leukocytosis
Less Common Causes		
Pancreatitis	Gallstone disease, alcohol use or recent binge, high triglycerides, medications	Postprandial, midabdominal, or diffuse pain radiating to the back Nausea and/or vomiting in 90% Grey Turner's or Cullen's signs if hemorrhagic; pain decreases with leaning forward
Cholangitis	Gallstone disease, pancreatic cancer, AIDS	Triad of high fever, RUQ pain, and jaundice
Bowel obstruction	Prior abdominal surgery, adhesions, hernia	Inability to pass stool or flatus Feculent emesis Distended, tympanitic abdomen

Condition	Clinical Features
Obstipation	Constipation Hard stool on abdominal/rectal exam
Diverticulitis	LLQ pain develops, usually over days Fever
Renal stone	Paroxysms of pain, writhing patient Pain radiating to the genitals Hematuria
Ruptured aortic aneurysm	Sudden onset pain radiating to the back May have loss of lumbar nerve functions Rapidly expanding abdominal size Pulsatile abdominal mass, shock
Ectopic pregnancy	Sudden, severe lower quadrant pain Significant pallor due to anemia
PID	Subtle to severe lower abdominal pain with fever shortly after menses Cervical motion tenderness Purulent cervical discharge May have abnormal bleeding High ESR, elevated WBC

Condition	Risk Factors
Obstipation	Elderly, narcotics, calcium channel blockers
Diverticulitis	Elderly, prior diverticulosis
Renal stone	Crohn's disease, prior renal stone
Ruptured aortic aneurysm	Elderly, atherosclerotic risk factors
Ectopic pregnancy	Sexually active women, prior PID, IUD
PID	Sexually active women, prior STD, IUD, douching

TABLE 7–2

Common Causes of Chronic Abdominal Pain, Associated Risk Factors, and Key Features

Cause	Risk Factors	Key Features
Gastroesophageal reflux	Obesity, calcium channel blocker use	Acid or food regurgitation
		Symptoms worse when supine
Peptic ulcer	NSAIDs, prednisone, alcohol, caffeine	Improved with antacids
		Worse with acidic or spicy food, NSAIDs
		Melena
Biliary colic	"Fat, forty, female"	Intermittent episodes of RUQ pain
		Pain may radiate to right shoulder
		Postprandial pain, especially after fatty food
Irritable bowel syndrome	Anxiousness	No nocturnal symptoms
	Female	Improves with defecation
	Young to middle-aged	Alternating constipation, diarrhea
		Mucus in stool
Inflammatory bowel disease	None known	Nocturnal pain, intermittent bloody stool
		Extraintestinal manifestations—arthritis, gallstones, erythema nodosum, pyoderma gangrenosum, episcleritis, uveitis, thromboembolism, sclerosing cholangitis
Obstipation	Elderly, narcotics, calcium channel blockers	Inability to pass stool
		Hard stool
Chronic mesenteric ischemia (ischemic bowel)	Atherosclerotic risk factors	Postprandial, diffuse abdominal pain (also called intestinal angina)
		Anorexia, weight loss
Atypical angina	Hypertension, family history of early MI, hyperlipidemia, smoking	Worse with exercise, eating
		Associated dyspnea, diaphoresis, nausea

hematoma or herpes zoster (shingles) may mimic an intra-abdominal process.

What causes of abdominal pain have associated back pain?

Cholecystitis can radiate to the back or shoulder. Pain from pancreatitis and aortic aneurysm often radiates to the back. Lower thoracic or upper lumbar nerve irritation, as with herpes zoster

BOX 7–1

Causes of Diffuse Abdominal Pain

Pancreatitis
Bowel obstruction
Early appendicitis
Ischemic bowel
Constipation
Peritonitis

BOX 7–2

Potential Abdominal Catastrophes

Cholangitis
Ischemic bowel
Bowel perforation
Appendicitis
Splenic rupture
Ruptured abdominal aortic aneurysm
Ectopic pregnancy

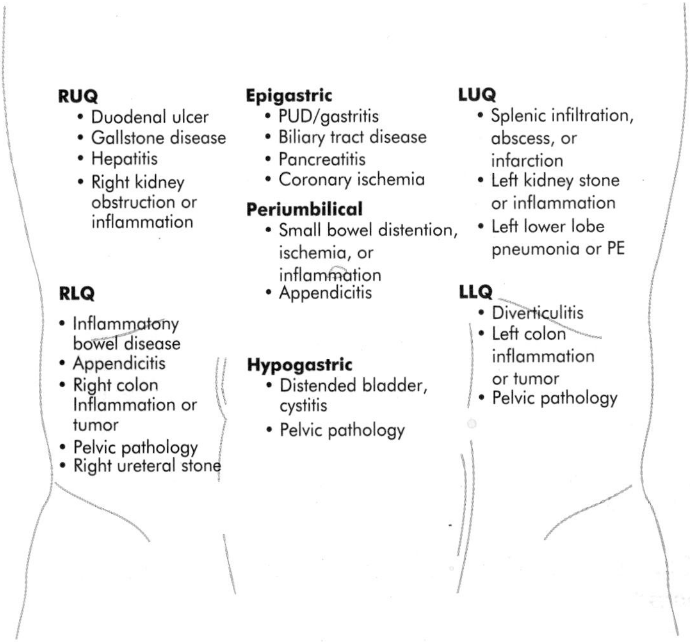

RUQ
- Duodenal ulcer
- Gallstone disease
- Hepatitis
- Right kidney obstruction or inflammation

RLQ
- Inflammatory bowel disease
- Appendicitis
- Right colon Inflammation or tumor
- Pelvic pathology
- Right ureteral stone

Epigastric
- PUD/gastritis
- Biliary tract disease
- Pancreatitis
- Coronary ischemia

Periumbilical
- Small bowel distention, ischemia, or inflammation
- Appendicitis

Hypogastric
- Distended bladder, cystitis
- Pelvic pathology

LUQ
- Splenic infiltration, abscess, or infarction
- Left kidney stone or inflammation
- Left lower lobe pneumonia or PE

LLQ
- Diverticulitis
- Left colon inflammation or tumor
- Pelvic pathology

Figure 7–1. Common causes of abdominal pain by location in the abdomen.

(shingles) or a ruptured disc, can cause pain radiating from the back to the abdomen.

What causes should I think of in elderly patients who have abdominal pain?

Cholecystitis, ischemic bowel, obstipation, diverticulitis, aortic aneurysm, and abdominal presentations of coronary artery disease are more common in elderly patients. It is also wise to remember that elderly patients may have a more subtle (altered mental status, vague symptoms), diffuse, or chronic presentation of a usually acute and focal process in the abdomen.

▶ EVALUATION

What are some "red flags" I shouldn't miss in evaluating patients with abdominal pain?

Beware that a prolonged evaluation can delay urgent intervention in a very ill patient. It is wise to do a quick initial survey for abnormal vital signs and peritoneal signs to get a sense of the urgency of intervention. In the acutely ill patient, dyspnea, pallor, diaphoresis, cyanosis, hypotension, tachycardia, or a rigid abdomen are worrisome signs of severe illness and warrant rapid evaluation by the most senior member of your team available. In such patients, it is also wise to involve the surgery consult team early as some conditions such as splenic or aortic rupture may require urgent intervention even before imaging is obtained. In patients with chronic pain, symptoms of fever, sweats, weight loss, melena, or cachexia are worrisome for a serious illness and usually warrant imaging by CT or endoscopy.

How do I approach history taking when there are so many questions I could ask?

Initially, ask open-ended questions to get a description of the onset and location of the pain in the patient's own words (e.g., "tell me more about your pain"). Listen for key information (Box 7–3). If necessary, ask more pointed questions to get as clear a picture as possible. Along the way, keep a running list of possible diagnoses and test them out by asking a few specific, key questions. For example, if you are thinking about appendicitis as a possibility, ask about loss of appetite, fever, and change of symptoms over time, as appendicitis usually causes profound anorexia, worsening fever, and progresses from diffuse or periumbilical pain to focal right lower quadrant pain over hours. Your write-up and presentations should reflect your differential diagnosis by pointing out the pertinent features on history and exam supporting and refuting

BOX 7-3

Key Information to Gather about Abdominal Pain from Patient History

Onset and duration
Character and severity of pain
Location and radiation
Progression of symptoms over time
Associated symptoms
Relation to meals, exercise, defecation
Change in stool or flatus
Exacerbating and relieving factors
History of recent travel, infectious exposure, alcohol use
Medications

the key illnesses you are considering. You will optimize your learning and improve your differential diagnostic skills by consulting a text after taking a history, and returning to the bedside to ask a few more questions based on what you learned from your reading.

What specific questions should I ask when patients have diffuse abdominal pain?

To assess for the likelihood of pancreatitis, ask about risk factors: gallstone disease, excessive alcohol use, hypertriglyceridemia, and certain medications such as antiretrovirals, prednisone, and hydrochlorothiazide, to name a few. Also ask about worsening of symptoms with eating and radiation of pain to the back or flank. To assess for the likelihood of bowel obstruction, ask about inability to pass stool or flatus. To assess for the likelihood of ischemic bowel or aneurysm, ask about atherosclerotic disease risk factors such as personal history of hypertension, hyperlipidemia, smoking, diabetes or family history of early MI. Also ask about postprandial symptoms and weight loss as these may accompany ischemic bowel disease. Ask about risk factors for chronic liver disease (country of origin, unprotected sexual exposures, and intravenous drug use) because cirrhosis with ascites can present with diffuse pain, and is a risk for spontaneous bacterial peritonitis.

What other historical clues are helpful?

Older men with benign prostatic hypertrophy may have painful bladder distention due to outlet obstruction. Prior gallstones put patients at risk for cholangitis, pancreatitis, and gallstone ileus. NSAIDs, cigarettes, oral steroids, caffeine or heavy alcohol use, are risks for peptic ulcer disease. Cigarette and significant steroid use are also risk factors for atherosclerotic disease, thus increasing the risk of angina, bowel ischemia, or aortic aneurysm. Patients with heavy alcohol use are at risk for gastritis, peptic ulcer disease, liver disease, and pancreatitis. Patients having unprotected intercourse or sharing needles are at risk for hepatitis. Women with unprotected sexual exposures are at risk for PID or ectopic pregnancy. Depression, anxiety, or sexual or physical abuse may be risk factors for functional abdominal pain without identifiable physical pathology.

What are helpful findings on physical exam in patients with abdominal pain?

Tachycardia or *hypotension* suggests a serious illness, requiring rapid assessment. Peritoneal signs of *involuntary guarding* or *rebound tenderness* are present when the peritoneal lining is irritated, usually by infection (e.g., with bowel rupture or appendicitis) or extravasation of blood into the peritoneum. Patients with peritoneal signs are usually lying very still to avoid irritating the peritoneum. *Turner's* and *Cullen's signs* are ecchymoses seen on the flank or around the umbilicus, respectively, in patients with retroperitoneal hemorrhage (usually due to hemorrhagic pancreatitis). Look for a hernia because a trapped piece of bowel can lead to bowel obstruction. *Shifting dullness* or a *fluid wave* may suggest ascites and a complication of liver disease. A *Sister Mary Joseph nodule* is an indurated nodule of metastatic cancer in the umbilicus, and is seen occasionally in patients with GI malignancy. The pelvic exam is very important in women with abdominal pain. *Cervical motion tenderness* and *purulent cervical discharge* suggest pelvic inflammatory disease. *Adnexal fullness* or tenderness may accompany ectopic pregnancy or tubo-ovarian abscess. Finger point tenderness at *McBurney's point* is used to confirm appendicitis. This point is located 1.5 to 2 inches from the anterior superior iliac spine (ASIS) on a line drawn between the ASIS and the umbilicus. *Carnett's sign* is used to determine if an abdominal wall process is causing pain. It is performed by examining patients in a half sit-up position; in this position, intra-abdominal pathology is usually less painful to deep palpation and abdominal wall pathology is more painful.

What work-up should I order in acutely ill patients with abdominal pain?

In patients with severe abdominal pain, standard lab work-up includes urinalysis, CBC, ABG, electrolytes, liver function tests, an amylase or lipase, and a pregnancy test. Blood cultures are warranted if fever is present. An abdominal x-ray series may detect bowel obstruction, or perforation (see Chapter 6). Don't forget the bladder or kidney as a potential source of pain. Bladder catheterization or ultrasound may reveal a bladder outlet obstruction.

Obtain a CT scan if you suspect cholecystitis, cholangitis, appendicitis, ischemic bowel, or abdominal aortic aneurysm, or if the cause remains unclear in a patient with severe abdominal pain. Ultrasound can be used to detect an ectopic pregnancy or biliary tree pathology. For patients with abdominal pain in shock (with unstable vital signs), urgent surgical exploration may need to occur before there is time for imaging. If you suspect an extra-abdominal source of pain, get a CXR and ECG.

What studies are warranted in patients with mild or chronic abdominal pain?

For patients with dyspepsia or reflux symptoms, a successful trial of antacid therapy can be used as a diagnostic test. For those with focal, episodic, right upper quadrant pain unresponsive to antacids, an ultrasound or CT scan may reveal gallstones. In patients with worrisome weight loss, bloody stool, melena, or change in bowel habits and abdominal pain, general lab studies including a CBC, electrolytes, glucose, and liver function tests are reasonable along with referral for endoscopy. A large percentage of patients with chronic abdominal pain have functional disease, meaning pain not associated with a discoverable pathologic abnormality. Such patients have often already undergone work-up without obtaining a clear diagnosis. A good psychosocial history is key and may reveal prior or current abuse or depression.

▶ TREATMENT

For specific treatments of common causes of abdominal pain, please see other relevant sections of this book (Dyspepsia, GI Bleeding, Gastroenterology, Hematology and Oncology, and Infectious Disease).

When should I hospitalize patients with abdominal pain?

Reasons for admitting a patient with abdominal pain include severe pain of unclear cause, peritoneal signs, unstable vital signs, suspected cholangitis, cholecystitis, bowel obstruction or perforation, appendicitis, aneurysmal leak, splenic rupture, ectopic pregnancy, tubo-ovarian abscess, and patients with pyelonephritis or PID with vomiting who need IV antibiotics. Part of treating a patient hospitalized for abdominal pain includes frequent serial examinations to assess for progression of disease, whether or not a diagnosis has been made. Patients with an unclear source of acute abdominal pain accompanied by peritoneal signs or shock may need urgent exploratory surgery, hence the importance of involving a surgical consult team early.

K E Y   P O I N T S

▶ Narrow the differential diagnosis of abdominal pain by acuity and location of the pain

▶ Order a pregnancy test and perform a pelvic exam in young women with lower abdominal pain of unclear cause

▶ A painful but soft abdomen in an elderly person is ischemic bowel disease until proven otherwise

▶ Myocardial infarction and pulmonary embolus can masquerade as abdominal pain

---

CASE 7–1. A 20-year-old college student is brought to the ED by a friend. She reports sudden onset right lower quadrant pain beginning three hours prior to arriving in the ED. She takes no medications and has been healthy without prior surgeries or hospitalizations. Her P is 110, BP is 90/60 and T is 99.6°F. Her exam reveals a diffusely tender abdomen with focal severe tenderness in the right lower quadrant.

    A. What is your differential diagnosis?
    B. What steps do you wish to take next in her evaluation and treatment?

CASE 7–2. A 70-year-old man with a history of hypertension, cigarette and alcohol use, and mild dementia is brought to the ED by his son. The patient reports severe, diffuse abdominal pain. His son also reports an associated 20-pound weight loss over the prior three months. He takes hydrochlorothiazide and aspirin. On exam, his P is 112, BP is 100/60, RR is 28, T is 98.9°F, and abdomen is scaphoid and soft but diffusely tender, without organomegaly, guarding, pulsatile mass, ecchymosis, or bulging flanks. Rectal exam reveals a diffusely large prostate and guaiac positive stool.

    A. What is your differential diagnosis for his abdominal pain?
    B. How will you evaluate him?

REFERENCES

Orient JM, Sapira JD: Sapira's Art and Science of Bedside Diagnosis, 2nd ed. Williams & Wilkins, Philadelphia, 2000.

Spiro HM: An internist's approach to acute abdominal pain. Med Clin North Am.96(2):63–67, 1993.

8

Anemia

What is anemia?

Anemia is a decrease in red cell mass. Because red cell mass is difficult to measure directly, we use hemoglobin or hematocrit (HCT) as surrogate measures. Hemoglobin of less than 12 in women and 13 in men defines anemia. HCT is roughly three times the hemoglobin. Hemoglobin and HCT measures are plasma volume–dependent. They are falsely elevated in dehydration and falsely decreased in volume overload, e.g., as in cirrhosis or CHF.

How does anemia occur?

Blood loss is the most common cause of anemia, usually from gastrointestinal bleeding or menses. Any disruption in the red cell life cycle will also cause anemia, including inadequate production or excessive destruction. Any of these causes may coexist. Red cell *production* is abnormal if the bone marrow does not have necessary building blocks, such as iron or vitamin B_{12}, or if the marrow is damaged due to drugs, fibrosis, or cancer infiltration. *Destruction* occurs by hemolysis, either within blood vessels (intravascular) or in the spleen (extravascular).

How do the reticulocyte count and MCV help determine etiology?

The normal bone marrow responds to anemia by releasing more reticulocytes (immature red cells). With hemolysis or acute blood loss, the reticulocyte count increases. A normal marrow response is reflected in a corrected reticulocyte index of greater than 2–3. Lower values, no matter what the cause of anemia, suggest that the bone marrow is not functioning normally, i.e., there is a production problem. In this case the MCV will help distinguish causes (Table 8–1).

What causes the changes in red cell size reflected in an abnormal MCV?

Enlarged red cells often develop when abnormal DNA synthesis delays nuclear maturation of erythrocyte precursors, as in B_{12} or

TABLE 8-1

Causes of Hypoproliferative Anemia by MCV

MCV	Common Causes	Less Common Causes
MCV <80 Microcytosis	Iron deficiency	Thalassemia Anemia of chronic disease Hemoglobin E
MCV 80–95 Normocytosis	Anemia of chronic disease Acute bleeding	Bone marrow suppression, fibrosis, or infiltration
MCV >95 Macrocytosis	Alcohol	Vitamin B_{12} deficiency Folate deficiency Hypothyroidism Reticulocytosis

folate deficiency. Alcohol may be the most common cause of macrocytic anemia. Between 40% and 90% of alcoholics have an MCV greater than 100, mostly due to a direct effect of alcohol on the bone marrow, though occasionally due to folate deficiency. Small red cells occur with problems in hemoglobin synthesis, as with iron deficiency or thalassemia.

How do people get deficient of folate or vitamin B_{12}?

Folate deficiency generally results from inadequate nutritional intake of leafy green vegetables and citrus fruits, and is especially seen in severely disabled patients. Folate deficiency is also common in alcoholics. Deficiency also results from problems with absorption (as with small bowel disease or the use of phenytoin or phenobarbital), or increased demand (as in pregnancy, psoriasis, chemotherapy, or hemolytic anemia). The body stores only a three month supply of folate so deficiency can develop after a short period of time. In contrast, the liver stores three to five years of B_{12} so a nutritional deficiency alone almost never occurs. Vitamin B_{12} requires binding to intrinsic factor from the stomach in order to be absorbed in the terminal ileum. B_{12} deficiency is usually caused by pernicious anemia, a destruction of the parietal cells that make intrinsic factor in the stomach. Achlorhydria, or loss of stomach acid, is common in older patients and also causes deficiency by preventing binding of B_{12} to intrinsic factor. Colchicine and neomycin can also block B_{12} absorption. B_{12} deficiency can cause any combination of nausea, heartburn, vague abdominal pain, depression, or subacute neurologic disease (dementia, dorsal and lateral column defects).

Why does chronic disease cause anemia?

Anemia of chronic disease, also known as inflammatory block, is a mild to moderate anemia resulting from an inability to utilize iron.

Inflammatory mediators prevent the normal transfer of iron from bone marrow stores into hemoglobin. This type of anemia is associated with chronic inflammatory conditions such as rheumatoid arthritis, systemic lupus erythematosus, and chronic infections such as osteomyelitis.

What causes hemolysis?

Hemolysis can be categorized according to where the hemolysis occurs. In *intravascular* hemolysis, red cells are broken down directly in the blood vessels. Examples include red cell fragmentation across mechanical heart valves or over fibrin strands in disseminated intravascular coagulopathy (DIC). By contrast, in *extravascular* hemolysis, abnormal red cells are lysed in the reticuloendothelial system (RES) of the spleen or liver. Red cells are recognized as abnormal by the RES due to attached antibodies, such as in autoimmune hemolysis or infection, or membrane or hemoglobin defects such as sickle cell disease or thalassemia.

What medications cause anemia?

Medications can cause anemia by a variety of mechanisms. Always review a patient's medication list in unexplained anemia. Common drugs associated with anemia are anticonvulsants, colchicine, trimethoprim, chloroquine, and certain antibiotics. Pioglitazone and rosiglitazone can cause a dilutional anemia. Other medications cause macrocytosis by altering DNA synthesis directly, e.g., chemotherapy agents, anticonvulsants, trimethoprim, and sulfasalazine.

> ▶ **EVALUATION**

In whom should I suspect anemia?

Mild anemia is asymptomatic and is often discovered accidentally as part of routine blood work. Asymptomatic patients should not be screened for anemia. Symptoms of anemia are nonspecific and reflect inadequate oxygen delivery. Symptoms are also dependent on the abruptness of onset, severity, age, and cardiopulmonary reserve of the patient. In general you should suspect anemia as a contributing factor in patients with fatigue, shortness of breath, dyspnea on exertion, dizziness, pallor, or tachycardia.

What should I look for when I evaluate patients with anemia?

A history of chest pain, lightheadedness, or shortness of breath indicates possible end-organ hypoxia, and should prompt rapid evaluation. Exam findings in patients with significant anemia include tachycardia, cardiac flow murmur, pale conjunctivae, and pale palmar creases and nail beds.

What tests are key in differentiating types of anemia?

Order an HCT or hemoglobin to confirm the diagnosis of anemia. Reticulocyte count, MCV, and peripheral smear will suggest a diagnosis or need for further testing (Figure 8–1).

If I suspect hemolysis, what tests are helpful?

Peripheral smear differentiates between intra- and extravascular hemolysis. Spherocytes are formed during extravascular hemolysis when abnormal red cell membrane is removed by the RES. Irregularly shaped red cell fragments, or schistocytes, are formed as red cells sheer across intravascular obstacles such as prosthetic valves and fibrin strands; they are only seen in intravascular hemolysis. Regardless of the site of hemolysis, red cell destruction results in reticulocytosis, elevated indirect bilirubin, elevated LDH and decreased haptoglobin. Measurable haptoglobin drops because it binds to the hemoglobin released from hemolyzed red cells.

If I suspect iron deficiency, what else should I look for?

Ask about heavy menses, bloody or black stool, fatigue, and pica (eating non-food items such as paper or clay). Pagophagia, or

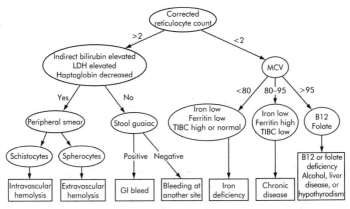

Figure 8–1. Diagnostic work-up for common causes of anemia. Sequence of testing may vary depending on the clinical situation.

pica for ice, is considered a specific symptom for iron deficiency. Spoon nails (koilonychia) or a smooth red tongue (atrophic glossitis) are uncommon signs of iron deficiency. Obtain serum iron, total iron binding capacity, and ferritin. Iron deficiency initially results in a low ferritin. Subsequently serum iron falls and TIBC rises. As deficiency progresses, hemoglobin falls and then microcytosis develops causing a low MCV. If the labs suggest iron deficiency, you need to find the source of blood loss. In addition to guaiac testing, endoscopy may be necessary.

What should I do next if my patient has normocytic anemia (MCV 80–95)?

Review the H & P for symptoms or signs of inflammation, which might cause anemia of chronic disease: 75% of anemias of chronic disease are normocytic. Since normocytic anemia can result from early iron deficiency, iron studies are helpful in differentiating iron deficiency from the anemia of chronic disease. Further, review medications that could suppress the bone marrow, such as antibiotics or chemotherapeutic agents. Additionally, check for signs or symptoms of neoplastic disease such as anorexia, weight loss, or night sweats. Peripheral smear may suggest hemolysis or sickle cell disease, or may show teardrops in the case of marrow fibrosis or infiltration. Other specific studies for hemolysis, chronic renal failure, or thyroid disease may be warranted. Bone marrow biopsy can rule out myelodysplasia, infiltration, or bone marrow fibrosis.

The MCV is low and labs have ruled out iron deficiency. What do I do next?

Iron deficiency is the most common cause of a low MCV. However, if laboratories rule-out iron deficiency, consider either anemia of chronic disease or thalassemia. In anemia of chronic disease, the ferritin, an acute phase reactant, is often high while TIBC and serum iron are low. Despite low serum iron, iron replacement is of no benefit because of the inflammatory block. Thalassemia is a genetic disease of globin chains seen in patients with Mediterranean, African, or Asian heritage. Patients with thalassemia have a very low MCV (in the 60–70 range), out of proportion to a mild anemia (HCT 33–40). Often target cells are seen on peripheral smear. Though β-thalassemia can be confirmed with hemoglobin electrophoresis, there is no confirmatory test for α-thalassemia. If the diagnosis remains unclear after full lab workup, consider a bone marrow biopsy and iron stain.

What tests should I order if my patient has macrocytic anemia (MCV greater than 95)?

Review history for alcohol or medication use, risk factors for and symptoms of vitamin B_{12} deficiency (gastric surgery, vitiligo, paresthesias in the feet), symptoms of hypothyroidism, or chronic liver disease. Also, look for signs or symptoms of acute bleeding or hemolysis because reticulocytes are larger than mature red cells and will raise the MCV. Examine the patient for signs of B_{12} deficiency such as beefy red tongue and decreased peripheral vibratory or position sense, or for findings of end-stage liver disease. Review the smear for hypersegmented neutrophils and macro-ovalocytes, megaloblastic changes that are caused by abnormal DNA synthesis, and delayed nuclear maturation of erythrocyte precursors. Red blood cell folate and serum B_{12} levels may reveal the cause. If no obvious diagnosis is apparent, consider ordering a bone marrow biopsy.

▶ TREATMENT

In general, the underlying cause of the anemia should be identified and treated. Rarely will outpatients need to be hospitalized or transfused for their anemia alone.

How do I treat iron deficiency anemia and what response should I expect from treatment?

The goals of treatment are: 1) identify and treat the cause of iron deficiency, and 2) give sufficient iron to correct the anemia and replenish stores. With few exceptions replace iron orally. Compliance can be difficult since about 25% of patients have side effects when they take iron on an empty stomach (nausea, epigastric pain, constipation, and diarrhea). Although absorption is decreased 40% when iron is taken with food, this may be a necessary compromise. Start with 325 mg of ferrous sulfate once a day and advance to twice a day as tolerated. Ferrous gluconate and elixir preparations are available as well. The HCT should increase by 2 points every three to four weeks. A reticulocytosis is the first sign of response and is evident after ten days.

When should I hospitalize a patient with anemia?

Hospitalize patients with anemia when they have a declining HCT due to ongoing blood loss or rapid hemolysis, or when cardiac or pulmonary symptoms occur.

K E Y   P O I N T S

▶ Anemia is never normal—seek a cause in all patients who are anemic

▶ History and exam are key in narrowing the differential diagnosis of anemia

▶ Carefully review medications for a cause of anemia

▶ Begin lab evaluation with an HCT, MCV, reticulocyte count, and smear

▶ For iron deficiency anemia, start with low dose iron replacement (325 mg PO qd)

CASE 8–1. A 75-year-old woman with history of a mechanical aortic valve replacement on chronic anticoagulation is brought to clinic for increasing confusion and shortness of breath. Her baseline HCT is 36 with rare schistocytes. She denies other medical problems or medications. On exam she is confused, pale, with a temperature of 100.5° F, RR of 30, P of 110, scleral icterus and palatal petechia. Labs reveal: HCT 28, MCV 102, corrected reticulocyte index of 8%, platelets 29K, creatinine 4.2, PTT INR 5.2.

    A. What are possible etiologies of her anemia?
    B. What should you do next?

CASE 8–2. A 70-year-old man reports fatigue. He denies other symptoms and takes no medications. He drinks alcohol two to three nights a week in moderation. He is found to have an HCT of 34 and MCV of 78. He is up-to-date on his colon cancer screening with a flexible sigmoidoscopy a year ago and is guaiac negative on examination. He is started on once a day iron and his fatigue improves.

    A. What would prompt you to evaluate this patient further?
    B. What tests would you do?

REFERENCES

Brill JR: Normocytic anemia. Am Fam Physician 62(10):2255–2264, 2000.
Davenport J: Macrocytic anemia. Am Fam Physician 53:155, 1996.

9

Chest Pain

What are the common causes of mild to moderate chest pain in clinic patients?

Angina, esophageal reflux, and musculoskeletal pain including costochondritis are common. Less common causes are panic disorder, esophageal dysmotility, and viral or bacterial infection causing pleural irritation. Rarely, biliary, gastric, or pancreatic disease causes chest pain.

What are life-threatening causes of chest pain I shouldn't miss?

Acute aortic dissection, unstable or acute angina pectoris, myocardial infarction (MI), mediastinitis, pericarditis, pneumothorax, and pulmonary embolus (PE) shouldn't be missed. Aortic dissection occurs when the aorta tears, allowing blood to dissect between layers of the vessel wall. Angina is chest pain due to insufficient oxygen supply to the heart muscle for the level of cardiac work (ischemia), seen particularly in patients with risk factors such as hypertension, diabetes, cigarette use, family history of early cardiac disease, or dyslipidemia. MI occurs if angina persists long enough to cause cell death (infarction). Mediastinitis is an infection of the mediastinum, usually caused by an esophageal rupture. Pericarditis develops if inflammation occurs in the pericardial sac. A pneumothorax involves air entering the pleural space. Pulmonary embolism occurs if clot from the venous circulation lodges in a pulmonary artery.

▶ EVALUATION

What pertinent history helps determine if chest pain is due to angina?

Ask all patients with chest pain about cardiac risk factors, character and distribution of pain, and associated symptoms. Angina is a heavy, tight, or squeezing retrosternal or left chest discomfort, which can radiate to the neck, jaw, shoulders, or left arm. Associated symptoms may include dyspnea, diaphoresis, nausea, or lightheadedness. Most angina is brought on by exertion, though stress or overeating can sometimes precipitate angina. Angina is typically relieved by rest or by sublingual nitrates. Atypical presentations are common, especially in women, the elderly, and in patients with diabetes. Atypical angina may present as burning or pressure in locations such as the arm, neck, jaw, shoulder, or abdomen, or with isolated dyspnea or nausea. Unstable angina refers to angina at rest, or to a substantial change in a previously stable angina pattern. MI causes similar but more severe pain and generally lasts longer than thirty minutes. Pain that is pleuritic, sharp, positional, or is exactly reproduced by palpation is unlikely to be due to ischemia. Pain lasting for only a few seconds is never due to ischemia. Findings that suggest specific noncardiac etiologies of pain can be found in Table 9–1.

How do patients with aortic dissection present?

Aortic dissection causes pain that is severe, sharp, or tearing, and often begins abruptly. Tears distal to the left subclavian typically radiate to the back while tears of the ascending aorta may radiate to the anterior chest or to the back. Pain can also radiate down the arms. Aortic dissection can cause neurologic deficits, decreased consciousness, or hoarseness. Complications can be life-threatening (Table 9–2).

What pertinent questions should I ask to explore the possibility of PE?

Ask about the triad of predisposing factors: 1) hypercoagulable states such as cancer or family history of hypercoagulability; 2) prolonged stasis as with airplane trips, surgery, or immobility; and 3) vessel injury with recent surgery or trauma. Ask about unilateral leg swelling since this may reveal the embolic source. Massive embolism can stretch a pulmonary artery, mimicking angina or causing actual right ventricular ischemia. Smaller PE's may produce lung infarcts at the pleural surface, causing sharp pleuritic pains. Isolated dyspnea without pain is the most common presentation. Syncope occurs in about 10% of PEs and is a sign of a larger embolus.

What pertinent history should I ask to reveal an esophageal source of pain?

Historical clues to esophageal pain from acid reflux include burning pain worsened with acidic or fatty foods or with lying down, relief with antacids, and absence of relation to exertion.

TABLE 9-1

Clues to Nonischemic Causes of Chest Pain

Diagnosis	History	Physical Exam	Diagnostic Tests
Costochondritis	Recent viral illness	Tender to palpation just lateral to sternum	None
Mediastinitis	Dyspnea, vomiting, recent esophageal instrumentation	Subcutaneous emphysema, "Hammon's crunch" = crepitus with heartbeat	CXR: mediastinal air, pleural effusion (usually left-sided)
Musculoskeletal pain	Worse with motion or breath, history of trauma or cancer with metastases	Pain reproduced by palpation	Physical exam, CXR
Pericarditis	Sharp pain improved by leaning forward; recent viral illness	Pericardial friction rub, JVD, pulsus paradoxus* (with large pericardial effusion)	ECG: diffuse ST elevation, PR depression
Pleurisy	Pleuritic pain, dyspnea, recent viral illness, autoimmune disease	Pleural friction rub	CXR: normal, +/− small effusion
Pneumonia	Fever, cough, dyspnea, purulent sputum, pleuritic pain	Crackles, egophony over involved lung	CXR: pulmonary infiltrate
Pneumothorax	Pleuritic pain, dyspnea	Hyperresonance over one lung field, decreased breath sounds, tracheal shift	CXR: loss of lung markings outside sharp pleural line
Pulmonary embolus	History of cancer, CHF, immobility, OCP use. Pleuritic pain, dyspnea, syncope	Tachycardia, pleural friction rub, unilateral swollen leg	ABG, D-dimer test, V/Q scan, Venous duplex

*Pulsus paradoxus is a drop in systolic blood pressure of more than 10 points with inspiration, caused by pericardial fluid compressing the right ventricle. You can palpate this at the radial pulse in dramatic cases of tamponade. To measure it more exactly, inflate a blood pressure cuff above systolic pressure, let air out slowly until you just begin to hear beats only during patient's expiration and remember that value. Then let out more air until you hear all the beats through both inspiration and expiration. Subtract this pressure from the first; if > 10 mm Hg, you have pulsus paradoxus, indicating cardiac tamponade. Significant pulmonary obstructive disease also causes pulsus paradoxus.

TABLE 9-2	
Complications of Acute Aortic Dissection in the Thorax	
Complication	**Mechanism**
Acute congestive heart failure	Aortic insufficiency due to valve involved in dissection
Acute MI	Dissection disrupts opening from aorta to coronary artery
Cardiac tamponade	Blood fills pericardium and compresses heart
Neurologic deficits	Flow to innominate, carotid, or spinal arteries disrupted

Esophageal spasms may closely mimic angina and often reverse with nitroglycerine. Cardiac catheterization is sometimes needed to distinguish coronary vascular disease from esophageal spasms.

How does pericarditis differ from angina in its presentation?

Pain from pericarditis is classically worse lying down, better leaning forward, and is unimproved by rest. Risk factors for pericarditis include recent viral syndrome, renal failure, connective tissue disease, or metastatic cancer.

What should I look for on exam?

Assess the patient's general appearance; patients with chest pain who appear to be in significant discomfort are likely to have ischemia or some other serious cause for their pain. Hypertension, though nonspecific, often accompanies angina and aortic dissection. Hypotension can be seen in patients with extensive or right ventricular MI, large PE, or tension pneumothorax. Tachycardia may accompany pulmonary embolism, MI, or hypoxia of any cause. Check blood pressure in both arms, as they are unequal (greater than 30 mm Hg) when a dissection interrupts vascular supply to one side. Listen for new murmurs: aortic insufficiency (diastolic murmur at the sternal border) suggests dissection involving the aortic valve; mitral regurgitation (systolic murmur at the apex) suggests an MI involving the mitral valve papillary muscle. Listen for rubs: a pulmonary friction rub timed with inspiration suggests viral pleuritis or pulmonary infarct due to PE; a rub with each heartbeat suggests pericarditis. Palpate the chest wall to assess for tenderness and ask if any tenderness exactly reproduces the patient's pain.

What diagnostic tests do I order in an outpatient with chest pain?

Obtain current and old **ECGs** and **CXRs** in all patients with acute chest pain. Look for the focal ST changes of angina or MI, or the diffuse ST elevations and PR depressions of pericarditis. CXR can reveal CHF, pneumonia, pulmonary infarction, pneumothorax, rib fractures, and lytic bone lesions. A widened mediastinum on chest film is a sign of possible aortic dissection, though 20% of dissections have a normal mediastinal width. **Therapeutic trials** in the clinic or at home may also aid in making a diagnosis: relief with antacids suggests GERD or PUD; relief with sublingual nitroglycerin suggests cardiac ischemia. Refer patients with stable episodes of angina-like symptoms for outpatient exercise treadmill testing (ETT) to assess for fixed coronary artery narrowing. For women (in whom ETT has low sensitivity) and for patients unable to walk, alternatives to ETT include nuclear medicine tests or stress echocardiogram.

What tests are appropriate for patients hospitalized due to chest pain?

In addition to ECG and CXR, obtain serial cardiac enzymes (see Ischemic Heart Disease section for details). Because of the high mortality of acute aortic dissection, obtain a transesophageal echocardiogram or chest CT if there is any suspicion for a dissection. Don't forget that CHF and MI can accompany aortic dissection. Thrombolytics for MI are likely fatal if given to patients with concurrent aortic dissection and can be fatal for patients with pericarditis. These diagnoses need to be carefully excluded before a patient is given thrombolytics. Obtain a CBC with differential to look for anemia or infection; platelets, PT and PTT time for coagulopathy; and a chemistry panel.

My clinic patient "ruled-out" for MI but still has pain. What other tests are useful?

Patients "rule-out" for MI when twenty-four hours of hospital monitoring and serial enzymes fail to reveal heart muscle damage. CAD is still possible even after "ruling-out" and can be diagnosed by ETT or other imaging (see Ischemic Heart Disease section). An outpatient GI evaluation may include a trial of proton pump inhibitors (PPIs), the more invasive esophagogastroduodenoscopy (EGD) to look for esophageal or gastric lesions, or twenty-four hour esophageal pH monitoring to confirm GERD. Further evaluation for esophageal dysmotility may include barium swallow or esophageal pressure monitoring.

▶ TREATMENT

When should patients be hospitalized for chest pain?

Patients with chest pain suspicious for ischemia, or with atypical chest pain and ECG changes consistent with ischemia are generally admitted. Patients with atypical chest pain, no ECG changes, and those who have cardiac risk factors are sometimes admitted, depending on the degree of suspicion that their pain could be due to ischemia.

What specific treatments are available for common causes of chest pain?

See Ischemic Heart Disease section for treatment of ischemia and Table 9–3 for treatment of other causes.

What is the prognosis for patients with "noncardiac" chest pain?

Normal angiography is associated with a 7-year mortality of less than 1%. Chest pain of unclear etiology can develop into a chronic pain syndrome, causing patients significant morbidity and cost. These patients are best managed by primary care physicians with continued vigilance for the possibility of CAD (especially in the elderly), selected evaluation for esophageal or psychiatric disease, judicious use of medications for symptom control, and reassurance.

TABLE 9–3

Therapeutic Options for Noncardiac Causes of Chest Pain

Cause of Chest Pain	Treatment Options
Acute aortic dissection	Blood pressure control, surgical repair
Costochondritis	NSAIDs or acetaminophen, time
Gastroesophageal reflux	PPIs, lifestyle modification, surgical fundoplication
Esophageal spasm	Antacids, calcium channel blocker, nitroglycerin
Musculoskeletal pain	Rest, stretching, physical therapy, NSAIDs or acetaminophen
Pericarditis	NSAIDs
Pneumonia	Antibiotics, oxygen, chest physiotherapy
Pneumothorax	If tension pneumothorax, urgent decompression by angiocatheter, chest tube

▶ Consider life-threatening causes in all patients with chest pain and use focused history, exam, and studies to rapidly find or exclude them

▶ After the initial evaluation, if ischemic cardiac chest pain is still a reasonable possibility, admit for monitoring and serial cardiac enzyme testing

▶ Consider a pulmonary embolus in any patient with unexplained chest pain, especially if the pain is associated with dyspnea or it has a pleuritic component

▶ Pericarditis causes diffuse PR depression or ST elevation on ECG and pain relieved by leaning forward

▶ Aortic dissection causes pain that begins abruptly and radiates to the back or chest, unequal pulses, a widened mediastinum, and may have associated neurologic deficits, CHF, or MI

CASE 9–1. A 36-year-old woman presents to the ED complaining of twenty-four hours of progressively increasing chest pain. The pain is 7/10, sharp, substernal, and pleuritic in nature. It is worsened by lying supine. She gives a history of fever and a nonproductive cough two weeks ago, which resolved one week ago. She denies dyspnea or calf pain. She takes oral contraceptives and smokes one pack a day. She is sitting on a stretcher, looking uncomfortable with vital signs of T 37.5°C, P 110, BP 125/80, and RR 18.

A. What are possible causes for her pain?
B. Which clinical features increase her likelihood of pericarditis? Which increase her likelihood of a pulmonary embolus?
C. The nurse hands you her ECG (Figure 9–1). What is the most likely diagnosis?
D. What would you expect to find on physical exam?
E. What is the most likely cause for this patient's syndrome?

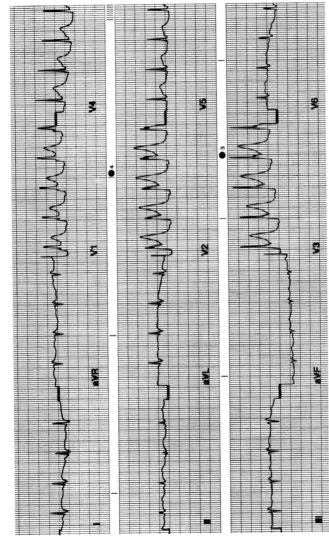

Figure 9–1. Electrocardiogram for patient in Case 9–1. (*From Davidson R*: Electrocardiography in Acute Care Medicine, *St. Louis, 1995, Mosby.*)

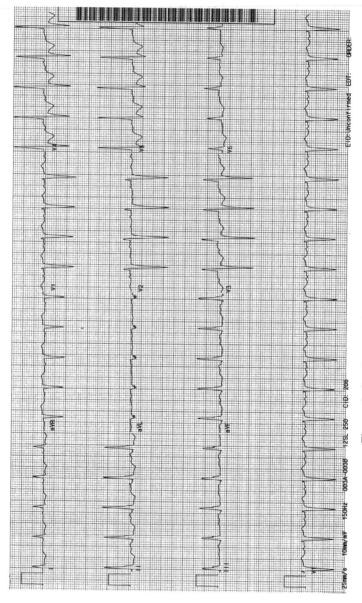

Figure 9–2. Electrocardiogram for patient in Case 9–2.

CASE 9-2.
A 60-year-old male presents with one hour of chest pain. The pain is a 7/10 substernal pressure radiating to the neck and left arm, associated with dyspnea. He has hypertension and hypercholesterolemia. His father had an MI at age 52. He has no prior history of similar pain and denies nausea, lightheadedness, a history of reflux or any pleuritic component to his pain. He takes hydrochlorothiazide, and simvastatin and smokes one pack a day. On exam, he is anxious and diaphoretic, his vital signs are T 36.8°C, P 112, BP 158/92, RR 22, his chest is clear and cardiac exam shows regular S_1-S_2 without murmurs, rubs, or gallops.

A. List this patient's CAD risk factors. What are other cardiac risk factors?

B. What are possible causes for his chest pain?

C. What are the significant findings on this patient's ECG (Figure 9-2). What is your diagnosis?

REFERENCES

American College of Emergency Physicians: Clinical policy for the initial approach to adults presenting with a chief complaint of chest pain, with no history of trauma. Ann Emerg Med 25(2):274–299, 1995.

Panju AA, Hemelgarn BR, Guyatt GH, Simel DL: Is this patient having a myocardial infarction? JAMA 280:1256–1263, 1998.

10

Cough

Acute cough = infection/irritant;
(< 3 wks)
Chronic cough = Asthma
(> 3 wks)   PND
*   GERD*

What are the most common causes of cough?

Acute cough, less than 3 weeks' duration, is almost always due to infection (usually viral) or irritants, such as cigarette smoke. *Chronic cough,* greater than 3 weeks' duration, is most commonly caused by the conditions listed in Box 10–1. Chronic bronchitis is defined as productive cough on most days for at least three months of two consecutive years and occurs almost exclusively in smokers. After acute viral infection, up to 40% of patients have persistent cough for several weeks due to transiently reactive airways. Up to 62% of cases of chronic cough have more than one cause. ACE inhibitors cause cough in approximately 10% of users.

What serious causes of cough should I not miss?

Cancer is always a concern in patients with chronic cough, particularly in smokers. About 80% of cancer patients have other symptoms such as weight loss or hemoptysis. CHF may present with cough. TB and pertussis, major public health risks, should always be considered. Up to 25% of adults with greater than 3 weeks of cough without another cause have serologic evidence consistent with recent pertussis infection. Previous vaccination does not exclude pertussis. Pulmonary embolism is an infrequent but serious cause of acute cough.

BOX 10–1

Common Causes of Chronic Cough

Cough-variant asthma 60%

PND 58%

Gastroesophageal reflux 41%

Chronic bronchitis/bronchiectasis 5–14% *(smokers)*

Single cause in 39%

Multiple causes in 62%

When cough is accompanied by hemoptysis, what should I consider?

Acute bronchitis is the most common cause of bloody sputum in the U.S. Consider cancer in smokers or patients over age 50. Other causes include pulmonary embolism and TB.

▶ EVALUATION

What historical points and exam findings are important?

Table 10–1 lists pertinent history and exam findings to explore for each of the common causes of chronic cough. Note medications such as ACE inhibitors. Inhaler or antacid use suggests asthma or GERD, respectively. Review constitutional symptoms and risk factors for cancer and HIV.

In puzzling cases, obtain an exposure history for work or hobby hazards such as contact with asbestos, persons with HIV, TB, or pertussis, and cats or birds.

TABLE 10–1

History and Exam Findings in Common Causes of Chronic Cough

Cause	History	Exam
Asthma	Recent viral infection Cold/exercise provoke cough Aspirin or NSAID sensitivity Family or personal history of asthma/allergies Wheezing	Eczema Wheezing (rare) Prolonged forced expiration
PND	Nasal drainage Early morning productive cough Throat clearing	Conjunctival irritation Pharyngeal cobblestoning Pale and boggy nasal mucosa Mucus in posterior pharynx
GERD	Heartburn Acid or food regurgitation Cough after meals Symptoms worse when supine Obesity Hoarseness Calcium channel blocker use	Obesity Hoarseness

What tests will help me determine benign causes of a chronic cough?

There is no standard work-up. If you suspect asthma, office spirometry is reasonably specific when FEV_1 is less than 80% predicted, or FEV_1/FVC ratio is less than 75%. Normal spirometry does not rule out asthma. Methacholine challenge, induction of bronchospasm in patients with cough-variant asthma, is the most sensitive test. If you suspect GERD, a barium swallow may show hiatal hernia or reflux (indicate that you suspect reflux on the radiology requisition). The standard is esophageal pH probe testing. In reality, most causes are suggested by history and confirmed by an empirical treatment trial.

How can I use therapeutic trials to diagnose these three common conditions?

With an empirical trial of therapy, the cough should improve significantly. These trials take time; allow four to six weeks before you assess the impact. If you suspect PND or allergic rhinitis, try decongestants, antihistamines such as diphenhydramine or chlorpheniramine that promote nasal mucosal drying, and/or nasal steroids, particularly if allergic rhinitis is suspected. If GERD is suspected, begin by eliminating substances that relax the GE sphincter such as cigarettes, alcohol, spicy foods, chocolate, and peppermint. Raise the head of the bed six inches with blocks or bricks (pillows don't work because bending at the waist increases pressure on the stomach). Prescribe empirical PPI therapy. These combined measures may be very effective but may take as much as six months to work. H_2 blockers are acceptable (e.g., ranitidine) but may be less effective. For patients with symptoms suggestive of cough-variant asthma (exacerbation with cold or exercise), treat with β-agonist inhalers. If the patient already uses β-agonists, add a steroid inhaler. Steroid inhalers can irritate airways, so do not start them during acute infection.

When should I obtain a CXR or other more specialized invasive tests?

Obtain a CXR in patients with acute cough with high fever, tachycardia, history worrisome for pulmonary embolism, abnormal lung exam, or hypoxia on pulse oximetry. For chronic cough patients, if history, exam, and empirical trial do not elucidate a cause, or if constitutional symptoms or cancer risk factors are present, obtain a CXR. Due to low sensitivity, sputum cytology cannot be used to rule-out cancer. A CXR should be considered early in the work-up if the patient has a history of cigarette use, occupational exposure, or risk for TB or HIV.

▶ TREATMENT

How do I manage acute infectious cough?

Sinusitis, bronchitis, and other viral respiratory infections often do not require antibiotic treatment. Community-acquired pneumonia should be treated with appropriate antibiotics (azithromycin, doxycycline, levofloxacin, or cefuroxime are good choices).

What are some ways to relieve symptoms for cough patients?

Prescribe β-agonist inhalers for cough due to postviral reactive airways. Eliminate irritants, especially cigarette smoke. Counsel about smoking cessation. Advise adequate hydration and humidity. Many patients expect a prescription for cough syrup, but only prescribe codeine if cough interferes with sleeping or eating. Start with 15–30 mg of codeine every two to four hours as needed. Otherwise, recommend over-the-counter preparations with only one or two active ingredients such as guaifenesin (expectorant) or dextromethorphan (suppressant). Cold and flu preparations are best avoided since the number of active ingredients may double or interact with other medicines.

When should I refer?

Refer to a pulmonologist when the cause of cough is unclear and/or empirical therapy has not helped, when bronchoscopy is indicated to rule-out TB, cancer or other rare disease, or when specialized intervention is required (e.g., interstitial lung disease, cancer). For suspected reflux that does not respond to PPI, refer to a gastroenterologist. In addition to your own counseling regarding cigarette use, smoking cessation clinics are helpful. If occupational exposure is a possibility, refer for occupational medicine evaluation.

K E Y   P O I N T S

▶ **The history and physical examination provide the key information for diagnosis**

▶ **Acute cough is almost always infectious or due to airway irritants**

▶ **Nonproductive chronic cough is often due to PND, GERD, or bronchospasm (postinfectious or asthma). Empirical therapy is often helpful**

CASE 10–1. A 37-year-old man is concerned about a cough that started three weeks ago with an upper respiratory infection. He has not had fevers or shortness of breath but describes a "barking" cough that produces scant yellow-green sputum, especially in the morning. He has a history of allergies treated with prescription antihistamines that he is taking now because it's allergy season. Over-the-counter cough syrup has not been helpful. Vital signs are T 37.0° C, BP 110/70, R 16, P 76.

A. What is your differential diagnosis?
B. What additional history and physical exam would be most helpful?
C. What tests should you order?
D. How will you treat him?

CASE 10–2. A 69-year-old man seeks your opinion about a cough he has had for 6 months. He was started on an ACE inhibitor three months ago for hypertension. He describes his cough as "loose" with a lot of sputum. He currently smokes ½ pack of cigarettes a day and has a 60-pack-year history. He has had several episodes of "bronchitis" this past year that have been treated with antibiotics without obvious relief. He is obese and does not have heartburn symptoms or wheezing.

A. What is your differential diagnosis?
B. What history or physical findings might help clarify the cause of his cough?
C. What tests or interventions will be helpful?
D. How would your answers change if examination shows an S_3 and lung crackles?

REFERENCES

Irwin, et al: Managing cough as a defense mechanism and as a symptom. A consensus panel report of the American College of Chest Physicians. Chest 114:133S–181S, 1998.
Gonzales R, Sande M. Uncomplicated acute bronchitis. Ann Intern Med 133:981–991, 2000.

11

Diarrhea

Does my patient really have diarrhea?

Diarrhea is an increase in stool water or a stool weight greater than 200 gm/day. If stool takes the shape of the container it is in, the patient probably has diarrhea. Chronic diarrhea lasts greater than one month.

Why does diarrhea occur?

Three main pathologic processes cause diarrhea (Table 11–1). In *secretory* diarrhea, intact intestinal cells produce excess fluid, usually from a toxin effect. In *osmotic* diarrhea, malabsorption of osmotically active agents increases stool volume. In *inflammatory* diarrhea, intestinal lining cells are destroyed so red and white blood cells are evident in the stool. Any of these processes may coexist. For example, inflammatory diarrhea can result in lactose intolerance (osmotic diarrhea).

TABLE 11–1

Patterns Suggesting the Underlying Pathologic Process in Patients with Diarrhea

Cause	Stool Pattern	Common Symptoms
Secretory		
Rotavirus	Watery	Low-grade fever, myalgias
Cholera	Watery, large volume	Severe dehydration
Hormone-producing tumors	Watery	Persists with fasting
Malabsorptive/osmotic		
Lactose intolerance	Loose	Bloating, cramping, flatulence
Pancreatic insufficiency	Loose	Greasy (floats like oil in water)
Inflammatory		
Ulcerative colitis	Bloody	Tenesmus, weight loss
Enteric pathogens	Bloody	Higher fever, myalgias, cramping

What are the common causes of acute diarrhea?

Viral infections cause most acute diarrhea (usually Norwalk agent or rotavirus). Bacteria or parasites are less common culprits. Transmission occurs via the fecal-oral route by ingestion of contaminated food or water, or by sexual activity. Less common causes of acute diarrhea include leakage around a fecal impaction, narcotic withdrawal, diverticulitis, and medications (Box 11–1).

What causes bloody diarrhea?

Bloody diarrhea indicates inflammation, most commonly from invasive enteric pathogens such as *Campylobacter, Shigella, Salmonella,* and *Escherichia coli* O157:H7. Inflammatory bowel disease (Crohn's and ulcerative colitis) may also present this way, usually in young adults. Other causes of bloody diarrhea include ischemic colitis, radiation injury, and rapid GI bleeding due to an ulcer or esophageal varices.

Is antibiotic-associated diarrhea always due to *Clostridium difficile* overgrowth?

Antibiotic-associated diarrhea is generally mild, dose-related, without a causative agent, and resolves when antibiotics are stopped. *C. difficile* causes 25% of antibiotic-associated diarrhea.

What are the common causes of chronic or recurring diarrhea?

Lactose intolerance, indolent infection, and irritable bowel syndrome are the most common causes. Lactose intolerance, an acquired lactase deficiency, occurs in greater than 75% of African- and Asian-Americans and up to 20% of whites. Undigested lactose

---

BOX 11-1

Common Medications That Can Cause Diarrhea

Alcohol
Antibiotics
Antihypertensives: β-blockers, furosemide, hydralazine
Anti-inflammatory medications: ibuprofen, colchicine
Caffeine
Digoxin
Laxatives
Magnesium-containing antacids
Serotonin reuptake inhibitor antidepressants
Sorbitol: cough drops, sugarless gum

following milk-product ingestion causes flatulence, bloating, and diarrhea. Infection with *Giardia lamblia* or *C. difficile* may be recurrent or chronic. *Giardia* is most notable for foul-smelling flatulence and steatorrhea. None of these conditions cause nocturnal diarrhea or bloody stool, so evaluate further if these symptoms are present.

What is the difference between irritable bowel syndrome and inflammatory bowel disease?

Irritable bowel syndrome (IBS) is a common alteration in intestinal motility with enhanced visceral sensitivity. Both IBS and inflammatory bowel disease can cause intermittent abdominal pain, cramping, and alternating diarrhea and constipation over many years. IBS has specific diagnostic criteria (Box 11–2). Inflammatory bowel disease (Crohn's disease and ulcerative colitis) is due to bowel wall inflammation of unclear cause, with peak incidence in 15–35 year-olds. In addition to diarrhea, patients with IBD may have bloody stool, tenesmus (if rectum is involved), or weight loss. Crohn's disease causes transmural inflammation and involves any part of the bowel from oral mucosa to rectum, in discontinuous patches. Ulcerative colitis causes more superficial inflammation of the bowel wall, begins at the rectum, and affects a continuous section of colon.

Why is malabsorption important?

Clinically significant malabsorptive syndromes can cause deficiencies of nutrients and/or vitamins. This can occur with intestinal

---

BOX 11–2

Criteria for the Diagnosis of Irritable Bowel Syndrome

Must have one of these for at least three months:
- Persistent or intermittent abdominal pain or discomfort relieved with defecation, or
- Persistent or intermittent change in stool frequency or consistency

Must also have two of these in addition to a criterion from list A:
- Altered stool frequency of greater than 3 bowel movements per day or less than 3 per week
- Altered stool form, either hard or loose
- Altered stool passage with straining, urgency, or feeling of incomplete evacuation
- Passage of mucus
- Bloating or feeling of abdominal distention

cell injury or loss of digestive enzymes. If fat is malabsorbed, due to bile salt depletion or Crohn's ileitis, fat-soluble vitamins A, D, E and K can become deficient causing vision problems (vitamin A), bone thinning (vitamin D), or coagulopathy (vitamin K). B_{12} deficiency can also develop with malabsorption in the terminal ileum.

▶ EVALUATION

What questions should I ask my patient with diarrhea?

Many patients cannot specifically characterize their diarrhea. Prompt them to describe frequency, volume, and appearance of the diarrhea to assess severity of their illness and identify likely causes. Categorize the diarrhea as acute or chronic based on duration of symptoms. Further, try to characterize the diarrhea as inflammatory by presence of blood and mucus, secretory by large volumes of watery stool, or malabsorptive by looseness without blood or water. Other pertinent details to ask about are included in Table 11–2.

What history suggests an infectious cause?

Acute onset, fevers, chills, or myalgias suggest infection. Patients at high risk include children in day care centers and their household contacts, travelers, patients institutionalized or hospitalized, immunocompromised or recently on antibiotics, and people who have anal sex.

What diagnostic tests should I order in a patient with acute diarrhea?

Most episodes of diarrhea are self-limited and require no tests. Although many tests are available, their indiscriminate use is

TABLE 11–2

Pertinent Questions Regarding Diarrhea

Question	Cause Suggested by Positive Answer
Bloody stool, mucus	Inflammatory cause
Fever	Infection (viral, bacterial), inflammatory bowel disease
Greasy stools	Fat malabsorption (sprue, pancreatic insufficiency)
Nocturnal symptoms	Concerning for pathologic cause, irritable bowel syndrome unlikely
Persistence with 24-hour fast	Secretory cause (VIP-oma)
Recent antibiotics, institutionalization	*Clostridium difficile*
Camping, day care exposures	*Giardia lamblia*

VIP-oma, vasoactive intestinal polypeptide secreting tumor.

unproductive and costly. For example, routine stool cultures for enteric pathogens in patients with diarrhea are positive only 2% of the time. Consider further testing only when the patient has any of the following: symptoms greater than three days, fever greater than 38.5°C, bloody diarrhea, severe volume depletion, severe abdominal pain, or immunocompromise (Figure 11–1).

When should I test for *C. difficile* or *Giardia*?

Obtain *C. difficile* toxin in those with recent antibiotic use, with recent hospitalization, or in chronic care facility. *C. difficile* toxin testing identifies clinical disease. Cultures will be positive with asymptomatic colonization, as seen in up to 20% of inpatients. The test for *Giardia* antigen has good sensitivity (greater than 92%) and specificity (95%) and should be ordered for campers and day care workers with persistent diarrhea.

What diagnostic tests should I order for chronic diarrhea?

Confirm the presence of diarrhea with a twenty-four hour stool collection since 40% of patients referred for diarrhea have fecal weights less than 200 g per day. Discontinue loperamide prior to testing. Consider irritable bowel syndrome in patients who do not have true diarrhea. Obtain CBC to look for infection or blood loss; ESR, electrolytes, albumin, stool guaiac, and fecal leukocytes to look for inflammation; and *C. difficile* toxin and *Giardia* antigen in patients at risk. If signs of malabsorption are present such as

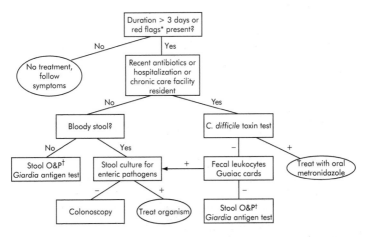

*Red flags: high fever, bloody diarrhea, severe volume depletion, severe abdominal pain, or immunocompromise. †In travelers.

Figure 11–1. Work-up of acute diarrhea.

weight loss, anemia, low albumin, ecchymoses, or neuropathy, obtain qualitative fecal fat and PTT (for vitamin K deficiency). A successful trial of a lactose-free diet diagnoses lactose intolerance. A twenty-four hour fast helps distinguish between malabsorption of ingested material (diarrhea abates) and secretory diarrhea (diarrhea continues). If parasitic infection is suspected, as in travelers or those engaging in anal sex, obtain 3 stool samples for ova and parasite studies.

How do I test for irritable bowel syndrome?

Irritable bowel syndrome is a functional disorder, meaning symptoms occur without objective abnormalities. Like many other clinical syndromes, there is no diagnostic test and clinical criteria assist in making the diagnosis.

When should I refer to a gastroenterologist?

Refer patients when the etiology of documented diarrhea is unclear, for endoscopic procedures (indicated in malabsorption, inflammatory diarrhea without infectious cause) and for treatment of advanced cases of inflammatory bowel disease.

▶ TREATMENT

Who needs antibiotics?

Antibiotics are not required for most acute infectious diarrhea. Treat *Giardia* and *C. difficile* with oral metronidazole. Refractory or recurrent *C. difficile* may require oral vancomycin (very expensive). Severe traveler's diarrhea, often due to an enteric pathogen, can be treated with a quinolone to reduce severity and duration. In patients with high fever, leukocytosis and frequent stool, test for enteric pathogens and treat if indicated. Do not use antibiotics for *E. coli* O157:H7 infection because antibiotics increase the risk of hemolytic uremic syndrome. *Campylobacter jejuni* and *Giardia* relapse in about 20% of cases, so consider re-treating for recurrent symptoms.

Which medications decrease the symptoms of diarrhea?

Treat volume depletion: for mild orthostasis, caffeine-free glucose-containing beverages are adequate; for more severe depletion, use oral rehydration solutions. Bismuth subsalicylate can reduce by 50% the number of unformed stools through antibacterial, anti-inflammatory, and antisecretory action. Opiate derivatives such as loperamide slow intestinal motility and reduce the number of stools by 80%. Beware, however, that antimotility agents can prolong the course of invasive bacteria and are not used in inflammatory bowel disease. Rule out *C. difficile* if this is a possibility before starting loperamide because of the risk of toxic megacolon and rupture.

How do I treat irritable bowel syndrome?

An effective physician-patient relationship is important for reassurance and for education about the chronic nature of symptoms, dietary modification (high fiber, low fat), and exercise. Treat the predominant symptom: hyoscyamine for abdominal cramping, loperamide for diarrhea, high fiber to even out alternating constipation and diarrhea.

When should I hospitalize a patient with diarrhea?

Hospitalize patients with severe dehydration (greater than 20% of volume lost), or significant emesis preventing oral rehydration, for intravenous fluids and electrolytes. Patients with severe GI bleeding, as from a flare-up of inflammatory bowel disease, may need hospitalization for stabilization and initiation of intravenous nutrition or steroids.

K E Y   P O I N T S

► Acute diarrhea is usually self-limited, requiring rehydration without further work-up.

► Take a thorough history to identify risk factors for acute diarrhea.

► Confirm the presence of chronic diarrhea by measuring stool volume first

► Use H & P to distinguish inflammatory, osmotic, or secretory chronic diarrhea.

► The presence of nocturnal symptoms suggests an organic, not a functional cause of diarrhea.

CASE 11–1.

A 78-year-old woman presents with diarrhea. She was healthy until four weeks earlier when she was hospitalized for angina. She started aspirin and atenolol and was treated for a urinary tract infection. Since discharge, she reports three to four soft, watery stools daily with mild left lower quadrant cramping. She denies fever, melena, or hematochezia. On exam she is afebrile, guaiac negative, and has mild abdominal pain to deep palpation of the left lower quadrant.

A. What are possible causes of her diarrhea?
B. What lab tests would you order, if any?
C. Would you start any treatment at this point?

CASE 11–2.

A 33-year-old man developed bloody diarrhea nine months ago. At that time sigmoidoscopy showed pancolitis consistent with an acute infectious process and his symptoms resolved spontaneously. Over the last three months he has had recurrent bloody diarrhea with 10–12 stools a day. He also reports mild dizziness, fatigue, and a 5 pound weight loss. He denies travel, anal sex, or HIV risk factors, or family history of bowel disease. On exam he is orthostatic, and has grossly bloody mucus in the rectal vault. The remainder of his exam is unremarkable.

A. What do you need to do for this patient today?
B. What is the next step in his work-up?

CASE 11–3.

A 56-year-old woman presents with four days of watery diarrhea. She has five to six nonbloody stools per day with lower abdominal cramping, malaise, subjective fevers, and dizziness when standing. She returned 3 days earlier from Mexico.

A. What are the possible causes of her diarrhea?
B. What lab tests would you order, if any?
C. What treatment would you start at this point?

REFERENCES

DuPont H: Guidelines on acute infectious diarrhea in adults. American College of Gastroenterology. Am J Gastroenterol 92(11):1962–1975, 1997.

Fekety R: Guidelines for the diagnosis and management of *Clostridium difficile*–associated diarrhea and colitis. American College of Gastroenterology. Am J Gastroenterol 92(5):739–750, 1997.

12

Dizziness and Syncope

How do I categorize causes of dizziness?

It is most useful to place dizziness into one of three broad cate-gories: vertigo, presyncope, or other. You can accomplish this by asking the patient to describe the sensation without using the word dizzy. *Vertigo* is an illusory sense that either the room or the patient is moving; this implicates the central or peripheral vestibular sys-tem. *Presyncope* is often described as being lightheaded, "see-ing stars," "blacking out," or impending faint. This sensation implies cerebral dysfunction due to decreased perfusion such as from low blood pressure or arrhythmia. One large study found that nearly half of the patients complaining of dizziness had more than one cause.

What are the causes of vertigo?

Vertigo is the most common type of dizziness, accounting for 40%–60% of all patients presenting with the complaint. Causes of vertigo are divided by anatomic source: *peripheral*, located in the eighth cranial nerve or inner ear, or *central*, located in the cere-bellum or brain stem (Table 12–1). Peripheral causes are very com-mon and usually benign; central causes are more worrisome. Certain features can help distinguish peripheral from central causes, including pattern of onset, latency (the time to onset of symptoms after an aggravating maneuver such as head movement), whether the symptoms are fatigable (get better with repeated maneuvers), and whether nystagmus is prominent (Table 12–2).

What are the causes of presyncope and syncope?

Presyncope and syncope are caused by decreased cerebral per-fusion. The main classes are *decreased intravascular volume* from bleeding, diarrhea, or diuretic overuse; *cardiac*, from intrinsic heart disease or arrhythmia; and *neurally mediated*, from loss of vas-cular tone and/or bradycardia. Neurally mediated causes may be

TABLE 12–1

Clinical Features and Frequency of Selected Causes of Vertigo

Location/Cause	Clinical Features	Frequency
Peripheral		
Benign positional vertigo (BPV)	Moderate to severe Brief spells (often < 1 min) Most pronounced with position changes Occurs after age 50, younger if history of head trauma Resolves in 3–10 days but may recur	25%–30% of all vertigo
Vestibulitis/neuritis	Severe, sudden onset Lasts days to weeks Often follows viral illness Can occur in clusters	10%–15% of all vertigo
Meniere's syndrome	Episodes with a triad of • vertigo • tinnitus • hearing loss Episodes last minutes to hours, not days	10% of all vertigo
Central		
Brain stem ischemia or lesion	Usually accompanied by other brain stem deficits: • diplopia • weakness • facial numbness or weakness • dysarthria	Rare
Cerebellar hemorrhage	**LIFE-THREATENING!** Abnormal finger-to-nose or heel-to-shin exam	Very rare
Central and Peripheral		
Acoustic neuroma	Unilateral hearing loss Tinnitus, headache Presents similarly to peripheral causes initially, then insidiously progresses to central pattern May involve 5th and 7th cranial nerves with facial weakness or numbness	Very rare

triggered by situations such as micturition, or a vasovagal response to pain. Common in patients younger than age 60, these reflex-mediated problems often have associated nausea and warmth prior to the lightheadedness or syncope. Elderly patients have a different set of neurally mediated causes, including an exaggerated carotid sinus reflex and autonomic neuropathy. Elderly patients are also more sensitive to medications (nitroglycerin,

TABLE 12-2

Features That Help Distinguish Peripheral from Central
Causes of Vertigo

Findings	Peripheral	Central
Initial onset of symptoms	Sudden	Insidious
Fatigability decreases with successive trials	Yes	No
Latency delay in onset of vertigo after exacerbating maneuver, i.e., moving the head	3–20 seconds	None
Nystagmus	Minimal Decreases with fixation	Marked Increases with fixation

antihypertensive agents, and antidepressants), which can lead to chronic postural lightheadedness or syncope.

What suggests a cardiac cause of syncope?

When symptoms occur without warning or with exertion, cardiac syncope is more likely. Cardiac syncope is more common at ages greater than 60. Syncope may be due to ischemia, arrhythmia, or structural problems such as critical aortic stenosis or hypertrophic cardiomyopathy. A pulmonary embolus (PE) can suddenly lower left ventricular filling and cardiac output, resulting in syncope. Consider PE when syncope occurs in patients with low cardiac risk and/or high deep venous thrombosis risk (e.g., pregnant women and oral contraceptive pill users).

What are some other important causes of dizziness?

Three other causes to keep in mind are early pregnancy, hyperventilation, and multiple sensory deficits. Hyperventilation is a common cause of a dysphoric lightheadedness, often accompanied by perioral or extremity tingling and numbness. Reproducing the symptoms after forced hyperventilation confirms the diagnosis and reassures the patient. A common mixed condition is hyperventilation exacerbating benign positional vertigo. Multiple sensory deficits are common in elderly patients with dizziness. Minor dysfunction in two or three of the spatial orientation systems (vestibular, visual, and proprioceptive) can cause significant lack of confidence and an unsteady sensation. In addition, polypharmacy can exacerbate problems with dizziness.

▶ **EVALUATION**

What questions should I ask the patient with dizziness or syncope?

- Timing, chronicity, onset, and prior episodes
- Effect of physical factors (position, movement, stress, or micturition)
- History of ear infections, head trauma, or barotrauma (suggests BPV)
- Medications causing hypotension or arrhythmias (nitroglycerin, antihypertensive agents, antidepressants) or ototoxicity (aminoglycosides, loop diuretics, salicylates, quinine, quinidine)
- Hearing loss, tinnitus (suggests Meniere's or acoustic neuroma)
- Brain stem ischemic symptoms (double vision, dysarthria, facial weakness or numbness)
- Palpitations, chest pain, or shortness of breath (suggest a cardiac cause or hyperventilation)
- Pregnancy risks

What should I look for on the physical examination?

Vital signs: irregular pulse, tachypnea, postural hypotension

HEENT: ear canals, carotid bruit, and upstrokes carotid sinus massage if older than age 60 to look for excessive bradycardic response from an exaggerated carotid sinus reflex (DO NOT perform carotid massage in patients with a bruit, a history of ventricular tachycardia, or recent MI or CVA)

Lungs: rales suggesting CHF

Heart: murmur, S_1/S_2, gallop, displaced point of maximal impulse (PMI), jugular venous pressure

Rectal exam: occult blood if patient appears volume-depleted

Neurologic: *cranial nerves,* especially hearing, visual acuity, diplopia, facial sensation, and symmetry; *cerebellar function* with finger-to-nose, rapid alternating movement, heel-to-shin; *sensation,* especially vibration and proprioception in feet; *strength and reflexes*

Other: 3 minutes of forced hyperventilation

Dix-Hallpike (also known as Nylen-Bárany) maneuver distinguishes peripheral from central causes of vertigo (Figure 12–1)

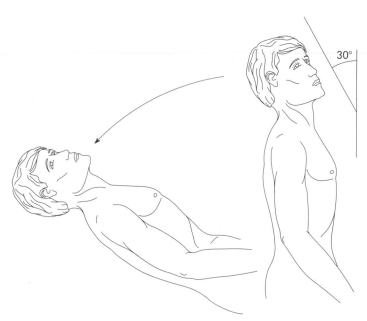

Figure 12-1. The Dix-Hallpike (or Nylen-Bárany) maneuver: Have the patient sit up with the head tilting back 45° and to the side 45°. Lie the patient rapidly backward while maintaining the same head position relative to the body (i.e., so the head ends up hanging off the edge, tipped 45° below the plane of the table). Have the patient keep eyes open. Look for nystagmus and reproduction of symptoms. Repeat the test, tilting the head to the other side. The side down when nystagmus is elicited is the affected side. Nystagmus onset will be immediate with the postural change for central causes and delayed by a few seconds for peripheral causes of vertigo. Nystagmus from a peripheral cause will be fatigable, meaning it decreases with repetition of the test.

What tests should be obtained routinely?

Obtain ECG when patients present with syncope or when you suspect a cardiac cause of dizziness. Echocardiogram, treadmill testing, or cardiac monitoring may also be warranted. Obtain HCT in patients with tachycardia, volume-depletion, or guaiac-positive stool. Obtain audiology if vertigo is accompanied by hearing loss. Obtain head MRI if documented sensorineural hearing loss accompanies vertigo.

▶ TREATMENT

What can I try before using medications?

Almost 50% of vertigo is from benign peripheral cause, either benign positional vertigo or vestibulitis. These conditions are fatigable, that is, they get better with repeated provocation. You can ask your patient to repeat whatever physical maneuver reproduces the vertigo until they no longer get symptoms (five to ten repetitions) about four times per day. If the patient can tolerate this, it is an excellent therapy. Hyperventilation is made better by breath-holding or bag-breathing exercises and therapy for underlying depression or anxiety. Particularly in the elderly, treat sensory deficits with eyeglasses, hearing aids, or a cane as needed. Wearing loose-necked shirts and avoiding neckties may help people with overactive carotid sinus reflexes.

What are useful medications for vertigo?

Antivertigo drugs treat symptoms and generally fall into four categories: neuroleptics (prochlorperazine, droperidol, promethazine), antihistamines (especially meclizine and cyclizine), anticholinergics (scopolamine and dramamine), and sympathomimetics (pseudoephedrine). Pseudoephedrine is useful in combination with antihistamines or anticholinergics because it helps to counter their sedative effects. Occasionally, a patient might need benzodiazepines (diazepam) for severe vertigo, antidepressants for hyperventilation, or thiazide diuretics for Meniere's disease.

When should I admit or refer patients with dizziness?

Consider hospital admission of a patient anytime you suspect one of the five life-threatening causes of dizziness: arrhythmia, critical cardiac outflow obstruction, cerebellar hemorrhage, pulmonary embolus, and significant blood loss (Table 12–3). This includes patients who have a first syncopal episode. Patients with suspected central cause of vertigo need admission when very ill or clinically unstable; these patients will likely need ENT or neurosurgery referral depending on audiology and MRI findings. Outpatients with vestibulitis or benign positional vertigo can be managed symptomatically and do not require referral unless the symptoms endure and do not improve over several weeks. Some patients with hyperventilation, especially those with associated panic symptoms, may benefit from psychiatric referral.

TABLE 12–3

Potentially Life-Threatening Causes of Dizziness or Syncope

Condition	Findings
Cardiac arrhythmia	History of palpitations Irregular pulse
Cardiac outflow obstruction such as aortic stenosis or hypertrophic cardiomyopathy	Exercise-induced syncope Systolic murmur Delayed carotid upstrokes Abnormal splitting of the S_2
Cerebellar hemorrhage	Abnormal cerebellar exam
Pulmonary embolus	Risk for deep venous thrombosis Tachycardia and hypoxia Loud S_2
Significant blood loss	History of bleeding Orthostatic hypotension Guaiac-positive stool Low hematocrit

K E Y   P O I N T S

► Dizziness is common, usually self-limited, and should be categorized by history as vertigo, presyncope/syncope, or other.

► Quickly screen dizzy patients for life-threatening causes: arrhythmia, cardiac outflow obstruction, cerebellar hemorrhage, pulmonary embolus, or significant blood loss.

► Use nonpharmacologic measures and medications such as meclizine to decrease symptoms of vertigo.

► Ask patients to call if symptoms get worse, if new symptoms develop, or if the symptoms have not resolved in two weeks.

CASE 12–1. A 20-year-old man presents for
evaluation due to a recent episode of syncope while
playing basketball. He relates some spells in the past of
lightheadedness with strenuous exercise. He has no other
significant history. On exam, blood pressure and pulse
are normal. His apical impulse is hyperdynamic and
displaced to the left. He has a grade II/VI systolic
murmur best heard at the left sternal border. The
murmur gets louder after standing from a squatting
position.

A. What is the likely cause of his syncope?
B. What test would you obtain to confirm your suspicion?

CASE 12–2. A 67-year-old man comes to the office
complaining of dizziness. He describes it as a feeling that
the room is spinning. It began when he got out of bed this
morning. It lasted about one to two minutes and has
recurred on and off all morning, especially when he
moves his head. He denies trouble speaking, weakness,
numbness, or headache. He has never had this before. On
exam he has normal pulse and blood pressure. His
carotid pulses are normal and he has no bruit. Cardiac
exam is normal. He has no edema. Finger-to-nose and
heel-to-shin functions are normal bilaterally. You lie him
rapidly down from a sitting position on the exam table.
After about four seconds, his symptoms are reproduced
and he has mild horizontal nystagmus. The symptoms are
less the second time you perform this maneuver.

A. What is the most likely diagnosis?
B. What test should you do to confirm this?

REFERENCES

Derebery MJ. The Diagnosis and Treatment of Dizziness. Med Clin North Am 83(1):163–177, 1999.

Kroenke K, et al. One-year outcome for patients with a chief complaint of dizziness. J Gen Intern Med 9:684–689, 1994.

USEFUL WEBSITE

http://www.teleport.com/~veda/
This is the home page of the Vestibular Disorders Association. It has many practical suggestions for patients and doctors.

13

Dyspepsia

What is dyspepsia?

Dyspepsia is pain or discomfort centered in the upper abdomen, which may be associated with other symptoms such as nausea, bloating, early satiety, or heartburn (substernal burning). Dyspepsia is very common and is one of the most frequent reasons for outpatient visits in adult medicine.

What causes dyspepsia?

Peptic ulcer disease (PUD), gastroesophageal reflux disease (GERD), and functional dyspepsia are the most common causes of dyspepsia. Uncommon causes include gastric or pancreatic cancer, gastroparesis from diabetes, atypical cases of chronic pancreatitis, and cardiac and biliary disease. Dyspepsia can be the result of medications including nonsteroidal anti-inflammatory drugs (NSAIDs), iron, antibiotics, theophylline, digitalis, and serotonin reuptake inhibitors. Functional dyspepsia, also called nonulcer dyspepsia, is the diagnosis given when no organic abnormality can be found to explain the dyspepsia. Functional dyspepsia is very common: 60% of patients with dyspepsia have functional disease.

► EVALUATION

What important points on history help distinguish the different causes of dyspepsia?

Obtain a history of the character and location of the pain or discomfort, as well as alleviating and precipitating factors. Patients who have associated regurgitation and heartburn most likely have GERD. GERD is often exacerbated by smoking, alcohol, large meals, and the supine position. Classic biliary pain is characterized by isolated attacks of moderate or severe epigastric or right upper quadrant pain, often associated with nausea. PUD and functional dyspepsia cannot be distinguished based on history alone. "Red flags" or alarm symptoms help identify patients with a serious problem, such as a complicated PUD or cancer. The red flags include dysphagia, bleeding, weight loss, and new onset of symptoms after age 45 (Box 13-1).

What evaluation is warranted for patients with alarm symptoms?

Patients with alarm symptoms should undergo prompt esophagogastroduodenoscopy (EGD) to rule out cancer and complicated PUD.

What evaluation is appropriate for patients with classic GERD symptoms?

Patients with uncomplicated GERD do not require further testing and should be treated as outlined below. The exception is the patient with longstanding GERD. Endoscopy should be considered in these patients to screen for Barrett's esophagus, a premalignant lesion (see later).

What evaluation is appropriate for patients with classic biliary symptoms?

For patients with uncomplicated biliary symptoms, order an abdominal ultrasound and if gallstones are found, refer the patient to surgery for cholecystectomy.

When should I test for *Helicobacter pylori* infection?

When alarm symptoms, classic GERD, biliary symptoms, and NSAID use have been excluded, many experts recommend testing young patients for *Helicobacter pylori* with a noninvasive test, though this remains controversial. Noninvasive methods to document infection include a serum antibody test (most commonly used), urea breath test (UBT), and stool antigen. Serology may remain positive for six to twelve months after eradication.

BOX 13-1

Alarm Symptoms of Serious Causes of Dyspepsia

Dysphagia
Bleeding
Weight loss
Age > 45 years

Serologies may be less reliable in elderly patients and those from areas of high prevalence. The UBT and stool antigen may be falsely negative in individuals treated with PPIs. These tests are generally more costly and are less widely available than serology.

Why test for *H. pylori* in patients with dyspepsia?

H. pylori infection and NSAID use are the most common causes of PUD. Eradication of *H. pylori* in patients with PUD leads to healing of the ulcer and a dramatic reduction in the risk of recurrent PUD. In the "test-and-treat" strategy (Figure 13–1), patients who are positive for *H. pylori* should be treated. Remember, while most patients with ulcers have *H. pylori* infection (or use NSAIDs), the converse is not true: Most patients with *H. pylori* infection do *not* develop ulcers. Eradication of *H. pylori* yields little or no benefit in patients with functional dyspepsia, and may actually worsen symptoms of GERD.

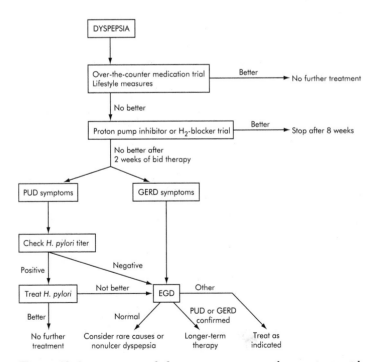

Figure 13–1. A recommended primary care approach to patients with dyspepsia.

What evaluation is appropriate when there are no alarm symptoms, no clear cause by history, and *H. pylori* serology is negative?

These patients should receive reassurance and a limited trial of antisecretory therapy, such as an H_2 receptor antagonist (H_2RA) or proton pump inhibitor (PPI). If they have persistent symptoms, they should be offered endoscopy.

What are the roles of EGD and upper GI series in the evaluation of dyspepsia?

EGD is used to rule out serious pathology in patients with alarm symptoms. Rarely used as an initial investigation in uncomplicated dyspepsia, it is used to investigate those who have persistent dyspepsia despite eradication of *H. pylori* and those without *H. pylori* infection who fail antisecretory therapy. Biopsy of the gastric mucosa during EGD is the gold standard to diagnose *H. pylori* infection. While EGD provides a superior evaluation (compared with an upper GI series), it is invasive and requires sedation. An upper GI series is less invasive, but is less sensitive for the detection of small ulcers and cannot detect Barrett's esophagus (see later).

What are the complications of GERD?

GERD can lead to esophageal ulceration and stricture formation. GERD can also exacerbate reactive airway disease. With chronic GERD, the squamous epithelium of the distal esophagus can be replaced by columnar epithelial cells, called Barrett's esophagus. Barrett's esophagus is a precancerous condition that can lead to esophageal adenocarcinoma. Most experts suggest that patients with longstanding GERD be screened with EGD for the presence of Barrett's esophagus, and that individuals with Barrett's esophagus undergo routine endoscopic surveillance.

What are the complications of PUD?

Gastrointestinal bleeding is the most common complication of PUD. In patients with upper gastrointestinal bleeding, prompt endoscopy is indicated for diagnosis and therapy. If a bleeding ulcer is visualized, therapy (injection and cautery) can be delivered to the ulcer. Rarely, gastric outlet obstruction and perforation can occur.

▶ TREATMENT

What are the treatment options for GERD?

Lifestyle modifications and/or antacids are the first line of therapy for milder symptoms (Box 13–2 and Figure 13–2). Patients with persistent symptoms require an H$_2$RA or PPI (Table 13–1). PPIs are the most effective treatment both for symptoms and healing of erosive esophagitis. Start with a single daily dose 30 minutes before breakfast. Increase to twice daily dosing if symptoms persist. Laparoscopic Nissen fundoplication is a surgical alternative for those who prefer not to take medications indefinitely, though many patients who undergo surgery still require medication for GERD symptoms. Prior to surgery, patients require esophageal pH

BOX 13–2

Lifestyle Modifications for Treatment of GERD

Elevate the head of the bed
Lose weight if obese
Avoid tobacco and alcohol
Avoid caffeine, mints, and fatty foods
Avoid eating two to four hours before bedtime

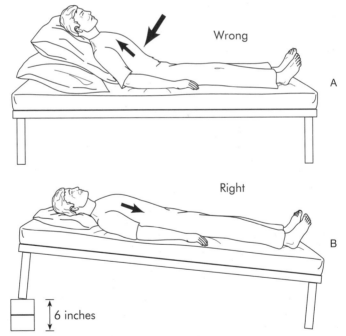

Figure 13–2. Appropriate bed elevation for GERD prevention. **A,** Sleeping on pillows actually increases intraabdominal pressure, leading to increased reflux. **B,** Elevating the head of the bed on blocks allows gravity to help reduce reflux.

TABLE 13–1

Drugs Used to Treat GERD

Class	Efficacy	Cost
Proton pump inhibitors[*]		
omeprazole 20 mg po qd to bid	++++	$$$$
lansoprazole 30 mg po qd to bid	++++	$$$$
pantoprazole 40 mg po qd to bid	++++	$$$$
rabeprazole 20 mg po qd to bid	++++	$$$$
H_2-receptor antagonists		
cimetidine 400–800 mg bid	++	$
ranitidine 150 mg po bid	++	$
nizatidine 150 mg po bid	++	$$
famotidine 20 mg po bid	++	$$

[*]Check with your local institution as many have negotiated lower contract prices for one or more PPIs.

testing and manometry to document abnormal esophageal acid exposure and to rule out esophageal dysmotility. Dysphagia and bloating are rare complications of Nissen fundoplication.

What are the treatment options for PUD?

NSAIDs should be discontinued. Treat patients who are positive for *H. pylori* to eradicate the organism (Table 13–2). A total of eight

TABLE 13–2

Two Possible Triple-Drug Treatment Regimens for *Helicobacter pylori*

Drugs	Doses
Omeprazole	20 mg po bid for 14 days
Amoxicillin	1 gm po bid for 14 days
Clarithromycin	500 mg po bid for 14 days
OR	
Ranitidine bismuth citrate	400 mg po bid for 14 days
Metronidazole	500 mg po bid for 14 days
Clarithromycin	500 mg po bid for 14 days

weeks of PPI therapy should be given to heal the ulcer. Bleeding secondary to PUD should be evaluated and treated endoscopically. If endoscopy fails to control the bleeding, surgical resection may be necessary.

What are the treatment options for functional dyspepsia?

Management of functional dyspepsia is challenging. A supportive physician-patient relationship is very important for patients with functional dyspepsia. Education and reassurance often lead to symptom improvement. A trial of H_2RA, PPI, or metoclopramide (a promotility agent) can be initiated. Without clear improvement in symptoms, the medication should be discontinued. Some patients with functional dyspepsia improve with antidepressant therapy.

K E Y   P O I N T S

▶ Dyspepsia is defined as pain or discomfort centered in the upper abdomen, with or without associated symptoms.

▶ Dyspepsia may be due to PUD, GERD, functional dyspepsia, and less common causes such as gastric cancer.

▶ Noninvasive testing for *H. pylori* is commonly recommended as an initial approach to guide management in younger patients with uncomplicated dyspepsia.

▶ Prompt endoscopy should be performed in older patients with dyspepsia and in patients with dyspepsia and associated symptoms of alarm.

CASE 13–1. A 60-year-old man presents with a two-month history of epigastric pain. He denies NSAID use or heartburn. His examination and labs are normal.

    A. What is the differential diagnosis?

    B. What investigation is warranted?

CASE 13–2. A 43-year-old woman complains of long-standing heartburn. She admits to smoking two packs of cigarettes and drinking two glasses of wine each day. Her heartburn is typically worse at night particularly after eating a late meal. She drinks Mylanta frequently and sleeps on three pillows to reduce her heartburn.

    A. What lifestyle modifications and medications do you recommend?

    B. Is any testing indicated?

REFERENCE

Talley N, Silverstein M, Agreus L, et al: American Gastroenterological Association Medical Position Statement: Evaluation of dyspepsia and AGA technical review: Evaluation of dyspepsia. Gastroenterology 114:579–595, 1998.

14

Dyspnea

What causes dyspnea?

A combination of mechanical receptors in the upper airway, lungs, and chest wall as well as chemoreceptors in the carotid arteries, aorta, and medulla appears to mediate the uncomfortable sensation of breathing experienced as dyspnea. Hypoxia, hypercapnea (elevated pCO_2), and increased work of breathing can all contribute to dyspnea.

What are common causes of chronic dyspnea?

While there are numerous causes for dyspnea, four conditions cause 70% of chronic dyspnea: asthma, COPD, CHF, and interstitial lung disease (Box 14–1). Deconditioning is another frequent cause for chronic exertional dyspnea. Less common causes for chronic dyspnea include anemia, neoplasms, hyperthyroidism, and recurrent pulmonary emboli.

What are common causes for dyspnea of recent onset?

Patients with recent onset dyspnea often have exacerbations of one of three chronic conditions: asthma, COPD, and CHF, or are found to have pneumonia (Box 14–2). Patients with bronchitis or other upper respiratory infections sometimes report dyspnea. This dyspnea is generally mild unless they have an underlying pulmonary

---

BOX 14-1

Common Causes of Chronic Dyspnea

Asthma
COPD
CHF
Interstitial lung disease

BOX 14–2

Common Causes of Acute Dyspnea

Exacerbations of
    Asthma
    COPD
    CHF
    Pneumonia

problem, such as asthma or COPD. Dyspnea is commonly associated with chest pain in patients with angina. Important and potentially life-threatening causes for acute dyspnea include PE, tachyarrhythmia, silent myocardial ischemia, and pneumothorax (Box 14–3). Dyspnea without chest pain can occur during myocardial ischemia or infarction and is called silent ischemia; this is more common in women and in patients with diabetes. Recurrent dyspnea associated with anxiety is often due to panic attacks. Tachyarrhythmias can also produce symptoms similar to panic attacks. Patients with anemia may present with dyspnea.

▶ EVALUATION

How helpful is the history in the evaluation of dyspnea?

In one study of 146 patients admitted with dyspnea, 74% were correctly diagnosed following a five to fifteen minute history. Important historical features in a dyspneic patient include character, duration, severity, exacerbating and relieving factors, associated symptoms; medication use with special attention to whether medications such as diuretics or inhalers have been used as prescribed; past medical history, particularly cardiac or pulmonary disease or environmental exposures; and any history of trauma. It can be helpful to ask patients how far they can walk or how many flights of stairs they can climb currently, and compare this to their exercise tolerance at some time in the past.

BOX 14–3

Life-Threatening Causes of Dyspnea

Arrhythmia
MI
Pneumothorax
PE

Which symptoms are commonly associated with important causes of dyspnea?

Symptoms provide clues to diagnosis (Table 14–1).

What are typical symptoms in a patient whose dyspnea is due to panic attacks?

Patients with panic attacks experience episodes in which they have some combination of dyspnea, chest pain, palpitations, dizziness, and anxiety. During an acute episode patients often benefit from reassurance and from advice to slow their breathing. Patients who fail to respond to this can be asked to breathe into a paper bag to increase the pCO_2 level that has been lowered by hyperventilation. Patients may have underlying symptoms of anxiety or

TABLE 14-1

Symptoms and Examination Findings in Important Causes of Dyspnea

Condition	Symptoms	Exam Findings
Congestive heart failure	Orthopnea (dyspnea when supine) Paroxysmal nocturnal dyspnea (awakening short of breath) Increase in leg edema Pink, frothy sputum	Elevated jugular venous pressure Crackles at lung bases Leg edema Third heart sound (S_3)
Asthma or COPD exacerbation	Productive cough Wheezing Chest tightness	Increased expiratory-to-inspiratory ratio Wheezing Supraclavicular retraction
Pneumonia	Fever Productive cough Pleuritic chest pain	Tachycardia Decreased breath sounds Rales and/or egophony
Pulmonary embolus	Abrupt-onset dyspnea Calf pain or swelling Pleuritic chest pain	Pleural rub Unilateral calf swelling Tachycardia
Cardiac ischemia	Chest pressure, heaviness, or discomfort Nausea or diaphoresis	Tachycardia and hypertension Diaphoresis
Pneumothorax	Abrupt-onset dyspnea Pleuritic chest pain	Deviated trachea Hyperresonance on affected side Decreased breath sounds on affected side
Hyperventilation	Anxiety Palpitations Paresthesias, distal extremities or perioral	Normal exam Depressed or anxious-appearing

depression so be sure to screen for these conditions. Patients with tachyarrhythmias may have similar symptoms; an event monitor, which records a tracing of a patient's heart during a period of symptoms, can be a useful way of distinguishing between the two.

Which elements of the physical exam are most important in evaluating a patient with dyspnea?

General appearance provides excellent information about the severity of the condition, including how hard the patient is working to breathe, the presence or absence of cyanosis, and the ability to speak a full sentence before taking a breath. Check vital signs for information about hemodynamic stability and the likelihood of infection. Measure the respiratory rate, because this is frequently recorded incorrectly. Inspect the conjunctiva and nails for evidence of anemia. Inspect the chest, looking for intercostal, subcostal, and supraclavicular retractions, for abnormalities of the chest wall, and for abnormal prolongation of the expiratory phase. Percuss, listening for dullness due to effusion or consolidation, or for the hyperresonance of a pneumothorax. Auscultate for wheezes, rales, rhonchi, or rubs, and for symmetry of breath sounds. Remember that patients with an exacerbation of congestive heart failure may have wheezes or "cardiac asthma" rather than rales. Be aware that the absence of wheezes in an acutely dyspneic patient with asthma or COPD may be an ominous sign of a serious limitation of airflow. Listen for murmurs and extra heart sounds, such as the S_3 gallop of severe congestive heart failure. Inspect the neck veins to determine the jugular venous pressure (JVP). Assess for edema and for unilateral calf swelling or tenderness. If a PE is being considered, measure calf diameters equidistant from the knee.

Which tests are most helpful in evaluating the patient with dyspnea?

Select appropriate testing to investigate your diagnostic hypotheses generated from H & P. A CXR is useful in patients with moderate or severe dyspnea, and in mildly symptomatic patients in whom the reason for their dyspnea is unclear. Oximetry at rest and/or with exercise can detect hypoxia, but does not detect hypercarbia. Arterial blood gas (ABG) provides accurate information about oxygen and carbon dioxide levels, especially useful in patients with suspected airflow obstruction or PE. Measures of airflow (spirometry or peak flow) provide information about the presence and severity of airflow obstruction. Pulmonary diffusion capacity (DLCO) can be used to determine if a patient has interstitial lung disease. Obtain an ECG in any patient who might have a cardiac cause for dyspnea. Order an HCT and thyroid stimulating hormone (TSH) in any patient whose diagnosis remains unclear after the initial H & P. A low HCT could be the cause of dyspnea; a very high HCT is evidence that a long-standing pulmonary problem is present. Cardiopulmonary exercise testing can be useful in some patients to clarify the cardiac and pulmonary components of their dyspnea and to determine the relative contribution of deconditioning. Order an echocardiogram when valvular heart disease or congestive heart failure is a concern. Pulmonary emboli (PE) can mimic many cardiac and pulmonary problems. Dyspnea is the most common symptom in patients with large pulmonary emboli, but patients with small emboli may present with pleuritic chest pain, tachycardia, or hemoptysis. See Chapter 34 for work-up when PE are suspected.

Why do I need an ABG when I can get pulse oximetry?

ABG gives a more accurate assessment of oxygenation, allows calculation of an alveolar/arterial oxygen gradient, and identifies patients at risk for cardiac or neurologic compromise due to hypoxia. Normal pulse oximetry in patients with obstruction does not exclude retention of CO_2 from obstruction and respiratory fatigue. In addition to the O_2 level, ABG measures CO_2, which indicates severity of airflow obstruction and likelihood of respiratory arrest in those who are becoming fatigued from the work of breathing.

▶ TREATMENT

How do I treat dyspnea?

Identify and treat the underlying cause. See relevant chapters for further details of treatment. Asthma and CHF often respond well to treatment directed at the underlying problem. Other causes of dyspnea such as COPD or interstitial lung disease may have a limited response to treatment. Opiates and benzodiazepines have been shown to reduce the feeling of dyspnea (without improving ventilation or oxygenation); they should generally be avoided due to the risk of dependence and of respiratory depression.

Which patients with dyspnea should receive supplemental oxygen?

Supplemental oxygen has been shown to improve survival for patients with chronic dyspnea and a pO_2 less than or equal to 55. Medicare currently will pay for supplemental oxygen if patients have
   pO_2 on ABG less than or equal to 55
   pO_2 less than or equal to 60 and a condition worsened by hypoxia, such as cor pulmonale (right heart failure associated with hypoxia)
   O_2 saturation by oximetry less than or equal to 88%

Patients with acute dyspnea who are moderately-to-severely symptomatic or who have oxygen saturations below 90%–91% should receive supplemental oxygen pending further evaluation and treatment. In chronic COPD, use oxygen cautiously because the respiratory force in these cases is driven by hypoxia.

Which patients with dyspnea should be hospitalized?

Patients with chronic dyspnea can be evaluated as outpatients unless the vital signs are unstable or the hypoxia is significant. Patients with acute dyspnea requiring supplemental oxygen or those who have potentially unstable cardiac or respiratory status should be hospitalized. Patients with acute dyspnea due to an exacerbation of asthma or COPD can be treated with inhaled bronchodilators and will often improve sufficiently to avoid hospitalization. These patients are often given a short course of steroids to decrease airway inflammation.

K E Y   P O I N T S

▶ **Most patients with dyspnea can be correctly diagnosed by taking a careful history.**

▶ **Common causes of chronic dyspnea are asthma, chronic obstructive pulmonary disease, congestive heart failure, and interstitial lung disease.**

▶ **Common causes of acute dyspnea are pneumonia and exacerbations of asthma, COPD, and CHF.**

▶ **Consider PE in any patient with recent onset dyspnea who doesn't have a clear explanation for his or her symptoms.**

CASE 14–1. A 60-year-old man with a ten-year history of diabetes reports two hours of dyspnea, worse with exertion but also present at rest. His symptoms began gradually and have worsened since their onset. He denies cough, a history of asthma, chest pain, nausea, melena, tobacco use, recent surgery or immobilization, or calf pain. He takes glyburide. On exam, BP 140/90, P 110, T 36.9°C, R 24. Skin is moist, chest is clear to auscultation and percussion, heart sounds are regular without murmurs, gallops, or rubs, JVP is normal at 7 cm. Stool is guaiac negative and extremities show no edema, cyanosis, calf swelling, or tenderness.

A. What is your differential diagnosis for this patient?
B. Which diagnostic tests would you order at this time?

CASE 14-2.

A 34-year-old woman presents with the abrupt onset four hours earlier of dyspnea and pleuritic left chest pain. She has had a nonproductive cough and nasal congestion for the last week. She denies positional changes in her pain, fevers, trauma, recent travel, or calf pain. She takes an oral contraceptive and smokes a pack of cigarettes daily. On exam T 37.3°C, BP 100/60, P 104, R 24. Chest is clear to auscultation and percussion, breath sounds are symmetrical, heart sounds are regular with no murmurs, gallops, or rubs, extremities show no calf swelling, tenderness, or cyanosis. Pulse oximetry is 90% on room air.

A. Which diagnoses would you consider?
B. Which clinical features make each of these diagnoses more or less likely?
C. Which diagnostic tests would you order?

REFERENCES

Jobe K: Dyspnea. In Fihn S, DeWitt D (eds): Outpatient Medicine, 2nd ed. Philadelphia, WB Saunders, 1998, pp 79–81.
Meek PM, Schwartzstein RM, et al: Dyspnea: Mechanisms, assessment, and management. ATS Consensus Statement. Am J Respir Crit Care Med 159:321, 1999.

15

Fatigue

How common is fatigue?

Fatigue is an extremely common patient concern in primary care practice. Though fatigue is the isolated concern in only 1%–3% of office visits, it is estimated that 20%–40% of patients would report significant fatigue if a thorough review of symptoms were obtained. Fatigue accounts for an estimated 7 to 15 million office visits yearly in the United States. Lifetime risk and point prevalence of fatigue are estimated at 25%.

What causes fatigue?

Over half of fatigue is due to a psychological cause, usually depression. Approximately 30% of fatigue is due to a diagnosable medical illness. No cause is found in about 20% of cases. Common physical causes include viral infection, metabolic disorders, and medications (Box 15-1). Duration is important: fatigue present for greater than 4 months is 75% psychiatric, while fatigue present less than 4 weeks has a physical cause determined in 70% of cases.

What are dangerous causes of fatigue I shouldn't miss?

Fatigue can be the presenting symptom for a vast array of diseases, including depression, infection (TB, HIV, hepatitis), cancer, renal failure, and endocrine (diabetes, thyroid disease), neuromuscular (multiple sclerosis), or inflammatory diseases (sarcoidosis, rheumatoid arthritis).

What is chronic fatigue syndrome (CFS)?

This is a symptom complex whose main feature is chronic or recurrent debilitating fatigue lasting more than six months. Only 5% of chronically fatigued patients meet criteria for CFS. The absence of a known medical illness, and presence of one or more other symptoms (impaired memory, sore throat, tender lymphadenopathy,

BOX 15-1

Common Causes of Chronic Fatigue

Endocrine and Metabolic disorders
 Uncontrolled diabetes
 Cardiopulmonary disease
 Renal failure
 Thyroid disease
Medications
 β-blockers
 Diuretics
 Sedatives
 Antidepressants
Pregnancy
Psychiatric
 Anxiety
 Depression
 Somatization
Viral infections
 Hepatitis viruses
 HIV
Sleep disorders
 Sleep apnea
Substance abuse

muscle pain, arthralgias, headaches, unrefreshing sleep, postex-ertional malaise lasting more than twenty-four hours) is required to make the diagnosis. The cause is unknown, and many etiologies have been proposed including chronic viral infection, hypo-thalamic dysfunction, and disordered autonomic regulation. A significant psychiatric component is often present, confounded by the fact that chronic fatigue can be depressing in itself.

▶ EVALUATION

What are key parts of the history for patients with fatigue?

Ask the patient what he or she thinks is causing the fatigue. This provides useful clues, as well as an opportunity to address fears. Have patients characterize what they mean by fatigue: some are sleepy, others short of breath with poor exercise tolerance, still others have muscle weakness. Determine the duration and progress of symptoms. Check for symptoms of depression: sleep disturbance, particularly early morning awakening, difficulty con-centrating, eating/weight changes, loss of the ability to enjoy anything (anhedonia), sadness, feelings of guilt or loss, or thoughts about death or suicide, as other clues to depression. Review medications, especially recent additions. With a careful review of systems, identify new neurologic, pulmonary, cardiac, or gastrointestinal symptoms. Pay particular attention to constitutional symptoms such as fevers, night sweats, or unexplained weight loss that suggest infection or tumor. Take a good sleep history, including initiation and maintenance of sleep, history of snoring, morning headaches, daytime sleepiness, or hypertension. Patients who frequently fall asleep during the day are at higher risk of having a sleep disorder.

In contrast to fatigue from physical causes, fatigue due to psychological causes is unimproved by sleep, worse in the morning, and improves through the day (Table 15–1). Ask a thorough social history, including questions about work, substance use, and sexual history, including history of physical or sexual abuse, HIV risk factors, and recent major stressors, such as career changes, deaths, or relocation. When patients answer yes to most questions, review again for abuse since a significant proportion of patients with multiple complaints have a history of domestic violence.

What is an appropriate physical exam?

Perform a complete exam, with special attention to the most bothersome associated symptoms. Be sure to note affect, to palpate for lymphadenopathy, thyroid abnormalities, and hepatosplenomegaly, and to perform a careful lung and heart exam. Although the diagnostic yield compared with history is low, exam may confirm suspicions raised by the history, and the exam itself reassures patients that their concerns are being taken seriously.

TABLE 15–1

Features of Fatigue from Psychological vs. Physical Causes

	Psychological	Physical
Diurnal pattern	Worse in AM Better as day progresses	Better in AM Worsens as day progresses
Duration	Chronic	Recent onset, parallels course of underlying disease
Effect of sleep	Sleep is nonrestorative	Relieved by sleep
Onset	Coincides with stress, psychological disruption, conflict	Coincides with onset of a physical disease (e.g., respiratory infection)
Progression	Fluctuates Worse with distasteful activity or stress May not progress	Progresses as disease worsens

What studies should I order?

Blood tests are appropriate when a nonpsychiatric cause is suspected (fatigue less than two to three months, worsening symptoms, worrisome findings on history or physical). In this case, order CBC with differential, electrolytes, calcium, glucose, renal function, ESR, liver transaminases, and TSH. Other tests may be indicated (CXR, ECG, urinalysis, other endocrine tests) as suggested by H & P. EBV titers are not useful and should not be ordered. With risk factors such as unprotected sex or intravenous drug use, test for HIV, hepatitis viruses, and syphilis (VDRL or RPR). For homeless, incarcerated, or HIV-infected patients, look for TB by placing a skin test (PPD) and consider ordering a CXR. Consider a pregnancy test in premenopausal women. Consider a sleep study if you suspect sleep apnea or another sleep disorder.

What if the results do not point to any specific abnormality?

Emphasize the positive—that there is no evidence of a life-threatening disease. Reassure the patient that you still are concerned about his or her symptoms, and want to schedule another visit. Help problem-solve to improve coping with symptoms. If there is personal turmoil, empathize that these upheavals can be exhausting. If you think your patient is depressed, find out what your patient thinks about this assessment. If he or she has trouble accepting this diagnosis, educate the patient about depression as a physical illness, and explain that the symptoms may show up in the body before people recognize its effect on their mood. Finally, recognize that you have begun to address a problem whose solution may be beyond the time frame of a single visit. You can ask patients to keep a diary of symptoms, activities, and degree of fatigue for review at the next visit.

▶ TREATMENT

Treat any underlying cause found. If no cause is identified, validate the patient's concerns, emphasize that the patient has gotten a thorough evaluation and no serious condition has been found, and express willingness to continue to care for them. If you suspect depression, recommend a trial of antidepressant therapy or psychiatry referral, emphasizing that even if depression is not the foundation of the problem, having fatigue for such a long time could by itself result in depression. Cognitive-behavioral therapy has been shown to be helpful in many somatic disorders. Set reasonable expectations: the goal of the chosen therapy will be to help the patient function with his or her symptoms, though the symptoms may not resolve entirely. Treatment of chronic fatigue syndrome includes adjustment of maladaptive coping strategies, treatment of concurrent depression, and low-level exercise.

K E Y   P O I N T S

▶ The duration, associated symptoms, progression, effect of sleep, and diurnal variation of fatigue help indicate whether the fatigue has a physical or psychiatric cause.

▶ Fatigue of recent onset or with new associated symptoms usually indicates physical disease.

▶ A trusting therapeutic relationship is the cornerstone of therapy for fatigue of unclear origin.

CASE 15–1. A 26-year-old woman reports two months of fatigue. She says in addition that she sometimes feels "chilly" but has never taken her temperature, has had mild lower abdominal pain, and feels out of breath when she goes upstairs. On further questioning, she says that she has had unprotected sex with two men.

   A. What features in this history suggest a physical cause of her symptoms?
   B. What other history would you like?
   C. What is your initial work-up?

CASE 15–2. A 45-year-old man reports he has felt "tired all the time" for the past five years. He has been to many physicians to try to find a cause for his symptoms and has a folder with his records. He says that since the onset of his tiredness he has had headaches, joint aches, "ups and downs" in his temperature between 96.4 and 99.2° F, feels unrefreshed after sleep, and feels "completely worn out" for more than a day after exercising. You review his records, which show an extensive laboratory, imaging, and cardiopulmonary evaluation, all within normal limits. He says that he is "tired of being told it's all in his head" and hopes that you'll find out "what's really going on."

   A. What further history should you obtain?
   B. What should be the focus of your physical exam?
   C. What further evaluation do you wish to order?

REFERENCES

Epstein KR: The chronically fatigued patient. Med Clin North Am 79:315–327, 1995.

Wessely S: Chronic fatigue: Symptom and syndrome. Ann Intern Med 134 (9-Part 2):838–842, 2001.

USEFUL WEBSITE

The National Center for Infectious Diseases Chronic Fatigue Syndrome website: *http://www.cdc.gov/ncidod/diseases/cfs/index.htm*

16

Gastrointestinal Bleeding

► ETIOLOGY

What are the most common causes of GI bleeding?

Divide GI bleeding into upper and lower, based on whether the bleeding originates above or below the ligament of Treitz in the distal duodenum. The most common causes of *upper GI bleeding* are peptic ulcer disease, gastritis, and esophageal varices related to cirrhosis and portal hypertension. Common causes of *lower GI bleeding* include diverticulosis and angiodysplasia, a condition of disordered vessel growth in the bowel wall (Table 16–1). In patients younger than age 50, bright red blood per rectum is often from hemorrhoids.

► EVALUATION

What pertinent history should I elicit when a patient has GI bleeding?

Use history to distinguish whether the source of bleeding is from the upper or lower GI tract. Generally, upper GI bleeds present with hematemesis or coffee ground emesis. The stool is usually melenic, i.e., black, due to oxidation of blood during the prolonged transit time through the bowel. By contrast, lower GI bleeding pro-

TABLE 16–1	
Common Causes of GI Bleeding	
Upper GI Bleeding	**Lower GI Bleeding**
Gastritis	Angiodysplasia
Mallory Weiss tear from retching	Brisk upper GI bleeding
Nose bleed	Colitis: infectious, inflammatory, or ischemic
Peptic ulcer disease	Colon cancer or polyp
Varices: esophageal, gastric	Diverticulosis
	Hemorrhoids

duces hematochezia (maroon stools) or bright red blood per rectum. The caveat to this distinction is that a brisk upper GI bleed can cause hematochezia due to the cathartic effects of fast bleeding. Patients with rapid, severe bleeding may report dizziness, weakness, confusion, or syncope related to volume depletion. A slow or chronic bleed from any source can lead to fatigue and dyspnea on exertion as anemia progresses. Most GI bleeding is painless, though bleeding from peptic ulcers may be preceded by days to weeks of burning epigastric pain. Risk factors for peptic ulcer disease include NSAID, steroid, or alcohol use. If tenesmus is present, rectal inflammation is likely, as from ulcerative colitis. Weight loss suggests neoplasm. Fever suggests infectious or inflammatory disorders.

Alcohol use and/or chronic liver disease are risks for esophageal varices. Older age is a risk factor for angiodysplasia or diverticulitis. Patients with diverticular bleeds may have a history of prior episodes of painful diverticulitis.

How does the physical exam help me evaluate my patient with bloody stools?

The exam should help you judge the severity of bleeding. Vital signs are key. Tachycardia and hypotension are worrisome for a large amount of bleeding. Orthostasis, i.e., an increase in pulse or drop in blood pressure of greater than 20 points from lying to standing, indicates volume loss of 20% or greater. Pallor, cool skin, and poor capillary refill are also signs of severe blood loss and volume depletion. Conjunctival pallor and pale palmar creases indicate an HCT in the low 20s or less. Suspect esophageal varices if signs of chronic liver disease are present. Exam findings suggesting liver disease include spider telangiectasia, ascites, jaundice, asterixis, hepato- and/or splenomegaly, palmar erythema, Terry's nails, or gynecomastia. Parotid or lacrimal gland enlargement, testicular atrophy, or Dupuytren's contractures of flexor tendons in the hand suggest alcohol abuse, which increases risk for gastritis, PUD, or cirrhosis-related esophageal varices.

When are anoscopy or nasogastric (NG) lavage helpful?

Perform anoscopy and digital rectal exam in patients with bright red blood per rectum to distinguish hemorrhoidal bleeding from other more proximal sources. Be aware that hemorrhoids on anoscopy do not necessarily rule-out other sources of bleeding, especially in older patients, because up to 20% may have another more proximal lesion. Perform lavage to confirm upper GI bleeding. Bloody NG aspirate diagnoses an upper GI bleed. The amount of saline lavage required to clear all blood from the NG aspirate correlates with the rapidity of bleeding. Rule-out a gastric bleed if the NG aspirate is clear but not a duodenal bleed because without bile you cannot be sure if the duodenum has been sampled.

What studies are standard in a patient with a GI bleed?

Repeat HCTs every four hours until you are sure the patient is not acutely bleeding. Remember, however, that a fall in HCT may lag behind blood loss by several hours. Order blood type, cross-match, and two to four units of blood to be kept "in house" in the event of catastrophic bleeding. Check chemistry panel for renal function and electrolytes. BUN may rise with upper GI bleeding due to absorption of blood in gut. Glucose may be low with severe liver disease and may provide a clue to presence of varices or gastritis. Check liver function values to screen for liver dysfunction, and check PT, PTT, and platelets for a coagulopathy that could worsen blood loss. Follow calcium in patients receiving transfusions because the citrate preservative may cause calcium levels to fall. In stable outpatients who have unexplained iron deficiency anemia or guaiac-positive stools, refer to a GI consultant for endoscopy.

Are x-rays or other diagnostic imaging studies useful?

Plain films are relatively unhelpful except to rule-out perforation with an upright view. Endoscopy for suspected upper bleeding often identifies the cause of bleeding, can be used to take biopsies for diagnosis of *Helicobacter pylori* or tumor, and may be used therapeutically to stop bleeding from a variety of causes. Selective arteriography or nuclear medicine-labeled RBC scan may identify the source of lower GI bleeding if the rate of bleeding is brisk.

▶ TREATMENT

Treat the underlying cause of bleeding (Table 16–2).

My patient is orthostatic and vomiting up blood. What should I do?

Begin with urgent resuscitation. Obtain rapid intravenous access, usually two IV catheters, 16 gauge or larger, or a central line. Administer normal saline to maximize the portion that stays in the intravascular compartment. Packed RBCs or whole blood are better than saline for expanding the intravascular volume but take longer to obtain. Replace factors or platelets as indicated by severe coagulopathy. Order two to six units of blood in-house (decide the number of units based on severity of bleeding) so you can quickly transfuse patients who are rapidly bleeding. Talk to

GI and surgical consultants early for almost all patients with GI bleeding. GI consultants can assist with diagnostic and possibly therapeutic endoscopy. Surgical colleagues prefer knowing as early as possible about patients who may require surgery if bleeding is refractory to medical therapy.

TABLE 16–2

Presentation, Diagnosis, and Treatment Options of Common Causes of GI Bleeding

Cause	Presentation	Diagnosis	Treatment Options
Angiodysplasia	elderly patients slow occult bleeding anemia and fatigue	colonoscopy; angiography if bleeding brisk	surgical removal of involved bowel if necessary
Colon cancer	elderly patients slow occult bleeding anemia and fatigue weight loss change in caliber of stool, new constipation	colonoscopy; if lesion extensive, CT scan for staging disease	surgical removal if cancer isolated to the bowel
Diverticulosis	acute, rapid bleed painless prior diverticulitis	colonoscopy, selective arteriography or labeled RBC scan if bleeding brisk	80% of bleeding resolves with bowel rest alone; surgical excision if persists
Ischemic bowel	elderly patients risk factors for atherosclerosis or emboli midabdominal pain postprandial pain pain out of proportion to exam acidemia	plain radiographs or CT scan to identify edematous bowel and to rule out perforation	surgical excision of infarcted bowel
PUD/gastritis	preceding episodes of epigastric pain NSAIDs, alcohol, caffeine, steroids, cigarette use	EGD with biopsy or serology for *Helicobacter pylori*	proton pump inhibitor, H_2 blocker, antibiotics for *H. pylori*, d/c NSAIDs, caffeine, alcohol
Mallory Weiss tear	retching preceding hematemesis usually painless	EGD	antiemetics, supportive care
Varices	hematemesis in patient with cirrhosis and portal hypertension usually painless	EGD	EGD banding, octreotide, Sengstaken-Blakemore tube, β-blockers for prophylaxis, TIPS

K E Y   P O I N T S

▶ Your evaluation should determine whether the bleed is from the upper or the lower GI tract to guide your differential diagnosis and further work-up.

▶ Call GI and surgical consultants early.

▶ Obtain adequate IV access, type and cross serial HCTs, and perform frequent reassessment.

CASE 16–1. A 68-year-old woman with a history of hypertension, osteoarthritis, and hypothyroidism reports an episode of hematochezia and associated dizziness, without abdominal pain or vomiting. Her medications include aspirin, benazepril, levothyroxine, rofecoxib, glucosamine, calcium, and vitamin D. On exam, BP is 90/60, P is 120, skin is cool and moist, mouth is without lesions, heart exam reveals a 2/6 systolic murmur at the right upper sternal border without radiation, abdomen is soft and nontender, and rectal exam reveals grossly bloody stool. Labs show HCT of 25, MCV 82, WBC count 11, BUN 45, creatinine 1.3, sodium 140, potassium 4.0, and chloride 102.

A. Does she have an upper or lower GI bleed?
B. What are the most likely causes of bleeding in older patients?
C. What can be done to prevent anti-inflammatory–induced ulcers?

CASE 16–2. A 47-year-old man presents with hematemesis, lightheadedness, and confusion. On exam, BP is 80/60, P is 140, skin reveals spider angiomata on the upper chest, abdomen is distended with bulging flanks, and extremities show palmar erythema and Terry's nails.

A. What is the most likely cause of this man's hematemesis?
B. What should you do to immediately stabilize this patient?
C. What is the most useful medication to administer?
D. What additional nonpharmacologic intervention might be useful?

REFERENCES

Fallah MA, Prakash C, Edmundowicz S: Acute gastrointestinal bleeding. Med Clin North Am 84(5):1183–1208, 2000.

Zuccaro G: Management of the adult patient with acute lower gastrointestinal bleeding. Am J Gastroenterol 93:1202, 1998.

17

Headache

What causes headaches?

Approximately 99% of all headaches are recurrent benign headaches and are either tension type, migraine, or cluster headaches. Rare causes not to miss are subarachnoid hemorrhage (SAH), meningitis, subdural hematoma, and cancer.

What features are associated with chronic daily headaches?

A subset of headache patients suffer from chronic daily headaches. Chronic daily headaches are often associated with the following features: family history of headaches (90%), sleep disturbance (close to 100%), analgesic overuse (NSAIDs, ergotamine, barbiturates, triptans, and particularly narcotics such as codeine), and depression.

What are cluster headaches?

These occur predominately in middle-aged men, are severe, unilateral, retro-orbital, and are often described as stabbing in quality. Often, cluster headaches are accompanied by ipsilateral nasal congestion or lacrimation. These headaches recur over consecutive days to weeks, and then remit, hence the term cluster headaches.

▶ EVALUATION

My patient has recurring headaches. What questions should I ask?

The basic goal of evaluation is to determine the type and severity of the headache. History should be directed at pattern and location, previous headaches and treatment, preceding and accompanying symptoms (nausea, vomiting, visual changes, photophobia), triggering factors, severity and progression, medication use, and family history.

What distinguishes tension-type and migraine headaches?

Patients with tension-type headaches classically describe a "band-like pressure" around the skull that is mild to moderate in severity, but does not prevent daily activities (Box 17–1). Migraines are usually unilateral, throbbing, may be associated with nausea and/or vomiting, and are frequently disabling, with sufferers often retiring to bed in a dark, quiet room. An aura may precede the headache, most commonly visual scintillations. Effective clinical criteria make the diagnosis (Box 17–2).

What are clues to ominous headaches versus benign ones?

While the etiology of most headaches is benign, it is important to recognize signs that suggest an ominous cause for headache (Box 17–3).

What should I look for on exam?

Perform a good general exam, with a complete neurologic evaluation including cranial nerve testing and mental status assessment. Conduct additional examination as suggested by the patient's history. For example, if you suspect meningitis, check

BOX 17–1

Features of Tension-Type Headache

Mild to moderate tightness, bandlike pressure
Lasts thirty minutes to seven days
Not worsened by daily activity
Lacks photophobia and phonophobia (one may be present)
Ten previous episodes

BOX 17–2

Clinical Diagnosis of Migraine Headache

Requires any two of the following:

▶ unilateral site
▶ throbbing quality
▶ nausea
▶ photophobia or phonophobia

BOX 17-3

Danger Signs Suggesting an Ominous Cause of Headache

History
▶ First headache, or marked change in chronic headache
▶ Onset after age 50
▶ Onset during exertion
▶ Sudden onset or "worst headache ever"

Exam
▶ Abnormal neurologic exam/mental status
▶ Fever
▶ Neck stiffness

vital signs, mental status, and nuchal rigidity. If you are concerned about sinus infection, look for maxillary tenderness, purulent discharge, and poor transillumination of the sinuses. If you are concerned about temporal arteritis, palpate the temporal arteries.

My patient requests a CT scan or an MRI. Should I order one?

Probably not. Headache is, for the most part, a clinical diagnosis. Several studies have demonstrated that imaging will not add anything to the diagnosis, as long as the person with a headache doesn't have any of the warning signs mentioned earlier and has a normal neurologic exam. Longitudinal care will help with diagnosis; if the patient develops suspicious symptoms, has a mental status change, or doesn't get better as you expect, go back and revisit your original diagnostic assumptions and reconsider further evaluation.

What test do I order if I suspect an SAH?

SAH usually presents suddenly, often as "the worst headache ever." The purpose of imaging is to detect the blood. The sensitivity of the CT scan depends on the presence of fresh bleeding. In the first twenty-four hours, CT detects 95% of SAHs. If the CT scan is negative, and you still suspect SAH, perform a lumbar puncture (LP) to detect the 5% of bleeds missed by CT scan. Look for xanthochromia, a yellow pigmentation to the spinal fluid indicating the breakdown of blood in the CSF. If the suspected bleed occurred more than a week before, then an MRI is more sensitive.

How will I know if my patient has a brain tumor?

This is often the patient's fear as well; it is good to ask patients what they are worried about to address this concern directly. While the headache of a brain tumor has been described as a morning headache associated with nausea and vomiting, in reality the majority of brain tumor–associated headaches do not fit this or any other typical picture. Use warning signs for ominous cause of headache to prompt further evaluation. If no warning signs are present, longitudinal care is the key to monitor for any progression of symptoms or neurologic changes, which would then warrant further evaluation.

▶ TREATMENT

How should I treat migraine and tension-type headaches?

Before adding a medication, make sure your patient isn't using any medications that might induce headaches, including birth control pills, caffeine, alcohol, antidepressants, H_2 blockers, nitrates, and many more. Headaches can also be due to daily withdrawal symptoms from medications initially used to treat headaches, including NSAIDs, acetaminophen (Tylenol), or aspirin. Have the patient look for other triggers (wine, cheese, too much sleep) and remove them. Tension-type headaches respond well to NSAIDs.

What medications are useful for treating migraine headache?

Medications to treat recurrent migraine headaches fall into two categories: abortive and prophylactic (Box 17–4). Abortive treatment is given at the time of the headache to try to stop it. Prophylactic treatment is used for headaches occurring more than four times a month. For abortive therapy, many people respond to aspirin, NSAIDs such as naproxen (500–1000mg effective about 60% of the time) or acetaminophen. Cafergot, a combination of ergotamine and caffeine, is effective 60% of the time, but because of frequent GI upset, this medication is not commonly used. Oral triptans are successful in 70% of cases with response rates of 80% with injectable sumatriptan, though relapse is common. Sumatriptan is available in injectable, nasal, and oral formulations. Ergotamines and triptans both can cause vasoconstriction and may induce angina or myocardial infarction, so do not use these in patients with atherosclerotic disease. Because gastroparesis accompanies headache, particularly migraine, concomitant use of pro-motility agents, such as metoclopramide, can improve the absorption and the effect of the analgesic medication.

BOX 17-4

Therapies for Migraine Headache

Abortive therapy
- NSAIDs, aspirin
- Acetaminophen
- Ergotamines (dihydroergotamine, cafergot)
- Triptans (sumatriptan, others)
- Narcotics (last resort)

Prophylactic therapy
- β-blocker (propranolol)
- Calcium channel blocker (verapamil)
- TCAs (amitriptyline)
- Riboflavin
- Antiseizure medications (valproate, gabapentin)
- Management of concurrent GI symptoms
- Antinausea agent (prochlorperazine)
- Promotility agent (metoclopramide)
- (Calcium channel blockers have been used historically but there is limited data to support their efficacy.)

If abortive therapy for migraine is not effective, what next?

Patients with severe migraines often come to the ED or to clinic having failed to get relief from the above therapies. For these patients, consider the following: sumatriptan is 80% effective when given SC but headaches recur in up to 50% of patients. IV prochlorperazine is particularly suited to patients with associated nausea, improving nausea and aborting 80% of headaches. Dihydroergotamine (IV or SC) is as effective as sumatriptan but may cause nausea. If a patient has received a triptan in the past twenty-four hours, dihydroergotamine should not be given. Narcotics, such as IV demerol, should be reserved as a last resort.

What should I do if the headaches are frequent?

If your patient has bothersome headaches more than four times a month, ensure that basic measures have been taken: regulate sleep patterns, avoid food triggers, and eliminate caffeine. Review medications to detect causes for withdrawal headaches. If these measures are to no avail, consider prophylactic treatment. A four month trial using the B-vitamin riboflavin in high-dose (400 mg) showed a marked effect on headache frequency (number needed to treat = 3) but less effect on severity similar to effects seen with other prophylactic agents. Its favorable risk-benefit ratio and tolerability make it a good initial choice. Low-dose tricyclic antidepressants (TCAs) are especially effective for tension-type headaches but also work for migraines. β-blockers, especially non-selective propranolol and nadolol, are effective for preventing migraine headaches. If possible, choose a medication that treats a concurrent medical condition. For example, in a patient with hypertension, β-blockers might be your first choice. The antiseizure drugs valproate and gabapentin are an option in patients who have failed β-blockers or TCAs.

How do I treat chronic daily headaches and cluster headaches?

The only treatment for chronic daily headaches is to get the patient off all analgesics and start from scratch. Unmedicated patients with chronic daily headaches may respond to TCAs. For cluster headaches, lithium, ergotamine, or 100% oxygen are effective.

How often should my patient follow-up and what should I review at appointments?

Headaches are a chronic condition. Have your patient keep a headache diary to track symptoms, medication use, response, and triggers. While you are initiating or changing therapy, follow-up every four to six weeks. Once stable, the frequency is dictated by the frequency of symptoms. At each appointment, review the headache diary for the type and frequency of headaches, triggers, compliance, and side effects. Strategize with the patient regarding avoidance or elimination of triggers. Review the treatment plan and change medications if the current regimen is ineffective. If a compliant patient is not getting better as you would expect, or develops a new, different headache, reassess your diagnosis and consider further evaluation or referral to a neurologist.

K E Y   P O I N T S

▶ **Most headaches are benign.**

▶ **The diagnosis of a headache is based on accurate history and exam.**

▶ **Look for warning signs suggesting an ominous etiology.**

▶ **Always review patients' medications for those causing headache as a side effect or by withdrawal reactions.**

CASE 17–1. A 25-year-old woman reports a unilateral throbbing headache, nausea, and phonophobia for twenty-four hours. She has had three previous episodes in the past two years. She has partial relief with extra-strength Tylenol. Her neurologic exam, including mental status, is normal.

A. What is your differential diagnosis?
B. What imaging technique do you recommend?
C. What treatment do you recommend?
D. If her symptoms recur every week, what treatment would you recommend?

CASE 17–2. A 72-year-old writer with a stressful year including the end of a 30-year relationship presents with a tingling headache over the right temple. She recently began exercising and eating a more healthful diet. Despite these efforts, she complains of muscle aches and increasing fatigue. She has difficulty getting out of bed in the morning.

A. Does she have any warning signs for ominous headache?
B. What testing will you order?

CASE 17–3. A 26-year-old orthopedic surgery resident presents with a sudden severe headache while weightlifting. Neurologic exam is normal including normal CT. He is fine until his next call night when he collapses with a severe headache.

A. What is his most likely diagnosis?
B. What testing do you recommend?

REFERENCES

Practice parameter: Evidence-based guidelines for migraine headache (an evidence-based review). Report of the Quality Standards Subcommittee of the American Academy of Neurology. Neurology 55:754–762, 2000.

Silberstein SD, Lipton RB: Chronic daily headache. Curr Opin Neurol 13:277–283, 2000.

18

Healthy Patients

What is preventive medicine?

Preventive medicine attempts to decrease disease and increase health. Prevention assumes that clinical disease is a cumulative process and that interventions can prevent, stop, or slow that process. The process includes three stages: 1) health prior to disease; 2) preclinical disease in which biological changes have occurred but disease isn't apparent; and 3) clinically overt disease. Examples of preventive interventions include screening tests, immunizations, counseling and behavioral changes, and chemoprophylaxis, for example, postmenopausal hormone replacement therapy to prevent osteoporosis.

Why is prevention important?

Many of the most common diseases can be prevented. It has been estimated that half of the deaths in the U.S. are related to preventable external factors, including diet and activity habits, tobacco, alcohol, illicit drug use, sexual behavior, and motor vehicles. Smoking alone contributes to one fifth of all U.S. deaths. In 1992, 41,000 deaths were attributable to not using a seat belt and driving while intoxicated.

What are primary and secondary prevention?

These terms refer to the stage of the disease process during which the intervention occurs. In *primary prevention*, interventions are begun in asymptomatic patients before disease is present to alter susceptibility or reduce exposure. Good examples are classes for smoking prevention or cessation, nutrition counseling, and immunization. *Secondary prevention* attempts to detect disease in preclinical or beginning stages. Examples include screening programs for cervical or breast cancer (pap smears and mammography, respectively). *Tertiary prevention* attempts to restore function and alleviate disability from disease, for example, cardiac rehabilitation after heart attack. The distinction is important because the risk/benefit ratio and cost effectiveness of an intervention differs depending on the stage of disease it targets. For example, lowering cholesterol in people who already have had an MI may be worth the cost and potential side effects of cholesterol lowering drugs. In comparison, primary prevention with medications in healthy people may be too costly, or may cause too many side effects for the smaller benefit gained.

Why do we screen for some diseases and not others?

Certain criteria must be met before screening is considered worthwhile. This varies according to the treatment of the disease, the test, and the patient population (Box 18–1).

Why are some screening tests controversial?

Prostate specific antigen (PSA) is an example of a screening test for prostate cancer that was clinically available before the implication of its use was clearly understood. There are several problems with it as a screening test. First of all, PSA has poor sensitivity and specificity: it can be elevated in the absence of prostate cancer or can be normal in cancer's presence. Second, cancer identified by an elevated PSA may not be clinically significant—that is, the patient may have cancer but may die from another cause. Third, the effectiveness of treatment for prostate cancer is debated. A Swedish study suggests that watchful waiting has the same mortality rates as surgery, without the perioperative risk or common postoperative complications of urinary incontinence or impotence.

BOX 18–1

Criteria for Judging Whether Screening is Worthwhile

Disease Characteristics

Prevalent and/or responsible for high burden of suffering
Detectable prior to symptom onset
Effective treatment available
Early detection improves outcomes

Test Characteristics

Accurate (good sensitivity, specificity, and predictive values)
Acceptable to patients
Benefits outweigh risks

Population Characteristics

Sufficient incidence to justify cost
Population screened will live long enough to benefit
Intervention acceptable to and used by population

Preventive health practices differ for age and gender. How can I know what to do?

In general, address the health issues specific to that age and gender. Some preventive measures apply to all adults: tetanus immunization, blood pressure screening, and counseling for healthful diet and exercise, smoking cessation, and use of seat belts. Other interventions are based on age and/or gender such as pap smears, mammography, or fecal occult blood testing. Certain measures are directed only to high-risk populations, for example, aspirin for heart disease. For more specific guidance, consult available references. One of the most widely used is the U.S. Preventive Services Task Force (USPSTF) Guide to Clinical Preventive Services (Table 18–1). This guide provides evidence-based recommendations for groups of people based on age, gender, and risk factors. The need to base recommendations on well-designed outcome studies is especially important in preventive medicine because you are recommending interventions to healthy patients and do not want to cause harm.

How do I track health maintenance/promotion?

One approach is to have a health maintenance/promotion section in the problem list or in the assessment/plan to prompt you. The use of reminders or prompts, especially computer-based, has been shown to increase the rate at which providers address health maintenance issues with their patients.

K E Y   P O I N T S

▶ Prevention saves lives, decreases disease, and increases health.

▶ Since prevention is aimed at healthy people, the evidence must be compelling that the benefits outweigh the risks.

▶ Evidence-based recommendations geared to specific age and gender are available, most notably in the USPSTF Guide to Clinical Preventive Services.

TABLE 18–1

Suggested Preventive Health Care for Adults

a. Periodic Health Exam

Height, weight, blood pressure, and symptom-focused examination	• Age 18-39: Every 3-5 years • Age ≥ 40: Annual

TABLE 18–1 *continued*

Suggested Preventive Health Care for Adults

b. Screening

Disease	Intervention	Recommended Schedule	Strength of Evidence
Breast cancer	Mammography	• annual for women aged 50-69 • consider for age 40-49 • reasonable to continue beyond age 69	Good
Cervical cancer	Papanicolaou smear	• every 1-3 years from age 18 or onset of sexual activity • stop after hysterectomy for benign disease or at age 65 if repeatedly normal	Good
Colorectal cancer	Fecal occult blood testing (FOBT) Flexible sigmoidoscopy Colonoscopy	• screen beginning at age 50 • annual FOBT and/or sigmoidoscopy every 3-5 years or • colonoscopy every 10 years, every 3 years if polyps	Fair
High blood cholesterol	Total cholesterol	• men aged 35-65 • women aged 45-65	Fair
Osteoporosis	DXA	• postmenopausal women at risk (see Chapter 37 for further discussion)	Fair
Pelvic inflammatory disease	*Chlamydia* screening	• women younger than 25 with multiple sexual partners at highest risk	Fair
Prostate cancer	Prostate specific antigen	• discuss possible benefits and known risks of screening with patient before testing • men aged 50-69 most likely to benefit	Poor

c. Counseling

Injury prevention	Use car lap/shoulder belts, wear bicycle helmets, install smoke detectors
Diet and exercise	Decrease fat and cholesterol intake, take adequate calcium and vitamin D, exercise aerobically regularly
STD prevention	Use safe sex practices
Substance use	Stop or abstain from smoking, moderate alcohol use, abstain from illicit drug use

Continued

TABLE 18–1 *continued*

Suggested Preventive Health Care for Adults

d. Routine Adult Immunization

Disease	Recommendation
Tetanus-diphtheria (Td)	Two booster strategies are equivalent: • Td boosters every 10 years throughout life • single booster at age 50 for individuals who received 3-dose pediatric series and teenage booster
Measles-mumps-rubella	• single dose for adults born after 1956 without proof of immunity or documentation of previous immunization • second dose for college students, health care workers, and foreign travelers
Hepatitis B	• recommended for all young adults and older adults at high risk • assess serologic response in persons older than 30
Hepatitis A	• recommended for adults at risk: foreign travelers, injection drug users, multiple sexual partners, day care workers, chronic liver disease
Influenza	• annually to all adults age 50 or older, younger if at risk, e.g., COPD, CHF, asthma, cancer, health care worker • consider for all healthy adults
Invasive pneumococcal disease	• recommended for all adults at age 65, younger if at risk • reimmunization recommended for: a) high-risk adults at age 65 who received vaccine >5 years earlier and b) asplenic and immunocompromised adults 5 years after first dose

---

CASE 18–1. A 22-year-old apparently healthy man is in clinic for a routine visit.

    A. What general counseling should I offer?
    B. What specific immunizations are indicated?
    C. Is prostate screening needed?

▶ CHANGING HARMFUL HEALTH HABITS

What are general guidelines to changing harmful health habits?

Studies of how people change provide a model that divides the process into clinically useful stages: 1) precontemplation, 2) contemplation, 3) determination, 4) action, and 5) maintenance. Relapse often occurs, reinitiating the cycle (Figure 18–1). By identifying which stage the patient has achieved, you can target your efforts to help the patient reach the next stage. Thus, the focus is on moving the patient closer to change rather than on an "all or nothing" outcome.

What is an example of using this model in patient care?

The example below follows a patient through smoking cessation.

Stage 1: Precontemplation. In this stage, the patient is not consciously thinking of quitting. Studies show that simple physician advice and encouragement to consider quitting have an effect, although the results are not immediately obvious. Maintain an empathetic and nonjudgmental approach while making a clear statement: "I think it is important for you to quit smoking. In fact, this is the most important thing you can do for your health."

Stage 2: Contemplation. The patient is now considering quitting smoking. Ask questions at each visit to help the patient identify reasons and barriers to quitting. Personalize the motivation: "You had one heart attack already—if you stop smoking, chances are higher you will be around to enjoy your new promotion." Make sure the motivation fits the particular age, gender, and individual. For example, adolescents tend to "bum" cigarettes so arguments about cost are ineffective. Rather, it may work to say "If you quit smoking, you may be able to breathe better, and that will help your soccer game."

Stage 3: Determination. The patient has decided to quit smoking. Problem-solve with the patient about what has worked in the past and what led to failure to quit. Address his or her concerns about possible negative consequences of quitting including weight

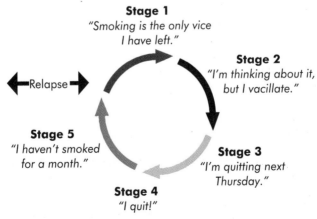

Figure 18–1. A model of change for smoking cessation.

gain, bad moods, and issues of peer nonsupport or other barriers. Offer support system: intensive smoking cessation program, nicotine replacement therapy such as gums, patch, or nasal spray, and/or other pharmacological aids such as bupropion.

Stage 4: Action. The patient quits! Schedule a series of biweekly or monthly visits, beginning one week after the quit date. Express continuing care and support.

Stage 5: Maintenance and Relapse. Congratulate the patient on his successes and reinforce the benefits of not smoking. Anticipate relapses, reframe these as positive learning experiences, and plan how to restart the cessation process.

What are specific guidelines in the use of medication and nicotine in smoking cessation?

Physician counseling, group counseling, and extended support groups all assist patients in smoking cessation and long-term maintenance. Nicotine replacement and the antidepressant bupropion, started a week before the quit date, double the successful smoking cessation rate to 35%. Given the great difficulty patients have in stopping smoking, this is encouraging. Nicotine can be administered by gum, inhaler, or most commonly, by transdermal patch. For the patch, a dose of 21 mg for ten to twelve weeks has shown the greatest success. Patients are advised not to smoke concurrently with the nicotine replacement, but studies of the patch have not revealed adverse cardiovascular outcomes. Extended release bupropion is dosed at 150 mg daily for three days, then increased to twice daily. This staggered start minimizes the initial agitation that many patients experience on this medication. Additionally, the quit date should be set for one week after starting bupropion to assure effective blood levels. Bupropion lowers the seizure threshold and so should not be used in patients with past history of seizure or alcoholism, or with ongoing eating disorders. A benefit of bupropion that may encourage patients in its use is that it may offset the weight gain and depression that can follow smoking cessation.

Is this model of change applicable to all behavioral changes?

Yes. Ambulatory medicine offers you a longitudinal relationship with a patient, allowing you to address these issues repeatedly, a little bit at a time. As you get to know your patients, you can help them recognize opportunities for and benefits of prevention that matter to them, whether it is being able to breathe easier when playing with their grandchildren since they quit smoking or their improved job performance since they quit drinking. Seeing the benefits of change is reinforcing for patients.

K E Y   P O I N T S

▶ There is a cycle of change that occurs in predictable stages: precontemplation, contemplation, determination, action, and maintenance.

▶ Providers can assist patients in moving from one stage to the next.

▶ Providers should inquire about harmful health habits, advise patients to change them, and offer continuing support in a nonjudgmental, empathetic manner.

CASE 18–2. A 35-year-old man wants to lose weight. He has tried several times in the past but failed and states he's "given up."

A. What stage of change is he in?
B. What questions should you ask?
C. He decides to try to lose weight. What follow-up should you plan?

USEFUL WEBSITE

Guide to Clinical Preventive Services, 2nd ed. (1996). Available online at *http://text.nlm.nih.gov*

19

Joint and Muscular Pain

JOINT PAIN

▶ ETIOLOGY

What causes joint pain?

The causes of joint pain can be divided roughly into two categories: mechanical and inflammatory (Figure 19–1). Mechanical processes are by far more common and arise from wear and tear on the joint or overuse syndromes affecting surrounding structures. Frequently a single joint is affected. Inflammatory causes of joint pain are autoimmune disease, crystal-induced disease, and infection. These can involve few or multiple joints, often in a characteristic pattern. The autoimmune arthropathies, systemic lupus erythematosus (SLE) and rheumatoid arthritis (RA) affect small and large joints as well as multiple organs. In gout, few joints are involved. Septic arthritis affects a single joint, unless disseminated gonococcal infection is present. Occasionally, patients and physicians confuse muscular pain with joint pain.

What serious causes of joint pain should I not miss?

Don't miss septic arthritis, malignancy, or osteonecrosis. Clues to these include rest pain, delayed response to therapy, risk factors

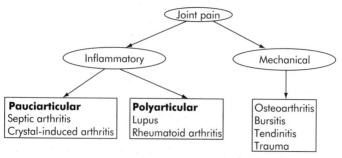

Figure 19–1. Classification of joint pain.

such as prior malignancy, or systemic signs like fever, chills, or weight loss. Osteonecrosis (death of bone due to vascular insufficiency) is seen in the hip or proximal tibia, particularly with long-term steroid use, sickle cell anemia, or vasculitis.

Why is septic arthritis important?

Septic arthritis is a medical emergency requiring rapid diagnosis and treatment, including possible surgical débridement to avoid joint destruction. Onset is acute, with marked synovitis, effusion, and extreme pain with movement. Eighty percent of cases involve one joint, usually the knee. Infectious agents in adults are *Staphylococcus aureus*, other gram positive organisms, and *Neisseria gonorrhoeae* (a gram negative coccus). *S. aureus* is especially common in septic arthritis superimposed on RA. This is particularly tricky, since a clinician may believe the inflammation is due to RA alone. Suspect gonorrhea in young, sexually active adults and remember that disseminated infection can rarely affect multiple joints.

What is osteoarthritis?

Synonyms include degenerative arthritis and mechanical arthritis. This condition occurs as a consequence of wear and tear on the joints which generates low grade inflammation. Prevalence is high in patients older than age 55, or when joints are heavily used, such as hip degenerative arthritis in a construction worker. Obesity or prior trauma also predisposes to early osteoarthritis.

Does patient age change the likely cause of joint pain?

Patients older than age 55 are much more likely to have degenerative arthritis, gout, or bursitis. Autoimmune arthropathies are more common in younger patients, as are trauma and overuse syndromes such as ligament injury or tendinitis.

For major joints, what are the common causes of joint pain?

Degenerative arthritis occurs predominately in high use joints such as the hands, and in weight-bearing joints, so knees and hips are frequently affected; the shoulder and elbow are often spared. Tendinitis and bursitis commonly occur due to overuse of any of the major joints (Table 19–1 and Figure 19–2).

What is rotator cuff tendinitis?

The rotator cuff is made of four muscles that rotate and stabilize the humeral head. The subacromial bursa lies between the cuff

TABLE 19–1

Common Conditions Afflicting Major Joints

Location	Condition	Findings
Hip	Degenerative arthritis	• pain in groin, medial thigh pain with internal and external hip rotation
	Trochanteric bursitis	• pain in lateral thigh point tenderness on greater trochanter
Knee	Degenerative arthritis	• pain deep to patella joint line tenderness effusion without heat
	Prepatellar bursitis	• pain over patella when kneeling heat, swelling anterior to patella
	Patellofemoral syndrome	• pain with deep knee bend, walking upstairs, prolonged sitting with knees bent
	Baker's cyst	• fullness behind knee, lower extremity swelling if ruptures
Shoulder	Rotator cuff tendinitis	• weakness if rotator cuff tear present pain rolling onto shoulder at night pain limits abduction and external rotation
	Frozen shoulder	• pain as above, markedly limited range of motion
	Trauma	• point tenderness, history of trauma, deformity with dislocation or fracture
Elbow	Lateral epicondylitis (tennis elbow)	• lateral elbow pain with wrist supination or extension
	Olecranon bursitis	• swelling and tenderness over olecranon process

muscles and the acromial process. Varying terms are used to describe a spectrum of disorders that affect this cluster of muscles and surrounding structures. These include rotator cuff tendinitis, subacromial bursitis, frozen shoulder syndrome, and impingement syndrome. A biceps tendinitis can occur simultaneously with any of these conditions. The primary symptoms of all of these conditions are shoulder pain and limited range of motion.

▶ EVALUATION

How can I distinguish mechanical from inflammatory causes of joint pain?

The presentation of these conditions can overlap. Aside from acute trauma, mechanical causes of joint pain tend to be gradual in

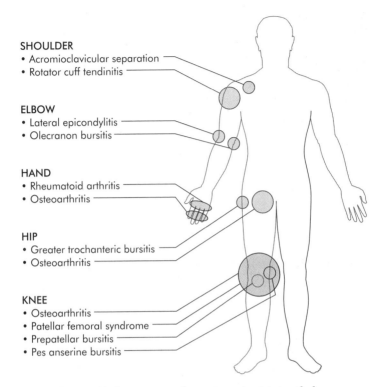

SHOULDER
• Acromioclavicular separation
• Rotator cuff tendinitis

ELBOW
• Lateral epicondylitis
• Olecranon bursitis

HAND
• Rheumatoid arthritis
• Osteoarthritis

HIP
• Greater trochanteric bursitis
• Osteoarthritis

KNEE
• Osteoarthritis
• Patellar femoral syndrome
• Prepatellar bursitis
• Pes anserine bursitis

Figure 19–2. Location of pain in major joint pathology.

onset with minimal obvious inflammation. By contrast, inflammatory causes of joint pain can come on rapidly or slowly, but synovitis is usually present with joint erythema, pain, swelling, and loss of function. These findings indicate either vigorous inflammatory arthritis such as gout or SLE, or possibly septic arthritis. Another key historical distinction is "gelling." In inflammatory arthritis, symptoms worsen with rest as the joint "gels" resulting in prolonged stiffness for more than one hour after a period of rest; in mechanical arthritis the pain improves with rest, and stiffness is worked out of the joint over minutes.

How is degenerative arthritis different from bursitis or tendinitis on exam?

The primary distinction is the anatomic location of the pain. A good example is the knee. In degenerative arthritis, the pain is localized behind the patella within the joint space. In prepatellar bursitis, the pain is localized anterior to the patella. Similarly, in the hip, degenerative arthritis symptoms are deep in the groin and anterior thigh and are reproduced with hip range of motion. Greater trochanteric bursitis produces point tenderness over the bursa with deep palpation over the lateral aspect of the hip. With a tendinitis, the tendon is tender to palpation and stretch, and active use of the tendon exacerbates pain.

When evaluating joint pain, what are key points on the physical exam?

Nothing will replace solid knowledge of the musculoskeletal system, with particular attention to the location of bursae. Focus on the following items:

Joints: Tenderness, range of motion, synovitis (heat, spongy synovial hypertrophy), deformity, crepitus, and effusions
Ligaments: Tenderness, laxity, pain with use against resistance
Tendons: Tenderness, laxity
Bursae: Tenderness, swelling, redness
Muscle: Tone, bulk, symmetry, strength, and tender points for fibromyalgia
Cartilage: Locking, clicking

How can I evaluate shoulder pain for presence of bursitis versus rotator cuff tear?

Patients with rotator cuff tendinitis and subacromial bursitis present with shoulder pain in the deltoid distribution, exacerbated at night when rolling over onto the affected shoulder. On exam, pain is reproduced with arm abduction in an arc between 80 and 120 degrees and with internal or external rotation (reaching hands behind the back). Range of motion is limited focally by maneuvers that cause impingement of the subacromial bursa, especially shoulder abduction and external rotation. In frozen shoulder, calcification of the tendon limits motion both passively and actively, and pain is more severe with any motion of the shoulder. Rotator cuff tear is distinguished by weakness, particularly with abduction, though passive range of motion is often pain-free. Pain and an inability to relax may make it difficult to assess strength. A lidocaine injection into the subacromial bursa may be necessary to allow evaluation for true weakness. Rotator cuff tears rarely occur in patients younger than age 40; patients can often identify a specific injury.

Is x-ray helpful in the diagnosis of joint pain?

Degenerative arthritis causes joint space narrowing and sclerosis (focal bone thickening seen as a bright whiteness at the joint surface). RA and gout cause characteristic erosions, which may be absent in the initial phases of disease (see Chapter 35). If the evaluation is consistent with a chronic mechanical cause, films do not add much information. If, on the other hand, recent trauma or concern for cancer are present, an x-ray can help rule out fracture or lytic disease. For suspected rotator cuff tear, obtain ultrasound or MRI to confirm diagnosis.

When is arthrocentesis required?

A synovial fluid tap is imperative if septic arthritis is suspected by presence of fever, monarticular synovitis in a young person, or worsening monarticular inflammation in the setting of stable polyarticular disease. Further, any patient with undiagnosed synovitis should have arthrocentesis. Send the fluid for culture, cell count, crystal evaluation, and glucose. This will distinguish between gout (birefringent crystals), inflammatory arthritis (WBC 2000–75,000), and septic arthritis (WBC greater than 75,000 with low glucose, though lower counts of 30,000–60,000 can occur).

What other tests should I order for patients with joint pain?

Given an H & P consistent with mechanical cause of joint pain, no further blood tests are needed. For suspected gout, obtain a serum uric acid test, though this may be normal. For any acutely inflamed single joint, or if disseminated gonococcal infection is suspected, obtain a CBC (elevated WBC in infection, anemia in autoimmune disease), electrolytes and creatinine (looking for abnormal renal function in autoimmune disease or gout), uric acid (gout), and C-reactive protein or sedimentation rate (general assessment for inflammation). If disseminated gonorrhea infection is suspected, swab the throat, cervix, penile urethra, and rectum for gonococcal cultures to confirm the infection. Use of ANA reflexive panel and rheumatoid factor are outlined in Chapter 35.

▶ TREATMENT

How are bursitis and tendinitis treated?

Maintaining range of motion and function is the overall goal. Instructions in strengthening exercises are helpful, either by handout, or through personal instruction from a physical therapist. Short-term use of nonsteroidal anti-inflammatories (NSAIDs) diminishes pain and inflammation. Most medication failures are due to insufficient or erratic dosing; NSAIDS must be taken at anti-inflammatory doses around the clock (e.g., ibuprofen 600–800 mg every eight hours). For severe cases, consider steroid injection into the inflamed bursa or tendon. Do not inject more often than every three months for a total of three shots as this can weaken tendons and muscles.

What is the appropriate treatment for osteoarthritis?

Avoid aggravating activities. Physical therapy and low-impact strengthening exercise have proved effective. Acetaminophen is first-line treatment for both pain and inflammation with fewer side effects than NSAIDs. The most common error is inadequate dosing; aim for up to 4000 mg per day, assuming normal liver function. NSAIDs are second-line therapy and have many more side effects, particularly gastrointestinal bleeding. Late data are favorable for chondroitin sulfate and glucosamine, cartilage derivatives. These are not FDA controlled (dosing depends on manufacturer's recommendations) and effects take six to eight weeks, so warn patients to expect delayed response. For severe pain at rest and/or severe limitation of daily activities, refer to an orthopedist for evaluation.

When does joint pain require referral?

Refer for orthopedic evaluation any patient with joint dysfunction such as locking or giving way, joint instability, or inability to weight-bear. These symptoms suggest significant meniscal tear, ligamentous injury, or unsuspected fracture or osteonecrosis. Suspected septic arthritis requires immediate orthopedic evaluation and treatment. For patients with degenerative arthritis and pain that significantly limits daily activities, an orthopedic evaluation for joint replacement is indicated. Rheumatologists are particularly skilled at the management of systemic arthropathies, particularly RA and SLE. Further, in any patient with persistent, unexplained symptoms, a subspecialty referral is indicated.

How should the inflammatory causes of joint pain be treated?

Septic arthritis is a surgical emergency. Treatment includes broad-spectrum antibiotics and joint space drainage. Once an organism is identified, the coverage can be narrowed. Repeated aspiration may be adequate, but often surgical drainage is required. For autoimmune processes like SLE and RA, standard of care is to treat aggressively before joint damage occurs by reducing inflammation with methotrexate or azathioprine. Acute gout responds to NSAIDs, prednisone, or colchicine. Allopurinol is effective for prophylaxis against repeat attacks, but may exacerbate an acute attack so should not be started until several weeks after an attack is resolved.

When should I hospitalize a patient with joint pain?

Any patient with acute monarticular synovitis with high fever needs immediate evaluation with a synovial arthrocentesis. If the patient is very ill, or if the tap confirms septic arthritis, the patient should be admitted.

K E Y   P O I N T S

▶ Mechanical causes of joint pain generally occur gradually and with minimal inflammation.

▶ Inflammatory causes of joint pain cause prolonged stiffness after rest and marked synovitis.

▶ Septic arthritis is a medical emergency.

CASE 19–1. A 64-year-old obese woman presents with bilateral knee pain, right greater than left. She has a sensation of fullness in her left knee. She currently does not exercise. She denies recent trauma, rash, fever, chills, weight loss, history of diabetes, or steroid use. Her exam shows mild joint line tenderness, a small effusion without erythema, and mild pain reproduced with range of motion. Anterior and posterior drawer signs (indicating ligamentous laxity) are normal. Prepatellar and pes anserine bursae are nontender.

    A. What is the most likely diagnosis?
    B. What further evaluation do you recommend?
    C. What treatment can you offer her?

CASE 19–2. A 32-year-old man presents with three day history of increasingly painful, hot and swollen joints, particularly in his hands and feet, low-grade fevers, and malaise. He has had no previous episodes and has been in excellent health with no history of preceding trauma or infections. Exam reveals multiple joints with marked synovitis and a rash on his face but no joint deformity.

    A. What is your differential diagnosis?
    B. What further questions should you ask?
    C. What tests will you order?

MUSCULAR PAIN

▶ ETIOLOGY

What causes diffuse persistent muscular pain?

Common causes are fibromyalgia, polymyalgia rheumatica (PMR), and hormonal conditions such as cortisol excess and thyroid aberrations. Less commonly, myositis with primary muscle inflammation is caused by autoimmune disease or as a medication side effect, for example with HMG CoA reductase inhibitors.

▶ EVALUATION

How are fibromyalgia, PMR, and polymyositis different?

All three conditions are characterized by muscle pain and aching. Muscle weakness and elevated creatine kinase (CK) are present in myositis only. *Fibromyalgia* is a syndrome of diffuse muscle and joint pain without any identifiable underlying pathology or inflammation. Criteria for diagnosis include widespread pain and presence of 11 of 18 tender points on exam (Figure 19–3). Stiffness and sleep disturbances are common. Patients with PMR also present with diffuse muscle pain, particularly in the proximal limb muscles. In contrast to fibromyalgia, PMR in patients older than age 50 causes elevated ESR, and is associated with temporal arteritis (TA), a vasculitis that can cause blindness or stroke. In both fibromyalgia and PMR, the muscle fibers themselves are not damaged, so muscle strength and enzymes are normal. *Myositis,* as the name implies, results in inflammation and destruction of muscle fibers with resulting weakness and elevated CK and aldolase. When polymyositis occurs with a heliotrope rash (violaceous discoloration of the eyelids) and Gottron's papules (scaly, plaquelike eruptions over the finger joints), the condition is called dermatomyositis. All three conditions are distinguished from arthritis by normal joint exams and tender muscles. Myalgias are quite common in patients on HMG CoA reductase inhibitors. Only a small minority of these patients have measurable elevations of creatine phosphokinase (CPK) warranting discontinuation of the medication.

▶ TREATMENT

Treatment depends on the underlying disorder (Table 19–2).

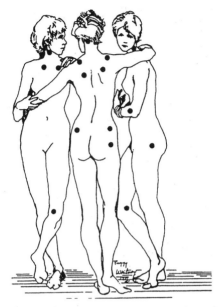

Figure 19–3. Tender points of fibromyalgia. (From Wolfe F et al: Arthritis Rheum 33:160, 1990.)

TABLE 19–2

Common Causes, Findings, and Treatment of Diffuse Muscular Pain

Cause	Findings	Treatment
Fibromyalgia	Nonrestorative sleep Tender points Normal blood tests Normal strength	Exercise NSAIDs Tricyclic antidepressants Improved sleep
Polymyalgia rheumatica	Diffuse aches, worse in AM Elevated ESR Associated temporal arteritis Jaw claudication Normal strength	Low-dose prednisone High dose if TA present
Polymyositis	Muscle weakness and tenderness on exam Elevated CPK and aldolase	Prednisone Methotrexate if needed
Hormones: Hypo- or hyperthyroidism	High or low TSH High 24 hour cortisol	Hormone replacement, or Identification and removal of site of overproduction

Continued

TABLE 19–2 *continued*

Common Causes, Findings, and Treatment of Diffuse Muscular Pain

Cause	Findings	Treatment
Cushing's syndrome	May have muscle weakness CPK elevated in hypothyroidism only	
Myalgias secondary to HMG CoA reductase inhibitor	Association with taking HMG CoA reductase inhibitor	Trial off meds to confirm Dx Monitor CPK and NSAIDs

K E Y   P O I N T S

▶ Fibromyalgia has no laboratory abnormalities and is based on clinical criteria.

▶ Fibromyalgia and PMR have normal muscle strength and enzymes.

▶ PMR occurs in the elderly, has elevated ESR, and may be associated with TA.

▶ Myositis results in elevated CK and muscle weakness.

CASE 19–3. A 45-year-old woman reports diffuse body aches and fatigue. She has a history of depression, poor sleep, and thyroid disease. Review of systems is otherwise negative. Exam reveals normal joints without pain on range of motion, normal muscle strength, and multiple tender points.

  A. What is your differential diagnosis?
  B. Would you order an ANA?
  C. What is appropriate therapy?

CASE 19-4. An 85-year-old woman presents with right shoulder pain. The pain is worse at night, and she has some morning stiffness that improves in half an hour. She can no longer brush her hair. She also reports 10 pound weight loss, but is otherwise in good health. Exam: decreased passive and active range of motion on right shoulder abduction; point tenderness under the acromial process on right.

A. What is the differential diagnosis?
B. What evaluation is indicated?
C. Does this patient have a rotator cuff tear?

REFERENCES

American College of Rheumatology Ad Hoc Committee on Clinical Guidelines. Guidelines for the initial evaluation of the adult patient with acute musculoskeletal symptoms. Arthritis Rheum 39:1, 1996.

Baker DG, Schumacher HR Jr: Acute monoarthritis. N Engl J Med 329:1013, 1993.

Dalakas MC: Polymyositis, dermatomyositis, and inclusion-body myositis. N Engl J Med 325:1487, 1991.

Goldenberg DL: Fibromyalgia syndrome a decade later: What have we learned? Arch Intern Med 159:777, 1999.

20

Low Back Pain

What causes acute low back pain?

Over 95% of all low back pain arises from relatively benign changes to musculoskeletal structures in the low back. Degenerative arthritis, lumbosacral strain, bulging vertebral discs, sciatic nerve irritation, and spinal stenosis all cause low back pain. Pinpointing the anatomic source of the pain is often difficult, and in fact does not correlate with prognosis. Fortunately, the great majority of low back pain will resolve with a conservative approach of brief rest, anti-inflammatories, and gradual return to previous activity. Your job is to reassure the patient and yourself that another condition doesn't exist, and to monitor the patient's progress.

What is sciatica?

Sciatica refers to pain radiating in the sciatic nerve distribution down the back of the leg. Although classically associated with a herniated disc, many other conditions can cause this pain syndrome (e.g.,spinal stenosis, sacroiliitis).

What are the "red flags" for dangerous causes of low back pain?

Warning signs for potentially serious causes of back pain are listed in Table 20–1.

► EVALUATION

Is the patient's description of the pain helpful?

Most back pain is nonspecific and does not lead reliably to a diagnosis. The following generalizations may be useful. *Radicular pain*, i.e., pain in a nerve distribution, extends from the back or buttock past the knee and suggests impingement of a nerve as it exits

TABLE 20-1	
Red Flags for Dangerous Causes of Low Back Pain	
Risk of cancer	Age older than 50
	History of cancer
Risk for infection	IV drug use
	Immunosuppression, including diabetes and corticosteroid use
Risk for fracture	Osteoporosis, primary or secondary to corticosteroid use
	Trauma, "severe" in all patients or "mild" if patient older than 50
Unusual course	Not improving as you would expect
	Progressive symptoms
Focal neurologic signs or symptoms	History of weakness, numbness, bowel or bladder dysfunction
	Exam findings of weakness, numbness, or diminished reflexes

the spinal canal. In contrast, back pain that extends to the thigh or hip but not past the knee is *radiating*, not radicular, pain and is less worrisome for a neuropathic cause. Rest pain and/or progressive pain may indicate cancer or abscess. Pain with cough, bowel movement, or sneeze is consistent with disc herniation, as increased pressure through Valsalva maneuver worsens this condition.

How is a history of spinal stenosis different from other causes of low back pain?

Spinal stenosis is narrowing of the spinal canal usually associated with arthritis. It causes pain in the thighs and buttocks with walking or standing that is relieved by sitting. In contrast, back pain from herniated disc or musculoskeletal strain worsens with hip and lumbar flexion, usually while sitting. Some patients with spinal stenosis have numbness in the legs without much pain.

What is an appropriate neurologic exam for low back pain?

For the evaluation of low back pain, a good neurologic exam is your best tool. This does not mean an exhaustive exam. Over 90% of neurologic sequelae of back disease occur in the L5-S1 region, so your exam can focus primarily on the foot. (The exception is patients with bowel or bladder symptoms, symptoms of possible acute cord compression. In those cases, you need to check perianal sensation and rectal tone.) The top of the foot allows you to test the three sensory distributions L4-S1. A helpful mnemonic is S1 = Small toe, L4 = Large toe. Reflexes are technically difficult to reproduce. This doesn't mean don't do them, but realize that they may not be accurate. Motor weakness should be obvious; a good screening test is great toe dorsiflexion (L5), and plantar flexion (S1) (Figure 20–1).

What is the best test for nerve impingement as the cause of acute low back pain?

The best examination maneuver is the straight leg raise. With the patient lying on his or her back, elevate the straight leg. A positive test reproduces radicular pain with the leg 70 degrees or less from horizontal, indicating tension in the L5/S1 nerve root. If raising the contralateral leg reproduces pain on the affected side, this is most specific for a disc herniation, and is called a positive crossed straight leg raise. Pain produced in the low back or hip does not qualify as a positive test.

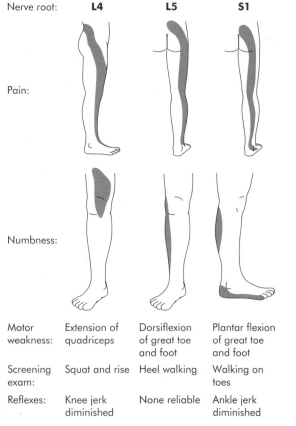

Nerve root:	**L4**	**L5**	**S1**
Motor weakness:	Extension of quadriceps	Dorsiflexion of great toe and foot	Plantar flexion of great toe and foot
Screening exam:	Squat and rise	Heel walking	Walking on toes
Reflexes:	Knee jerk diminished	None reliable	Ankle jerk diminished

Figure 20–1. Findings localizing lumbar nerve root compromise.

If the neurologic exam is abnormal, what should I do?

This is a red flag. Major motor weakness, such as absent dorsi-flexion of the great toe, traditionally requires imaging. However, here is a refinement on this rule: a patient with mild disc hernia-tion may have slight numbness or even weakness by H&P. This mild degree of symptoms can be managed conservatively for two to four weeks. If the patient's numbness persists, obtain a CT and EMG as evaluation for potential surgery.

How do red flags help me decide what further studies to order?

If no red flags are present, no further work-up is needed. When any red flag is present, start with an ESR and lumbosacral spine film. If history suggests infection, obtain a CBC and/or urinalysis. Although you may be tempted to obtain a CT or MRI scan early in your evaluation, remember that CT and MRI are very sensitive modalities but they are extremely nonspecific. These studies reveal disc bulging in up to 60% of the normal population. In the asymp-tomatic elderly, frank disc herniation is seen in 30%. Reserve these studies for symptoms/signs of cord compression (see later), when you suspect spinal stenosis, when there is an abnormal x-ray or sedimentation rate, or for preoperative evaluation.

What are potential low back pain emergencies?

The spinal cord sits within a confined space, defined by the sur-rounding vertebral bone structure. If the cord is compressed, paralysis can occur. The main causes of acute spinal cord com-pression are epidural abscess (an infection in the epidural space surrounding or next to the cord), encroaching tumor, and, rarely, massive disc herniation. Acute neurologic change or progres-sive neurologic symptoms, particularly in high risk patients with IV drug use or known cancer, should alert you to this possibil-ity. If you suspect one of these conditions, the patient requires emergent imaging and neurosurgical evaluation. The quicker the treatment, the more complete the recovery.

What is the cauda equina syndrome?

The cauda equina is the "horse's tail" of sacral nerves that travel in the distal spinal canal. This syndrome is a description of acute cord compression, such as with disc herniation, of these distal sacral nerves, causing bowel and bladder dysfunction of either marked constipation or incontinence, and sacral nerve numbness in the "saddle" distribution.

▶ TREATMENT

How do I treat acute low back pain?

When red flags are absent, conservative therapy is indicated. First, prescribe nonsteroidal anti-inflammatories on scheduled three-times-a-day dosing; no evidence exists that any one NSAID is better than another. Second, have the patient return to previous activities as soon as tolerated, with the exception of heavy lifting. Initially, some patients may require two to three days of bed rest, but with longer inactivity, outcomes worsen. Third, physical therapy and back exercises should be started as soon as tolerated (Box 20–1).

Do I manage acute and chronic low back pain differently?

A repeat episode of acute low back pain is managed in the same manner as the first episode. Chronic back pain present for several months is a different problem. First, review your H&P for red flags and consider further studies if the patient has not responded as you would have expected. Second, screen your patient carefully for depression. This condition is common among patients with chronic pain. Antidepressants serve a dual function in these cases, improving both chronic pain and depression. Pending legal action predicts poorer prognosis.

How do I fill out disability forms?

Describe objectively what you see on exam. You do not have to determine disability; that is the job of the Department of Labor and Industry. Often there is a section asking how many pounds the patient can lift. A general guideline follows symptom severity (Table 20–2).

Is there a role for the chiropractor? Acupuncture?

In a nonblinded study, 400 men with acute back pain improved over controls with chiropractor intervention in the first two weeks after acute back pain. There is no evidence supporting more frequent weekly chiropractic intervention or acupuncture. Nonetheless,

---

BOX 20-1

Elements of "Conservative Therapy" for Acute Low Back Pain

Nonsteroidal anti-inflammatory medications
Return to previous activities after minimal bed rest
Physical therapy/back exercises

TABLE 20–2

Weight Lifting Limitations by Symptom Severity

Symptom severity	Women (lbs)	Men (lbs)
moderate to severe	20	20
mild	35	60
none	40	80

many patients anecdotally report relief from chiropractors and acupuncture.

What if my patient has a true disc herniation?

If the patient has acute radicular pain and a positive straight leg raise, and none of the historical red flags, he or she most likely has a herniated disc. However, 80%–90% of patients with disc herniation will be back to normal after one month without any specific intervention. So unless the patient has significant neurologic symptoms or signs, you can watch and wait. If symptoms persist, it is reasonable to obtain a CT or MRI and refer to a neurosurgeon.

What surgeries are done for back pain? Do they work?

With the exception of catastrophic herniations, most disc herniations resolve on their own. Although initial response to surgery may be good, at four years, there is little difference between conservative and surgical management. Various surgical techniques have been developed. They range from open discectomy, where the surgeon exposes the disc space and removes herniated disc material, to endoscopic discectomy (analogous to laparoscopic gallbladder removal: less invasive, leaves smaller scar). The least invasive procedure is chymopapain injections, where a proteolytic enzyme is injected into the disc and causes reduction in the disc size. Unfortunately, this has been associated with anaphylaxis and transverse myelitis, so is out of favor in the U.S.

Surgery should only be considered if the patient meets appropriate criteria (Box 20–2).

BOX 20–2

Criteria for Surgical Intervention in Back Pain Patients
Epidural abscess
Cauda equina syndrome
Cord compression
Persistent nerve root compromise
Severe spinal stenosis

K E Y   P O I N T S

▶ Most back pain, although bothersome to patients, is benign and self-limited.

▶ Red flags for pathology will dictate when to order further studies.

▶ With few exceptions, conservative therapy is the appropriate first step.

CASE 20-1. A 47-year-old nurse has severe low back pain after turning a patient. She has never had back pain before. She exercises regularly, doesn't smoke, and takes no medications. On exam, she has paraspinal tenderness and normal lower extremity strength and sensation. Her straight leg test is normal.

    A. Do you want any further tests, and if so, what tests?
    B. What do you recommend for treatment?
    C. When can she return to work and does she require any lifting limitations?
    D. How soon should she feel better?

CASE 20-2. A 76-year-old woman comes in with low back pain after working in her garden this weekend. She reports chronic back pain which has worsened somewhat over the past six months, particularly at night. Her other medical problems include mild anemia and low grade chronic renal failure. Her pain is steady and has not improved with ibuprofen.

    A. What are the red flags in her history?
    B. Do you want any further tests, and if so, what tests?

REFERENCES

Atlas SJ, Deyo RA: Evaluating and managing acute low back pain in the primary care setting. J Gen Intern Med 16:120, 2001.

Bigos S, Bowyer O, Braen G, et al: Acute low back problems in adults. Clinical practice guideline No 14. AHCPR Publication No. 95–0642, Agency for Health Care Policy and Research, Public Health Service, U.S. Department of Health and Human Services, Rockville, MD, December 1994. Also available on the world wide web at http://text.nlm.nih.gov. Go to archived AHCPR guidelines.

21

Lower Extremity Pain, Swelling, and Ulcers

LOWER EXTREMITY PAIN

▶ ETIOLOGY

What are common causes of lower extremity pain?

Common causes are peripheral vascular disease (PVD, also known as arterial insufficiency), peripheral neuropathy (PN), radiculopathy, venous obstruction (also called venous stasis), and nocturnal cramps.

Are there any emergencies that cause lower extremity pain?

Compartment syndrome and arterial occlusion from thromboembolism are rare emergencies. Compartment syndrome occurs when tissue swelling or hematoma in a muscle compartment raises pressures above arterial pressure, occludes blood flow, and causes tissue necrosis. Arterial occlusion causes acute onset of the five "Ps": pain, paresthesias, paralysis, pulselessness, pallor.

▶ EVALUATION

How are symptoms different from the common causes of leg pain?

Patients with PVD report claudication with exertion: muscle aching or cramping that occurs predictably with exercise and resolves with rest. Pain from spinal stenosis, also called pseudoclaudication, can be very similar. Unlike true claudication, spinal stenosis may be accompanied by back pain, does not resolve with standing still, but requires sitting for several minutes. PN pain occurs in a stocking-glove distribution and is described variably as burning, tingling, perceived swelling, "pins and needles," or numbness. It is often worse at night. Radiculopathy is often worse with sitting and is relieved by standing. Pain from venous obstruction may be worse when legs are dependent, and improved with leg elevation. Nocturnal muscle cramps occur only at night and are sudden, nonexertional, and relieved with massage or stretching.

What physical findings help with diagnosis?

With PVD you may hear bruits, find weak or absent pulses, and see loss of leg hair, dependent rubor, pallor with elevation, or delayed capillary refill. With PN look for decreases in proprioception, light touch, sharp sensation, and deep tendon reflexes. PVD and PN are usually bilateral, but are sometimes worse on one side. Radiculopathy is usually unilateral, and may give focal loss of a reflex or strength or shooting pain down the leg with straight leg raise (see Chapter 20).

What does the ankle/brachial index (ABI) mean?

The ABI assesses severity of PVD, as estimated by ankle systolic pressure divided by brachial artery systolic pressure. To measure ankle systolic pressure, inflate a cuff around the calf and palpate the systolic pressure at the dorsalis pedis or posterior tibialis artery. Normal values are 0.9–1.2. ABI greater than 0.9 generally rules out arterial insufficiency. An ABI of 0.6–0.8 usually correlates with one-block claudication. A ratio less than 0.4 indicates limb-threatening ischemia; these patients often have leg pain at rest and/or ischemic nonhealing ulcers. Obtain an arterial duplex ultrasound when the ABI is less than 0.9. ABIs may be falsely elevated and unreliable in diabetic patients due to noncompressible, calcified arteries.

What tests are appropriate for patients with PN?

Most patients with PN have diabetes and require no further workup. If diabetes is absent, you need to consider other causes (Box 21–1). A complete history including alcohol use, diet, toxic exposures, medications, and family history helps direct evaluation. In patients without diabetes, start with CBC, vitamin B_{12}, TSH, creatinine, serum protein electrophoresis, and ANA (looking for vasculitis). EMG and nerve conduction studies confirm PN and assess its severity. Nerve biopsies are rarely indicated.

▶ TREATMENT

(See Table 21–1.)

BOX 21-1

Causes of PN

Common causes

Metabolic: diabetes, alcohol use

Medications: DDC, D4T, DDI, INH (if B_6 not replaced), amiodarone

Less common causes

Metabolic: malnutrition, hypothyroidism, renal insufficiency, B_{12} deficiency

Medications: metronidazole, pyridoxine, simvastatin, hydralazine, colchicine

Infections: HIV, Lyme disease, syphilis, leprosy

Immunologic: multiple myeloma, paraneoplastic syndromes, vasculitis

Toxins: lead, arsenic, solvents (toluene, hexane)

TABLE 21-1

Treatment Strategies for Common Causes of Lower Extremity Pain

Cause	Treatment
Peripheral neuropathy	Tight glycemic control in diabetes Tricyclic antidepressants, SSRIs Anticonvulsants (gabapentin, carbamazepine) Topical capsaicin Foot care for prevention (shoes, lanolin to prevent cracks) Lidocaine patches
Peripheral vascular disease	Risk factor reduction (smoking, hypertension, lipids, diabetes) Antiplatelet drug Exercise Angioplasty or surgery for claudication at rest
Nocturnal cramps	Quinine, calf stretching during day

LOWER EXTREMITY SWELLING

▶ ETIOLOGY

What causes swelling in the lower extremities?

Swelling is due to edema, i.e., the accumulation of fluid in the interstitial tissue. Edema is pitting when skin remains indented after pressure has been applied. Nonpitting edema does not indent, and implies inflammation, infiltration, or chronic edema of any cause. Edema may signal significant systemic illness.

What diseases cause unilateral lower extremity edema?

This depends on how rapidly the edema develops. Acute edema occurring over hours to days is often associated with pain and inflammatory signs such as increased warmth and erythema. Common causes of acute unilateral edema are deep venous thrombosis (DVT), cellulitis, Baker's cyst rupture, superficial thrombophlebitis, and trauma. Chronic unilateral edema accumulates over weeks to months without accompanying inflammatory signs, and is usually caused by venous insufficiency or lymphatic obstruction. Lymphatic obstruction, also called lymphedema, may be idiopathic or secondary to tumor, infection, or scarring from previous surgery or radiation.

What is a Baker's cyst?

A Baker's cyst is accumulation of excess synovial fluid in a pouch of synovium that extrudes from the knee joint into the popliteal fossa. It is related to underlying joint inflammation (osteoarthritis, rheumatoid arthritis, meniscal tear, trauma, or crystalline arthropathy).

What diseases cause bilateral lower extremity edema?

Causes of bilateral edema are venous insufficiency or systemic diseases that cause fluid retention or low albumin. Medication is a common cause of edema unresponsive to diuretics (Box 21–2).

▶ EVALUATION

What features of the H & P and work-up distinguish a DVT?

All causes of acute unilateral edema can present exactly the same way (erythema, swelling, and pain developing over hours). Because DVT can cause life-threatening pulmonary embolism, it is imperative to exclude this first. Ask about DVT risk factors (oral contraceptive pills, recent period of prolonged inactivity, pregnancy, postpartum, recent major surgery, family history of hypercoagulability, paresis, history of DVT). On exam of the leg, look for a palpable cord (indurated vein) or positive Homans' sign (pain elicited in popliteal region with ankle dorsiflexion of

BOX 21-2

Systemic Causes of Bilateral Lower Extremity Edema

Conditions associated with fluid retention

Congestive heart failure
Cushing's disease
Hypothyroidism
Menstrual cycle fluid retention
Pregnancy
Renal insufficiency

Conditions associated with hypoalbuminemia

Hepatic cirrhosis
Malnutrition
Nephrotic syndrome
Protein-losing enteropathies

Medications

Clonidine
Corticosteroids
Estrogen, progesterone, testosterone
Hydralazine
Nifedipine, felodipine, amlodipine
Nonsteroidal anti-inflammatory agents

the flexed knee), though neither finding is very sensitive or specific. Exam may be normal or only reveal mild unilateral calf swelling confirmed by measuring bilateral calf diameters. Duplex ultrasound can be highly sensitive (98%) and specific (greater than 97%) for clots above the knee.

How do I distinguish Baker's cyst, DVT, cellulitis, and superficial thrombophlebitis?

A Baker's cyst presents as a bulge on the medial aspect of the popliteal fossa and often is diagnosed by exam alone. Cyst rupture may create ankle or foot ecchymoses differentiating it from a DVT. With cellulitis, pain, lymphangitis (red streaking along a lymph vessel), ipsilateral groin lymphadenopathy, chills, or fever may be present. About 50% of the time, a portal of entry for bacteria can be identified, usually maceration from tinea pedis infection. Superficial thrombophlebitis causes a localized tender vein, without lymphangitis, adenopathy, or palpable cord. If you are not convinced that it isn't a DVT, obtain duplex ultrasound to be sure.

When should I look for a systemic cause of edema?

Bilateral lower extremity or generalized edema suggests a systemic cause. Obtain a thorough H & P. Ask about signs of CHF:

fatigue, dyspnea on exertion, orthopnea, and paroxysmal nocturnal dyspnea. Exam findings suggesting left heart failure include tachypnea, tachycardia, rales, and S_3. Signs of right heart failure include distended neck veins and hepatojugular reflux (see CHF section in Chapter 24). Renal insufficiency and nephrotic syndrome may not be apparent from history or exam. Hypothyroidism and low albumin states such as nephrotic syndrome can cause periorbital edema. Hypothyroidism is usually accompanied by other symptoms such as fatigue, weight gain, cold intolerance, and hair, voice, or skin changes (see thyroid disease section in Chapter 26).

What laboratory tests or imaging studies are helpful?

Obtain a serum TSH, creatinine, BUN, and albumin looking for hypothyroidism, renal insufficiency, or low albumin states in patients with new bilateral edema. If creatinine is high, obtain renal ultrasound to distinguish acute from chronic insufficiency. If albumin is low obtain a urinalysis to screen for the nephrotic syndrome. A low albumin without proteinuria suggests malnutrition, malabsorption, or liver disease, so reexamine for ascites and consider liver function tests, abdominal imaging, or a GI referral to exclude a protein-wasting enteropathy. If you suspect heart failure, obtain CXR, ECG, and echocardiogram. Obtain a 24-hour urine cortisol when you suspect Cushing's syndrome.

▶ TREATMENT

How do I manage fluid retention in the legs?

General treatments include lower extremity elevation, salt restriction, elastic support stockings, and low dose diuretics (hydrochlorothiazide 12.5 mg/d). Avoid medications that cause edema. Treat underlying Cushing's, CHF, thyroid, renal, or liver disease when present.

How do I treat a DVT?

Clot at or above the popliteal fossa increases risk for pulmonary embolus. Identify and address any underlying risk factors and if none are found, screen for a hypercoagulable state before starting anticoagulants (see Chapter 29). Hospitalize for IV heparin. Start oral warfarin to overlap with heparin (duration of overlap is debated). Goal of warfarin is to raise the protime INR to a therapeutic range of 2–3. Some physicians now use low molecular weight heparin (LMWH) in place of standard heparin. LMWH is given subcutaneously and can be used at home without monitoring, so it eliminates hospitalization. Continue anticoagulation for six months. Anticoagulation is not indicated for clot isolated to the calf since these are unlikely to embolize; however, these require serial duplex ultrasounds to monitor for proximal migration.

How do I treat a Baker's cyst?

Observe smaller cysts. Aspirate cysts when large or interfering with knee function. Submit synovial fluid for crystal analysis and cell count. NSAIDs and intra-articular steroids can decrease inflammation. Recurrent problems may warrant MRI to look for a meniscal tear.

Is there an effective treatment for lymphedema?

Address treatable obstructive processes (pelvic mass, infection). Treatment options are limited when lymphedema is idiopathic or due to postsurgical scarring or radiation. Compression garments and home Lymphapress machines may be helpful. Diuretics are ineffective. Cellulitis worsens lymphatic obstruction, so prevent it by moisturizing skin and treating tinea.

How do I treat cellulitis and superficial thrombophlebitis?

Treat cellulitis with oral dicloxacillin or cephalexin. Patients with diabetes may need broader coverage. Arrange close follow-up. Hospitalize for IV antibiotics if response is inadequate. Treat superficial thrombophlebitis with warm compresses, elevation, and NSAIDs. Symptoms should resolve or improve significantly within a week. If not, obtain a duplex ultrasound.

LOWER EXTREMITY ULCERS

▶ ETIOLOGY

What predisposes patients to ulceration?

Main causes of lower extremity ulcers are venous insufficiency (90%), sensory PN, and arterial insufficiency secondary to PVD. Pyoderma gangrenosum is an unusual cause associated with inflammatory bowel disease.

▶ EVALUATION

What distinguishing exam features help with diagnosis?

Venous insufficiency ulcers usually are painless, abrupt in onset, located on the medial malleolus, and accompanied by edema, stasis dermatitis, and superficial varicosities. Neuropathic ulcers are painless, sharply marginated, and found at plantar pressure points (metatarsal heads, distal phalanges, heels). Ulcers from arterial insufficiency/ischemia occur distal to the ankle joint (often at the tips of the toes), have a punched-out appearance, and are exquisitely painful. Associated findings include dependent rubor, nonpalpable pulses, delayed capillary refill, and loss of hair growth. Pyoderma gangrenosum ulcers are sharply demarcated, exudative, and have heaped-up, boggy, violaceous edges that are often undermined.

How do I know if the ulcer or underlying bone is infected?

This can be difficult to determine. All ulcers are colonized with bacteria and therefore cultures are unhelpful. A yellow/green discharge is common, even in noninfected wounds. Débride and probe all ulcers to determine their depth. If the bone can be probed osteomyelitis is likely. If there are systemic symptoms (fever, chills, sweats) or local signs of cellulitis (warmth, erythema, and swelling) presume the ulcer is infected and give antibiotics. X-ray may be helpful to screen for a foreign body, gangrene (gas), or late osteomyelitis (periosteal elevation). If you are highly suspicious for osteomyelitis, check ESR and obtain MRI, bone scan, or bone biopsy.

▶ TREATMENT

Are all ulcers treated the same?

Some general wound care measures pertain to ulcers of many causes: saline wet to dry dressings, whirlpool treatment for débridement, synthetic occlusive dressings (DuoDerm), or Unna boots. Ulcers due to PN require nonweight-bearing to heal. Other specific treatment depends on the cause (Table 21–2).

TABLE 21–2

Treatments for Common Lower Extremity Ulcers

Cause	Treatment
Ischemic ulcers	Vascular surgery referral
Peripheral neuropathy/neuropathic ulcers	Non–weight bearing Good shoes Avoidance of foot trauma Meticulous foot care
Venous insufficiency/stasis ulcers	Edema reduction (improves healing) 　elevation 　compressive stockings Skin lubrication (prevent cracks, cellulitis) Topical steroids for stasis dermatitis
Pyoderma gangrenosum	Oral steroids

K E Y   P O I N T S

▶ Rule out DVT in a patient with acute unilateral peripheral edema.

▶ Bilateral lower extremity edema warrants an investigation for systemic diseases.

▶ Patients with diabetic PN and ulcers require nonweight-bearing to heal.

▶ Lymphedema will not respond to diuretic therapy.

CASE 21–1. A healthy 65-year-old woman presents with symptoms of bilateral ankle swelling for one month. It is not associated with erythema or pain. On further questioning, she has had some puffiness in her fingers and around her eyes in the morning and mild fatigue. Otherwise she feels well. Medications include daily conjugated estrogen and medroxyprogesterone and ibuprofen as needed. Exam is normal except for mild pitting edema of both ankles.

A. What is your differential diagnosis?
B. How would you manage her care?

CASE 21-2.
A 34-year-old man with type 2 diabetes mellitus and hypertension reports a two-year history of left leg pain with exercise. This occurs predictably walking two blocks. It originates in his left hip/buttock and radiates down the lateral aspect of his leg to the bottom of his foot. The pain resolves with standing after a few minutes. He does not have back pain, paresthesias, or motor weakness. Exam of the lower extremities shows negative bilateral straight leg raise, symmetrical deep tendon reflexes, normal motor strength, posterior tibialis pulse intact on the right but diminished on the left, and sensation intact to light touch and pinprick.

A. What could be causing his pain?
B. What test(s) would you order?
C. What risk factors should be addressed?

REFERENCES

Powell AA, Armstrong MA: Peripheral edema. Am Fam Physician 55(5): 1721–1726, 1997.
Sumio BE: Primary care: Foot ulcers. N Engl J Med 343(11):787–793, 2000.

22

Lymphadenopathy

Is lymphadenopathy always pathologic?

Lymph nodes increase in size in response to infection, inflammation, medications, and cancer. Some lymphadenopathy can be normal. In the neck and groin, small, shotty nodes less than 1.0 cm are common and are of no consequence in someone who feels well. Reactive nodes, which occur in response to infection, are tender, enlarge quickly, and regress in four to six weeks. Some reactive nodes do not regress completely; they may remain small and palpable, but are nonetheless benign.

When should I be concerned about pathologic causes of adenopathy?

Node size and risk factors for cancer and infection help determine whether adenopathy is likely to be pathologic (Box 22–1). Nodes larger than 1.5×1.5 cm^2 suggest malignancy in an adult. Lymphadenopathy is more likely to be pathologic in patients who have risk factors or symptoms suggesting malignancy or protracted infection: weight loss, night sweats, fatigue, fevers, tobacco abuse, family history of cancer, excessive alcohol use, high risk sexual activity, TB exposure. Although age is a risk factor for most malignancies, the preponderance of lymphadenopathy is likely to be benign even at later stages of life. While it is true that in patients sent for node biopsy who are older than age 50, malignancy is found in 60%, these numbers reflect a selection bias in that the

---

BOX 22–1

Lymphadenopathy Requiring Further Evaluation
Node greater than 1.5 cm
Age older than 40–50 years
Smoking or drinking history
Constitutional symptoms (fever, sweats, weight loss)

---

patients had been referred for biopsy. A retrospective study of a family practice clinic looked at unexplained adenopathy in patients older than age 40; cancer was detected in only 4%. In patients younger than age 40, cancer was found in 0.4%.

What is meant by generalized or localized lymphadenopathy?

Generalized adenopathy is present when two or more noncontiguous sites have enlarged nodes, e.g., right neck and left axilla. The most common causes are infectious (Table 22–1). Localized nodes occurring contiguously suggest an inflammatory process or malignancy in the corresponding area of drainage. A single source of infection may explain several clusters of nodes, e.g., a chronic nonhealing ulcer of the left hand causing forearm, epitrochlear, and axillary adenopathy.

What causes lymphadenopathy in the neck?

The neck is the most common site of lymphadenopathy. Unilateral cervical adenopathy in the younger patient is most likely to be mononucleosis or pharyngitis. Bilateral cervical adenopathy in younger patients is due to infectious mononucleosis, pharyngitis, or dental infections. Other less common causes of cervical adenopathy with a mononucleosis-like illness (fever, fatigue) include primary HIV infection, cytomegalovirus infection, toxoplasmosis, primary herpes simplex infection, and secondary syphilis. Although cervical adenopathy in a young patient is likely to be benign, more than half of patients with Hodgkin's disease present initially with adenopathy in the neck. In older patients, cancer is more likely. Submandibular and anterior cervical nodes suggest head and neck cancer. Anterior cervical nodes can also arise from metastatic lung, breast, or thyroid cancer. Preauricular

TABLE 22–1

Causes of Generalized Lymphadenopathy

Commonly Seen	Less Commonly Seen
Infection	Drugs
Mononucleosis	Phenytoin
HIV or AIDS	Hydralazine
Tuberculosis	Allopurinol
Hodgkin's lymphoma	Sarcoidosis
Non-Hodgkin's lymphoma	Secondary syphilis
Leukemia	Lupus/rheumatoid arthritis
	Serum sickness
	Hyperthyroidism
	Castleman's disease

adenopathy is seen with conjunctivitis and cat-scratch disease (a self-limited disease seen mostly in children) while postauricular adenopathy is common with scalp infections or inflammation, such as seborrheic dermatitis.

What is Virchow's node?

Supraclavicular nodes are often pathologic and the side of presentation suggests the cancer of origin. Virchow's node refers to any left supraclavicular node and is usually due to a gastrointestinal, renal, testicular, or ovarian malignancy. A right supraclavicular node may herald a pulmonary, mediastinal, or esophageal tumor.

What are the common causes of axillary lymphadenopathy?

The most common cause is ipsilateral injury or infection in the arm or hand. The axilla is a common spot for adenopathy due to cat-scratch disease, because the hands and arms are the most common site for cat scratches. In a woman with unilateral axillary adenopathy, breast cancer must be considered. Lymphomas such as Hodgkin's disease also present in the axilla. When a linear, inflamed set of nodes leads from an open wound, group A streptococcal skin infection is the usual cause.

What causes epitrochlear lymphadenopathy?

Unilateral epitrochlear nodes suggest infection in the hand. Bilateral epitrochlear adenopathy is uncommon, but is a clinical clue suggesting lupus, secondary syphilis, or sarcoidosis.

What causes hilar lymphadenopathy on CXR?

Causes of bilateral hilar adenopathy include lymphoma, bronchogenic carcinoma, sarcoidosis, and infection such as primary TB, coccidioidomycosis, and histoplasmosis. If a mediastinal mass, pleural effusion, or pulmonary mass is associated with bilateral or unilateral adenopathy, then a diagnosis of cancer should be pursued. If a patient has bilateral hilar adenopathy and is asymptomatic, the diagnosis is most likely sarcoidosis.

What causes inguinal lymphadenopathy?

Chronic, shotty, inguinal adenopathy is common. This may be due to subclinical or low-grade infections in the lower extremities or perineum. A femoral hernia may masquerade as a single, large inguinal node. More marked inguinal adenopathy often accompanies acute lower extremity infection or sexually transmitted diseases: herpes, syphilis, gonorrhea, chancroid, and lymphogranuloma venereum. A persistent or large node can result from rectal, vaginal or cervical cancer, or melanoma.

What causes lymphadenopathy in patients with HIV infection?

In HIV infection, persistent generalized lymphadenopathy occurs often before the CD4 counts drop below 200. Nodes are rarely larger than 1.5 cm. Larger nodes or asymmetrical distribution should be evaluated further. Non-Hodgkin's lymphoma, Hodgkin's disease, Kaposi's sarcoma, and TB are more common in HIV positive patients. They can occur when the CD4 is only modestly suppressed, i.e., 200 to 500. If the CD4 is less than 100, *Mycobacterium avium* complex and fungal and suppurative infections need to be ruled out.

▶ EVALUATION

Is this lump a lymph node?

Your exam for lymphadenopathy must include careful palpation of the occiput, around the ears, the entire neck, supraclavicular fossa, axillae, epitrochlear space, abdomen, and groin. Pay attention to the quality of the node: size, mobile or matted, tender or painless, rock-hard or rubbery. Cancer tends to be painless and may or may not be matted. Infection is tender, mobile, and occasionally rubbery. The cervical node exam may be most problematic due to overlying muscle, tendon, thyroid, carotids, and salivary glands. The parotid and submandibular salivary glands can be nodelike. If their respective ducts are obstructed, inflammation or infection can occur. Parotid gland enlargement can occur with a number of conditions such as pregnancy, eating disorders, Sjögren's disease, sarcoid, diabetes mellitus, alcoholism, mumps, and HIV. Any distinct mass should be referred for biopsy. Similarly, submandibular glands may be the site of infection, but masses here are even more likely to be cancer. Other findings may mimic lymphadenopathy, such as rheumatoid nodules, lipomas, sebaceous or ganglion cysts, and even less commonly, thyroglossal and branchial cleft cysts.

If I suspect an acute, self-limited, infectious cause of lymphadenopathy, how can I be sure?

A follow-up exam is required, particularly in patients with constitutional symptoms such as ongoing fever, weight loss, or fatigue, risk factors for prolonged infection or cancer, or if the nodes are greater than 1.5 cm.

What are pertinent clues from the history in patients with generalized lymphadenopathy?

The causes of generalized adenopathy are limited, so a focused history can quickly narrow your differential. Epidemiologic clues may provide the diagnosis before any laboratory tests return. Ask about symptoms of acute viral syndrome vs. longer-term weight loss, night sweats, and fatigue. Explore risk factors for HIV exposure. Patients with secondary syphilis have constitutional symptoms and a history of a painless, genital ulcer that has healed. Review drug or serum exposure, symptoms of hyperthyroidism, rheumatoid arthritis, and lupus.

What physical exam findings are useful in the evaluation of generalized lymphadenopathy?

Skin: Rash on the palms and soles (syphilis); tender subcutaneous nodules seen on the lower extremities in sarcoidosis or TB (erythema nodosum); malar rash (lupus).
Oropharynx: erythema or exudate of pharynx (mononucleosis); oral hairy leukoplakia (HIV).
Abdomen: splenomegaly (lymphoma, leukemia, or mononucleosis).
Musculoskeletal: Synovitis (lupus, rheumatoid arthritis, serum sickness); tremor (hyperthyroidism).

What laboratory and imaging tests are helpful?

When the clinical picture is confusing, order a CBC, WBC differential, ESR, PPD, and CXR. The presence of hilar adenopathy points to granulomatous disease in a young patient and malignancy in an older patient. Atypical lymphocytes suggest mononucleosis, other viral infections, or toxoplasmosis. A CT scan is helpful to confirm lymphadenopathy, identify other nodal enlargement, or to seek masses or abscesses. Extensive testing is rarely needed (Table 22–2). The list of causes of lymphadenopathy, however, includes many uncommon ones. For discussion of persistent lymphadenopathy or unusual symptoms see the references at the end of the chapter.

When should I pursue a biopsy?

If no cause is found and the node is enlarging, refer to a surgeon. Do not delay if cancer is suspected. When H & P suggest a viral infection, a biopsy may be confusing because the histology may mimic lymphoma. In this case, watchful waiting for four to six weeks is advisable before referral for biopsy.

TABLE 22-2

Recommended Testing According to Clinical Presentation of Lymphadenopathy

Clinical Scenario	Recommended Testing
Cervical adenopathy and pharyngitis	Throat culture for strep +/– gonorrhea Monospot
Cervical adenopathy and mono-like syndrome	Monospot (Negative in 10% of EBV mono); if negative consider EBV IgM, HIV RNA, CMV, and Toxo serology
Cervical adenopathy in a patient older than 40, or with history of tobacco or alcohol use	Refer for biopsy
Adenopathy and HIV risks	HIV test
Inguinal adenopathy, marked	HIV test, RPR Culture for herpes simplex and gonorrhea Chlamydia LCR Culture for *Haemophilus ducreyi*
Hilar adenopathy	PPD testing

K E Y   P O I N T S

▶ A complete H & P will narrow your differential diagnosis for lymphadenopathy.

▶ Laboratory testing need not be extensive.

▶ When the diagnosis is uncertain and the risk for malignancy is low, careful observation for one month is appropriate.

CASE 22-1. A 55-year-old woman comes to your clinic reporting a lump in her armpit. She otherwise feels well. She thought it was just an inflamed hair follicle but it has persisted for several weeks. She has received yearly pap smears and mammograms, most recently eight months ago. On exam you find a firm 2 × 2 cm node in the left axilla. The remainder of her exam, including her breasts, is normal.

A. What are the most likely diagnoses?
B. How do you evaluate her further?

CASE 22–2. A 68-year-old man is seen for an initial evaluation. He has noted mild fatigue but is quite active. He denies fever, weight loss, or anorexia. He has not seen a physician in many years and has no past medical history. Exam reveals enlarged bilateral cervical, axillary, and inguinal lymph nodes, and splenomegaly.

A. What is your differential diagnosis?
B. How do you proceed?

CASE 22–3. A 21-year-old male complains of chills, anorexia, fatigue, myalgias, sore throat, and headache for one week. Many residents in his dormitory have the flu. On exam he appears ill. Vital signs: T, 102.8, RR, 114, BP, 122/84. A faint maculopapular rash over his torso is seen. His eyes, ears, chest, and abdomen are normal. Oropharynx is injected but without exudate. Neck, axilla, and groin show bilateral adenopathy.

A. Does he have influenza? What is your differential diagnosis?
B. What other questions would you ask him?
C. What test would you order? Should he be admitted?

CASE 22–4. A 24-year-old woman comes to clinic complaining of fatigue, fever, and sore throat for one week. She reports she has been otherwise healthy without weight loss, night sweats, or high-risk sexual activity. On exam, she is a vigorous woman. On her head and neck exam you note pharyngeal erythema and bilateral cervical adenopathy. The nodes are boggy and tender; the largest is 2.5 cm.

A. Do you need to examine her further?
B. What lab testing will you order, if any?
C. If she improves fully, does she require a follow-up visit?

REFERENCES

Habermann TM, Steensma DP: Lymphadenopathy. Mayo Clin Proc 75:723–732, 2000.

Pangalis GA, Vassilakopoulos TP, Boussiotis VA, Fessas P: Clinical approach to lymphadenopathy. Semin Oncol 20:570–582, 1993.

23

Sleep Disorders

▶ ETIOLOGY

What is a sleep disorder?

The sleep disorders are a heterogeneous group of conditions (see Table 23–1 for a partial list) characterized by sleep that is abnormal or disrupted and thus not restorative. Insomnia, defined as self-reported dissatisfaction with the quality, quantity, or timing of sleep obtained, is one type of sleep disorder. People with sleep disorders other than insomnia are typically unaware that their sleep is abnormal and often do not recognize feeling chronically sleep-deprived. Some medical conditions and medications can disrupt sleep (Table 23–2), but these are not considered sleep disorders.

How common are sleep disorders?

Sleep disorders are common (Table 23–1) but underdiagnosed. In middle-aged adults, airflow obstruction occurs during sleep in 24% of men and 9% of women, most of whom report no daytime symptoms. Requiring excessive daytime sleepiness to make the diagnosis of obstructive sleep apnea syndrome (OSA syndrome) in those with obstructive apneas reduces this prevalence to 4% in men and 2% in women. The prevalence increases with age and body mass index (BMI). It is highest among those who are obese, hypertensive, and who snore. More than a third of patients in typical primary care internal medicine practices have at least one risk factor for OSA. Over 80% of men and 90% of women with moderate-to-severe OSA syndrome have not had the condition diagnosed.

▶ EVALUATION

How do patients with sleep disorders present?

Consider the possibility of a sleep disorder in a patient presenting with fatigue or nonspecific changes in mood, memory, or cognition. A pattern of job loss or accidents can suggest a sleep

TABLE 23–1

Features of Selected Sleep Disorders

Disorder	Common Presentation	Prevalence in Adults	Causes, Contributing Factors
Insomnia (includes multiple disorders)	Difficulty falling asleep or staying asleep	Up to 19% chronically, 67% episodically	Multiple; can become self-perpetuating (conditioned insomnia)
Narcolepsy	Unplanned daytime sleep (sleep "attacks")	0.04%–0.09%	Familial Associated features: cataplexy sleep paralysis hypnagogic hallucinations
Obstructive sleep apnea (OSA)	Daytime symptoms from repeated sleep disruption, due to repeated obstructions to airflow in upper airway	4% of men, 2% of women	Increases with body mass index and age, supine position
Periodic limb movement disorder (PLMD)	Daytime symptoms from repeated sleep disruption due to repetitive flexor movements of limbs; sleep study makes diagnosis	Prevalence unknown; significant overlap with RLS	Similar to restless legs syndrome (see Box 23–4)
Restless legs syndrome (RLS)	Difficulty falling asleep or staying asleep due to restlessness or paresthesias in limbs occurring in evening or bedtime; history makes diagnosis	5%–15%	Primary familial idiopathic Secondary (see Box 23–4)

TABLE 23-2

Other Factors That Can Impair Sleep

Medical Conditions	Psychiatric Conditions	Medications	Substances
Asthma/COPD	Anxiety, panic disorder	Antidepressants	Alcohol
CHF	Bipolar disorder	bupropion	Caffeine
GERD	Depression	SSRIs	Nicotine
Hyperthyroidism	Post-traumatic stress	β blockers	Stimulants
Menopause	disorder	(nonselective)	
(via hot flushes		Bronchodilators	
and night sweats)			
Nocturia (BPH)		Corticosteroids	
Pain		Decongestants	
Pregnancy		Quinolones (some)	
		Stimulants	
		Theophylline	

disorder (or substance abuse). People with undiagnosed OSA have motor vehicle accidents at 2 to 7 times the rate of the general population. Patients with severe OSA and obesity-hypoventilation syndrome have morbid obesity, marked somnolence, obvious apneas, chronic pedal edema, chronic hypoxemia, and respiratory acidosis. Patients with milder OSA may experience unrecognized effects on daytime functioning, including safety and quality of life. Some patients may report being told that they snore loudly, choke, or stop breathing during sleep. OSA may present with complications of nocturnal hypoxia (Box 23–1), most commonly hypertension. Most patients with insomnia do not mention the problem to their doctors. Insomnia does not necessarily result in daytime sleepiness. Restless leg syndrome (RLS) may not be mentioned by the patient, or may not be recognized by a physician who is not familiar with the syndrome. Patients with RLS who bring the condition to medical attention report an average of two years after first description of symptoms before the diagnosis is made.

BOX 23-1

Signs and Symptoms of Nocturnal Hypoxia in OSA
Hypertension
Morning headaches
Edema (via pulmonary hypertension)
Nocturnal arrhythmias
Nocturnal angina

What aspects of the history may be helpful?

Take a screening sleep history (Box 23–2). If possible, query the sleep partner about loud snoring, apneas, and movements during sleep.

What are helpful findings on physical examination?

Most sleep disorders are not associated with abnormalities on exam. OSA can contribute to hypertension, a common finding among internal medicine patients. Physical examination of the neck, face, and oropharynx (Box 23–3) can suggest a predisposition to OSA.

Is lab testing useful?

Most sleep disorders are not associated with lab abnormalities. RLS and periodic leg movement disorder (PLMD) can arise in the setting of several common medical conditions (Box 23–4), for which blood work can be helpful. Hypoxia and hypercarbia on an ABG in the setting of suspected OSA indicate prompt diagnostic evaluation with an overnight sleep study.

BOX 23–2

Screening Sleep History
How have you been sleeping lately?
How well have you been sleeping?
How much sleep have you been getting?
How is your energy level during the day?
Do you feel refreshed when you wake up?
Do you nod off during the day? Ever do so while driving?
Have you been told that you snore?
Do you know if you snore loudly and often?
Have you ever been told that you choke or stop breathing?

BOX 23–3

Features Most Suggestive of OSA
Habitual loud snoring
Observed apneas
Neck circumference more than 17 in/43 cm (men) or 16 in/41 cm (women)

BOX 23-4

Medical Conditions Associated with RLS and PLMD

Folate deficiency (possible)
Iron deficiency
Medications (tricyclics, SSRIs, MAO inhibitors, OCPs, others)
Peripheral neuropathies, including
  diabetes
  B_{12} deficiency
  lumbosacral radiculopathies
Pregnancy
Renal failure
Rheumatoid arthritis
Sjögren's disease

What is the next step if a sleep disorder seems likely?

If you suspect a sleep disorder but the history and physical do not strongly suggest OSA, screen for depression. Do bloodwork to evaluate for other causes of fatigue, and for medical conditions that might cause RLS or PLMD (Box 23-4). If the patient is not allowing enough time for sleep, advise that he or she increase sleep time to eight hours (or more, if needed). If symptoms persist despite adequate sleep time, arrange consultation with a sleep medicine specialist, who will review the sleep history in more detail and may order sleep studies.

What is a sleep study?

An overnight sleep study, or nocturnal polysomnogram (PSG), quantitates specific aspects of sleep, including amount of time spent in each sleep stage (by EEG and by measurement of eye movements and chin muscle tone), respiratory effort and airflow, oxygen saturation, and limb movements (by leg EMG). A PSG can be diagnostic for a variety of disorders, including OSA, central sleep apnea, and PLMD. A multiple sleep latency test (MSLT) monitors the patient by sleep EEG while he or she attempts to nap 4–5 times over the course of a day. The MSLT gives an objective measure of daytime sleepiness and can be diagnostic for narcolepsy. It is usually done the day following a PSG. Sleep studies can be influenced by a number of factors, including recent sleep deprivation, alcohol or benzodiazepine use, psychiatric disorders, and medications. They are rarely used to evaluate insomnia. Sleep studies may not be diagnostic on the first attempt and may need to be repeated for diagnosis, or to assess response to treatment.

BOX 23-5

Sleep Hygiene Measures—Advice for Patients

Keep the same bedtime and wake time every day.
Sleep in comfortable conditions in a quiet, darkened room.
Use the bedroom only for sleep and sex.
Get up out of bed if unable to sleep. Return when sleepy again.
Avoid alcohol, caffeine, and nicotine four to six hours before
  bedtime.
Exercise daily, but not within four to six hours of bedtime.
Get exposure to daylight or other bright light each day.
Avoid daytime napping (unless elderly or narcoleptic; then
  keep stable nap schedule).

► **TREATMENT**

What are some treatment approaches for insomnia?

Advise good sleep hygiene (Box 23–5). For short-term insomnia (e.g.,in the setting of stress or grief), sedating medications can be helpful and can lessen the chance that insomnia will become conditioned behavior and thus a long-term problem. Diphenhydramine, trazodone, and low-dose tricyclic antidepressants can help patients fall to sleep. Benzodiazepines are popular sedatives, but are also potentially addicting so should be avoided. For chronic insomnia, cognitive behavioral therapy is more effective and safe.

What are some general medical treatment approaches for OSA?

Obese patients with OSA benefit from weight loss. All patients with OSA should avoid sedatives and alcohol, which worsen airway obstruction. Most patients with OSA have more apneas in the supine (rather than lateral decubitus) sleep position; you can suggest that the patient attach a tennis ball to the back of his or her nightclothes, to encourage side-sleeping. Specialty treatments include nocturnal continuous positive airway pressure (CPAP), which is the best and most rapidly effective treatment for OSA, but one that is not tolerable for some patients. For mild OSA, an oral appliance fitted by a dentist can reduce apneas. Palate surgery reduces snoring but not apneas. Protriptyline, a tricyclic antidepressant, increases pharyngeal muscle tone and can reduce apneas.

What are some treatments for RLS and PLMD?

Treat the underlying cause, if one is found. Dopamine agonists (pramipexole, carbidopa/levodopa, and pergolide) are usually effective. Clonazepam and other benzodiazepines reduce the sleep loss but not the limb movements. Opiates are effective but should be reserved for refractory cases.

K E Y   P O I N T S

▶ Sleep disorders are common but underrecognized and underdiagnosed.

▶ Take a screening sleep history when patients report fatigue or daytime sleepiness, or when physical findings suggest obstructive sleep apnea.

▶ Restless legs syndrome is a common, treatable cause of insomnia that can be diagnosed by history and that may be due to an underlying medical condition.

CASE 23–1. A 38-year-old woman with
long-standing menorrhagia from fibroids presents with new-fatigue. She is taking an iron supplement intermittently. Recently, she has begun falling asleep at her desk at work. On examination, she is a slender, fatigued-appearing woman with normal skin color and pink mucous membranes. Pelvic exam is unchanged and consistent with known fibroids. Remainder of exam is normal, including thyroid. HCT is 38 with MCV 81. Ferritin is low at 8.

    A. What do you think is causing her fatigue?
    B. What further history might you ask?
    C. Read answer to B. What do you think is causing these symptoms?
    D. What treatment would you suggest?

CASE 23–2. A 57-year-old man with hypertension
presents with minor abrasions of his face, sustained when
his airbag deployed in a low-speed, rear-end motor
vehicle accident (MVA). He was driving and struck
another car without braking. He cannot remember the
moment of the accident but reports no other memory loss,
loss of consciousness, or head injury. On questioning, he
thinks he might have fallen asleep at the wheel. This is
his third MVA in two years. His only medication is an
antihypertensive. On physical exam, he is obese. BP is
154/98. He has superficial abrasions over his face. His
neck circumference is 44 cm and his oropharyngeal
opening is narrowed by a large tongue and long soft
palate. Remainder of exam is normal.

A. What medical conditions can increase the chance of a motor
vehicle accident?
B. What further questions might you ask the patient or his wife?
C. Read answer to B. What advice might you give him?
D. Would you refer him for any further evaluation?

REFERENCES

National Heart, Lung, and Blood Institute Working Group on Sleep Apnea.
Sleep apnea: Is your patient at risk? Am Fam Physician 53:247–253,
1996.
National Heart, Lung, and Blood Institute Working Group on Restless Legs
Syndrome. Restless legs syndrome: Detection and management in pri-
mary care. Am Fam Physician 62:108–114, 2000.
Poceta JS, Mitler MM, eds: Sleep Disorders: Diagnosis and Treatment.
Totowa NJ: Humana Press, 1998.

Patients Presenting with a Known Condition

24

Cardiology

COMMON CARDIAC ARRHYTHMIAS

▶ ETIOLOGY

How should I categorize arrhythmias?

Categorize abnormal heart rhythms by their ventricular rate and the origin of the rhythm disturbance. Rhythms with a rate greater than 100/min are called tachycardias, while those less than 60/min are called bradycardias. The origin of the abnormality may be in the atria, nodes, or ventricles (Figure 24–1). Close inspection of the ECG will usually allow specific localization (see later).

What causes a fast heart rate?

Tachycardia can originate anywhere within the heart. Fast rhythms that are initiated in the atria or AV node are collectively referred to as *supraventricular tachycardias*. Common causes include sinus tachycardia and atrial fibrillation. Less common causes are atrial flutter, AV nodal re-entrant tachycardia (AVNRT), and multifocal atrial tachycardia. *Ventricular tachycardia* (VT) originates below the AV node within abnormally functioning ventricular tissue. It occurs most commonly with cardiac ischemia, but is also seen with electrolyte abnormalities, cardiomyopathy, and drug intoxication (Table 24–1). Sustained VT can rapidly deteriorate into ventricular fibrillation (completely disorganized ventricular electrical impulses), a precursor to cardiac arrest (see Figure 24–4).

What is the significance of sinus tachycardia?

In sinus tachycardia, the ECG shows a normal P wave before each QRS (sinus rhythm), but at a rate faster than 100 beats/minute (Figure 24–2A). It is often due to hypovolemia, anemia, hyperthyroidism, hypoxia, fever, or pain. Unexplained sinus tachycardia requires a search for a cause.

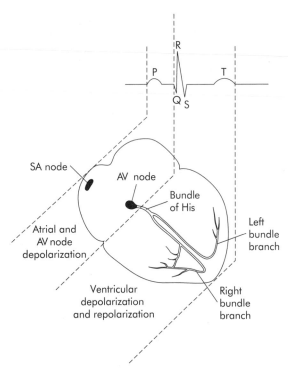

Figure 24–1. How the ECG reflects the normal sequence of heart muscle depolarization. Normal depolarization begins in the SA node and travels through the atria, causing a P wave. There is a slight delay as depolarization funnels through the AV node, reflected in the P-R interval. The QRS reflects rapid depolarization by way of the bundle of His and bundle branches. The T wave reflects ventricular repolarization to resting potential.

TABLE 24–1

Causes of Tachyarrhythmias

Type and Origin	Common Causes	Less Common Causes
Supraventricular tachycardia Originates above or in AV node	Sinus tachycardia Atrial fibrillation	Atrial flutter Multifocal atrial tachycardia AV node reentry

Ventricular tachycardia
 Originates below AV node
	Cardiac ischemia	Electrolyte
		  abnormalities ($\downarrow$Mg, $\downarrow$ or $\uparrow$ K)
		 Cardiomyopathy
		 Drug intoxications
		  tricyclic antidepressants
		  quinolones

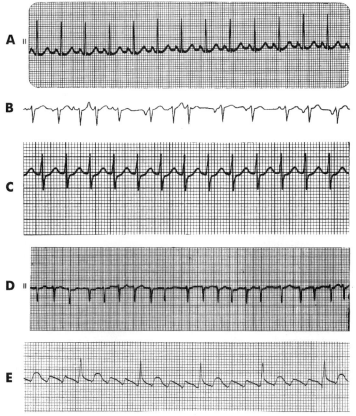

Figure 24–2. Atrial arrhythmias. **A,** *Sinus tachycardia*: rate >100 and regular, QRS is narrow, each P wave is associated with a QRS, each QRS has a P wave, P–R interval is normal in length. **B,** *Multifocal atrial tachycardia*: irregular rhythm with a P wave before each QRS and at least three different p-wave morphologies reflecting three or more atrial foci initiating beats. **C,** *Supraventricular tachycardia*: rate >100 and regular, QRS is narrow, P waves may be absent so P–R interval cannot be determined. Cause is likely an AV nodal reentry loop (see text). **D,** *Atrial fibrillation*: rate irregularly irregular, QRS is narrow, P waves are absent so P–R interval can't be determined. Atrial fibrillation can be fast, regular or slow, depending on how refractory the AV node is to passing on the erratic atrial electrical activity to the ventricles. **E,** *Atrial flutter*: regular rate with a saw-toothed baseline of P waves going at a rate of about 300/minute (one per large box), conducting every 4th P through to the ventricles (4:1 conduction). Atrial flutter can be associated with a fast or slow ventricular rate depending on refractoriness of the AV node. (*From Goldberg AL*: Clinical Electrocardiography: a simplified approach, *6th ed, St. Louis, 1999, Mosby.*)

What is atrial fibrillation and what causes it?

Atrial fibrillation results from completely disorganized electrical activity in the atria causing the atrial muscle to quiver, or fibrillate. On ECG, "a fib" shows an irregularly irregular rhythm without identifiable P waves. Atrial fibrillation may exist in isolation, but usually occurs secondary to longstanding hypertension, CHF, hypoxia, valvular heart disease, hyperthyroidism, alcohol use, or high catecholamine states such as acute MI or surgery. Atrial flutter, a related rhythm, occurs when an organized circuit of electrical activity causes a fast atrial rate. The ECG shows a regular oscillating ("saw-toothed") baseline on the ECG. Atrial flutter often degenerates into atrial fibrillation. A third atrial rhythm, multifocal atrial tachycardia (MAT), is an irregularly irregular rhythm that is often confused with atrial fibrillation. In contrast to atrial fibrillation, the ECG in MAT shows P waves before each QRS. To be diagnostic, there must be at least three different P-wave morphologies reflecting the multiple atrial foci (Figure 24–2B, D, and E).

What is AVNRT?

AVNRT (atrioventricular nodal re-entrant tachycardia) is a cyclic, or re-entrant, loop of electrical activity within the AV node that is conducted into the ventricles. It produces a regular tachycardia usually at a rate of 160 to 180 beats/minute (Figure 24–2C). Though not a sign of underlying heart disease, AVNRT may produce ischemia, hypotension, or heart failure.

What are the causes of a slow heart rate (bradycardia)?

Bradycardia refers to any rate less than 60 beats/minute. Sinus bradycardia is the most common cause and is frequently seen with advanced age, athletic training, myocardial infarction, hypokalemia, hypothyroidism, and drugs such as β-blockers, calcium channel blockers, and digoxin. Sinus bradycardia is simply sinus rhythm with beats less than 60/minute. Less common causes of bradycardia are AV node block or SA node failure. In complete AV block and SA node failure, an ectopic ventricular focus (idioventricular rhythm) or area in the AV node (junctional rhythm) may take over pacing the ventricular beats.

What is AV node block?

AV block occurs when there is impaired conduction of atrial impulses though the AV node. Cardiac ischemia and medications such as β-blockers, calcium channel blockers, and digoxin are the most common causes. AV block is subcategorized into 1st, 2nd, or 3rd degree based on the severity of the conduction abnormality (Figure 24–3).

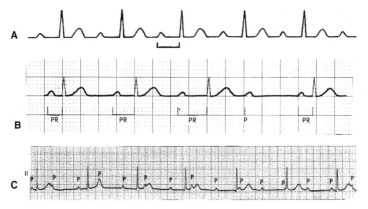

Figure 24–3. AV node blocks. **A,** *First-degree block*: P-R interval uniformly prolonged longer than one big box (>0.2 sec). **B,** *Second-degree block* type 1 (Wenckebach): a cycle of P-R widening culminates in a dropped QRS, then cycle begins again. **C,** *Third degree block*: no atrial impulses pass through the AV node, causing complete atrio-ventricular dissociation. AV node or ventricle may beat independently, usually at a rate far slower than 60/sec giving AV dissociation as seen above. (*From Goldberg AL*: Clinical Electrocardiography: a simplified approach, *6th ed, St. Louis, 1999, Mosby*.)

My patient is reporting "extra heartbeats." What could be causing this?

Patients frequently report the sensation of extra heartbeats, or palpitations. These are usually due to premature atrial or ventricular contractions (PACs and PVCs). Though common, only a minority of patients notice them. PACs occur when atrial tissue outside of the SA node initiates an early beat. The ECG shows an early P wave that appears different from the preceding beats. Episodic PACs do not indicate cardiac pathology. PVCs result from the same phenomenon, but the beat is initiated in the ventricle. The ECG shows episodic wide QRS complexes without associated P waves (Figure 24–4A) superimposed on the patient's baseline rhythm. When frequent (greater than 5/minute), PVCs are indicative of ischemic or structural heart disease.

▶ EVALUATION

What symptoms suggest a cardiac arrhythmia?

In general, arrhythmias cause the heart to function poorly or work harder. As a result, patients with arrhythmia often present with syncope, dizziness, chest pain, palpitations, shortness of breath, or

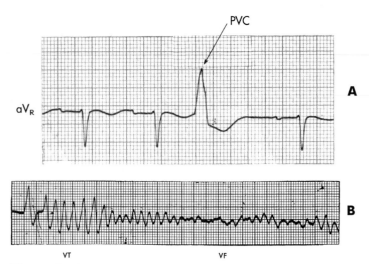

Figure 24–4. Ventricular arrhythmias. **A,** *Premature ventricular contraction*: an isolated wide QRS superimposed on the baseline sinus rhythm. **B,** *Ventricular tachycardia*: a rapid regular rhythm >100/sec with wide QRS degenerates to *Ventricular fibrillation*: distorted, unrecognizable complexes. (*From Goldberg AL*: Clinical Electrocardiography: a simplified approach, *6th ed, St. Louis, 1999, Mosby.*)

exercise intolerance. Some patients are asymptomatic and an arrhythmia is only identified when an abnormal pulse is noted on exam.

How do I evaluate an abnormal pulse?

Ensure clinical stability with a quick assessment of vital signs. Look for signs or symptoms of cardiac ischemia or shock. Get help immediately if the patient is unstable. If the patient is stable inquire about prior heart problems and cardiopulmonary symptoms. A quick exam focusing on signs of cardiopulmonary disease, anemia, and thyroid abnormalities is appropriate. Characterize the pulse by rate and pattern and obtain an ECG.

Now that I have this ECG, how do I identify the rhythm?

First, determine the *rate*: greater than 100/min=tachycardia; less than 60/min=bradycardia. Second, measure the *QRS width*. A narrow QRS (less than 3 small boxes or 120 msec) indicates that the rhythm originates in the atria or AV node and is traveling through the ventricles via the His-Purkinje system. Conversely, a wide QRS indicates a ventricular origin. Occasionally, very rapid supraventricular rhythms will not conduct normally through the His-Purkinje system due to incomplete recovery of bundle tissue between the rapid beats. This is called aberrancy, or intraventricular conduction delay, and can make distinguishing ventricular tachycardia from supraventricular tachycardia difficult. Third, compare *R-R intervals* with a pair of calipers to decide if the rhythm is regular. Regular rhythms have equal distances between each QRS complex. An irregular rhythm with no pattern to the irregularity is termed *irregularly irregular* and is almost always atrial fibrillation. Fourth, look for *P waves*. If absent, and the rhythm is irregular, atrial fibrillation is likely. If P waves occur in no relation to the QRS complexes consider AV dissociation with VT (fast wide QRS) or AV block (with a slow ventricular escape rate). Examine the *P-R interval* for prolongation, variability, or intermittently dropped QRS complexes suggestive of AV block. Algorithms to aid in identifying common rhythm disturbances are suggested (Figures 24–5 and 24–6).

Is this ventricular tachycardia (VT)?

VT is a potentially lethal rhythm requiring rapid identification and intervention. The rate is usually 160–200 and regular. The QRS is always wide (greater than 120 msec). The SA node continues to produce independent P waves that may be buried or appear as irregularities on the wide QRS complexes. When sustained VT occurs, evaluate for ischemia, magnesium, and potassium disturbances.

How do I evaluate an irregularly irregular rhythm?

Although atrial fibrillation is by far the most likely cause, obtain an ECG to confirm the rhythm. If atrial fibrillation is present, obtain electrolytes, cardiac enzymes, a TSH, and a CXR to look for pulmonary disease or signs of LV failure. An echocardiogram may be useful to identify valvular heart disease or left ventricular dysfunction. Pulmonary embolism is an unusual but potential cause, so ask about leg swelling, dyspnea, previous clots, and medicines (e.g., estrogens and tamoxifen).

My patient has bradycardia. What evaluation is indicated?

Study the ECG carefully to identify the rhythm. If ischemia is suspected, or the patient is symptomatic with syncope or presyncope, hospitalize the patient for cardiac monitoring, serial cardiac enzyme testing, and possible pacing. A list of medications may identify possible precipitants (digoxin, calcium channel-blockers, β-blockers).

How do I evaluate a patient with palpitations?

Get a clear description of what the patient is sensing. Often it is helpful to have patients tap out the rhythm of abnormal beats. Ask

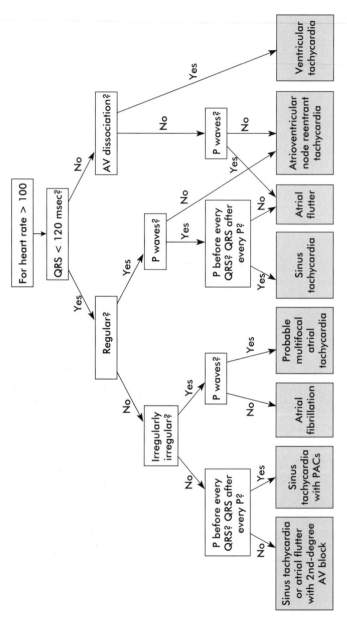

Figure 24-5. Algorithm for identifying tachycardias.

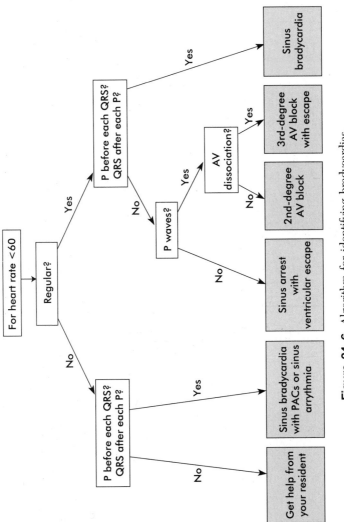

Figure 24-6. Algorithm for identifying bradycardias.

about prescription and nonprescription medications, caffeine, and substance abuse. Occasional "extra beats" without associated symptoms are almost always PACs or PVCs. An ECG alone is usually adequate evaluation. A history of associated dizziness, syncope, chest pain, or shortness of breath are concerning for SVT, VT, ischemia, or structural problems and require an ECG, electrolytes, and TSH as well as ambulatory or inpatient monitoring.

▶ TREATMENT

My patient has atrial fibrillation. What should I do now?

The three main treatment goals are conversion to normal sinus rhythm, rate control, and anticoagulation. Unstable patients should undergo conversion to normal sinus rhythm immediately using electrical cardioversion. Stable patients are treated initially with β-blockers or diltiazem to bring the ventricular rate to less than 100. Digoxin may be used, but not as the sole agent since it does not maintain rate control with physical activity. If the atrial fibrillation onset is clearly within the past 48 hours, cardioversion using electricity or medications may be indicated. Since patients with atrial fibrillation for greater than 48 hours have a significant risk of atrial clot and embolism, they should receive anticoagulation for three weeks prior to cardioversion. Patients with persistent atrial fibrillation require anticoagulation to reduce embolic events. If there are no signs of heart failure, cardiac ischemia, or pulmonary emboli, hospitalization is not required. Check a thyroid function test as hyperthyroidism can appear as atrial fibrillation.

How do I treat ventricular tachycardia?

Patients with sustained VT should undergo immediate electrical cardioversion to prevent deterioration of the rhythm into ventricular fibrillation. The only exceptions to this rule are patients with sustained monomorphic VT who have stable blood pressure and no angina. These patients can be treated with an antiarrhythmic drug (lidocaine or amiodarone) or synchronized (low energy) cardioversion. Supraventricular tachycardias (atrial flutter, AVNRT) with aberrancy may look like VT. In the setting of hypotension or chest pain, assume the rhythm is VT and cardiovert immediately.

How do I treat AVNRT?

Hemodynamically unstable patients require immediate electrical cardioversion to restore sinus rhythm. In clinically stable patients, adenosine is the agent of choice to terminate AVNRT. β-blockers or calcium channel blockers may decrease recurrence. Refer patients with recurrent AVNRT to a cardiologist for catheter directed ablation of abnormal conduction pathways.

How do I treat bradycardias?

In patients without symptoms, intervention is not necessary. Associated dizziness or syncope usually requires hospitalization to initiate cardiac pacing. Stop medications likely to slow the rate. Unstable patients should be given atropine and considered for cardiac pacing.

K E Y   P O I N T S

► When reading ECGs, look systematically at the rate, QRS width, R-R interval, P waves, and P-R intervals to determine the rhythm.

► An irregularly irregular rhythm is usually atrial fibrillation.

► Electrically cardiovert any patient who has an unstable arrhythmia.

► Assume any wide complex tachycardia is ventricular in origin and treat as VT.

CASE 24–1. A 67-year-old man reports increasing shortness of breath and fatigue on exertion. He denies associated chest pain, diaphoresis, or nausea. He has noted an intermittently rapid heart rate. He has a history of myocardial infarction and mild compensated congestive heart failure. Exam is significant for a fast irregular heart rate but is otherwise normal. His rhythm strip is as shown in Figure 24–7.

  A. What is the rhythm?
  B. How will you treat this patient?

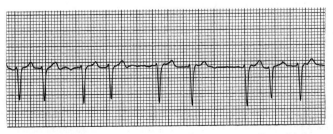

Figure 24–7. Electrocardiogram for patient in Case 24–1.

CASE 24–2. A 52-year-old man is admitted to the hospital for an acute myocardial infarction. He is treated with aspirin, thrombolytics, and heparin. On hospital day two, he suddenly becomes short of breath and then loses consciousness. His rhythm strip is shown in Figure 24–8.

A. What is the rhythm?

B. How should this patient be treated?

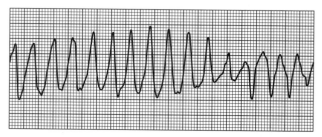

Figure 24–8. Electrocardiogram for patient in Case 24–2.

CONGESTIVE HEART FAILURE

▶ ETIOLOGY

What is congestive heart failure and what are the common causes?

Congestive heart failure (CHF) is a clinical syndrome including dyspnea, fatigue, and fluid overload that occurs as a final pathway in various cardiac diseases. Left and/or right ventricles (RV and LV) may be involved. CHF affects 1% of all people in the U.S. and 10% of those over 75 years of age. Hypertension and coronary artery disease account for 50%–75% of left ventricular failure. Right ventricular failure is usually due to failure of the left ventricle (Table 24–2).

How do I classify a patient's heart failure?

CHF is classified as right or left ventricular failure, with systolic or diastolic dysfunction. In systolic dysfunction, ejection fraction is low due to poor ventricular contraction. In diastolic dysfunction, ejection fraction is normal, but cardiac output is low due to poor filling of a stiff ventricle during diastole. Functional status is classified as I through IV (Table 24–3). These functional categories guide treatment and prognosis.

▶ EVALUATION

What are classic findings in left ventricular failure?

LV failure increases pulmonary venous pressure and causes pulmonary manifestations (Table 24–4): decreased exercise tolerance (dyspnea on exertion), shortness of breath while supine (orthopnea), or awakening from sleep short of breath (paroxysmal nocturnal dyspnea). You may hear an S3, an early diastolic filling sound over the left ventricular apex, and crackles in the lungs due to pulmonary edema. Characteristic CXR findings include: enlarged heart, pulmonary edema, pleural effusion, Kerley B lines, or redistribution of pulmonary blood flow against gravity to upper lung zones. LV failure can overload the right ventricle and create signs of RV failure.

TABLE 24–2

Causes of Systolic Dysfunction in Left and Right Heart Failure

	Common Causes	Less Common Causes	Rare Causes
LV failure	Ischemia Hypertension Valvular disease Idiopathic dilated- cardiomyopathy	Chronic alcohol use Hypothyroidism Toxins (chemotherapy)	Viral myocarditis (including HIV) Chest irradiation Hemochromatosis* Amyloidosis*

RV failure	LV failure
	RV ischemia
	
	COPD
		Sleep apnea
		Recurrent pulmonary
		  emboli
			Interstitial pulmonary diseases
			Primary pulmonary hypertension
			  (PPH)

*Commonly present with diastolic dysfunction.

TABLE 24–3

New York Heart Association (NYHA) Functional Classification

Functional Class	Symptoms
Class I	No limitation with ordinary physical activity
Class II	Mild symptoms, slight limitation with ordinary activity
Class III	Marked symptoms of fatigue, dyspnea, palpitations, or angina with minimal activity
Class IV	Symptoms at rest; symptoms increase with any activity

TABLE 24-4

Symptoms and Signs of Left and Right Ventricular Failure

	History	Exam
LV failure	Orthopnea	Leg edema
	Dyspnea on exertion	Rales (crackles)
	Paroxysmal nocturnal dyspnea	S_3 over left ventricle
	Cough	PMI >3 cm and displaced laterally
	Frothy hemoptysis	Cool, mottled lower extremities
		Abnormal abdominojugular reflux
RV failure	Exercise intolerance	Leg edema
	Dyspnea	JVP >8 cm H_2O
	Increasing abdominal girth	Right ventricular parasternal heave
	RUQ pain	S_3 over right ventricle
	Anorexia	Abnormal abdominojugular reflux
		Ascites

What are classic findings in right ventricular failure?

RVF increases systemic venous pressure. Isolated RVF does not cause lung symptoms but because most RVF is due to LVF, the presence of lung findings helps determine if LVF is the cause. Pertinent findings are listed (see Table 24–4). To evaluate jugular venous pressure (JVP), elevate the head of the bed to 30–45 degrees and observe for venous pulsations in the neck. Measure the height of the pulsations vertically up from the angle of Louis (where the second rib meets the sternum). Add 5 cm to your measurement to estimate the vertical height in cm of H_2O above the right atrium. To evaluate for abdominojugular reflux, apply pressure to the abdomen for ten seconds while you watch the JVP. If JVP rises more than 4 cm for the duration of pressure, this implies high right heart filling pressures. Chest films may reveal underlying lung disease (usually pulmonary hypertension).

What diagnostic tests should I order in a patient with new left-sided systolic heart failure?

Standard work-up includes chemistry panel, cholesterol, ECG, CXR, and echocardiogram. Echocardiogram estimates ejection fraction (EF) and evaluates ventricular wall motion and valve function. An EF of less than 40% is considered systolic dysfunction. An ejection fraction of greater than 40% does not rule out CHF because LV diastolic dysfunction, seen in up to one third of patients with clinical CHF, presents with normal EF. Focal wall motion abnormalities suggest ischemic injury. If standard work-up does not reveal a diagnosis, review the history for alcohol use, then consider further testing for ischemia, thyroid disease, hemochromatosis, amyloidosis, or HIV.

> ▶ TREATMENT

What are the treatment goals in CHF patients?

Management goals are to reduce symptoms, prevent complications, and improve survival.

What can patients do to improve symptoms?

Patients can restrict salt intake to 3–4 gm/day, stay as active as possible and avoid cigarettes and alcohol. They can follow home blood pressures and daily weights and notify their physician of major changes so medications can be adjusted. Recognize that nonadherence with medications is common in CHF patients (20%–60%) so counsel patients to take medications as prescribed.

What medicine is best for left ventricular systolic failure?

Angiotensin-converting enzyme inhibitors (ACEIs) are the first line agents for LV systolic dysfunction. They reduce LV afterload and decrease morbidity and mortality, particularly in patients with decreased ejection fraction from recent myocardial infarction. Increase the ACEI dose as tolerated to maximum dose or systolic BP 90–100 mm Hg. Monitor the serum creatinine and the potassium frequently as both may rise with initiation of ACEI. Common side effects include hypotension, worsening renal function, hyperkalemia, cough, rash, or taste disturbance. The side effect of angioedema is an absolute contraindication to continuing ACEIs. About 10% of patients develop intolerable ACEI cough. Cough is common from CHF itself, but if clearly due to ACEI, consider changing to angiotensin II receptor blockers (ARBs). ARBs also decrease afterload and mortality and do not cause cough. The combination of hydralazine and isosorbide, also used to decrease afterload, is less effective in reducing mortality, but should be used when angiotensin-blocking agents are not tolerated.

When do patients need diuretics?

Most patients with CHF have sodium and water overload. Start a diuretic if ACEI alone does not resolve volume overload. Titrate diuretics to achieve a jugular venous pressure less than 8 cm H_2O. Dose diuretics once a day unless higher doses are required (e.g., furosemide greater than 160 mg/day). Hypokalemia requires replacement if the potassium level is below 4.0 mEq/L; use potassium cautiously in patients on ACEIs. Low dose spironolactone

(25 mg/day) decreases mortality and the need for potassium sup-
plementation. Close monitoring of K^+ is necessary if spironolactone is used with an ACEI, because both can raise serum K^+ level.

When should I use β-blockers for CHF?

Increased plasma norepinephrine levels in patients with CHF are
strongly associated with worsening CHF and increased mortality.
β-blockers block this effect and improve LV function, decrease
hospitalization, and delay need for heart transplant. Most importantly, β-blockers decrease CHF mortality significantly, especially
in post-MI patients. Use carvedilol (an α- and β-blocker with antiox-
idant properties), metoprolol, or bisoprolol. Because of negative
inotropy with these agents, symptoms may initially worsen; start
with low doses and monitor for fluid overload suggesting the need
for a temporary increase in diuretics.

When should digoxin be used? Digoxin are good for peeps c CHF : A-fib

Add digoxin when patients remain symptomatic on full dose ACEI
and diuretics, and when β-blockers are not an option. Digoxin is
a good choice for patients with atrial fibrillation and CHF. Digoxin
increases exercise tolerance and improves functional class.
Withdrawal of digoxin results in worsening CHF and increased risk
for hospitalization. Digoxin has not been shown to decrease mortality. Digoxin toxicity causes arrhythmias, confusion, visual disturbances, anorexia, nausea, and vomiting. Levels do not reflect
clinical digoxin toxicity, so follow symptoms and ECG changes.
Renal insufficiency, hypokalemia, hypothyroidism, and drug interactions increase the risk of digoxin toxicity.

How is treatment for diastolic dysfunction different?

β-blockers and calcium channel blockers are first line therapy, ACEIs
are second line. These agents increase cardiac output by increasing diastolic filling time for patients with diastolic dysfunction.

What are the major prognostic indicators in patients with CHF?

Poor prognostic indicators include symptoms at rest, poor ejection
fraction, hyponatremia, and ventricular arrhythmias. Major causes
of death include progressive CHF (40%) and sudden death (40%).
One-year mortality for patients with class IV CHF exceeds 50%.

How do I prevent complications?

Up to 90% of CHF patients demonstrate complex ventricular
ectopy. Amiodarone suppresses ventricular arrhythmias. Automatic

implantable cardiac defibrillating devices (AICDs) can help to resuscitate patients with frequent ventricular fibrillation. Thromboembolism is more common when left ventricular ejection fraction is less than or equal to 25%, so warfarin is often used. Depression decreases medication adherence. Since tricyclic anti-depressants increase the risk of arrhythmias, use a serotonin reuptake inhibitor.

When should I hospitalize patients with CHF?

Hospitalize patients with newly diagnosed CHF of unclear etiology to rule-out ischemic disease and begin work-up and treatment. Admit patients for clinical exacerbations with hypoxia or hypotension, or if ECG suggests new ischemic injury. Admit orders should include daily weights, fluid intake and output records, and a low salt (2–4 gm) diet. Monitor clinical volume status using daily exam, serum chemistries, and renal function. Daily exam should include vital signs (including orthostatics), weight, JVP, cardiovascular exam for S_3 sounds, lung exam for crackles or effusions, and extremity exam for edema. For significant volume overload, give oxygen, intravenous diuretics, or even a furosemide drip if necessary. Swan-Ganz catheters are used in refractory CHF for careful volume management or when inotropic agents are used. Intravenous dobutamine, an inotropic agent, may be given to increase cardiac output and lower afterload. Some patients require intermittent hospitalization for intravenous dobutamine therapy while they await cardiac transplant.

K E Y   P O I N T S

▶ Patients presenting with CHF should be classified by type of heart dysfunction and by functional class to guide treatment strategies.

▶ All patients with systolic dysfunction should be treated with ACEIs unless contraindicated.

▶ Treat volume overload with diuretics.

▶ β-blockers should be considered for all patients with CHF, especially those with ischemic CHF.

▶ ACEIs, β-blockers, and spironolactone all have been shown to reduce mortality in patients with CHF due to systolic dysfunction.

CASE 24–3. A 65-year-old woman with diabetes treated with insulin, an ACEI (enalapril 10 mg po qd), and aspirin presents with twelve hours of chest pain and is diagnosed with an acute MI. After coronary angioplasty she does well and is discharged on the same medications. Two months later she presents saying she cannot climb stairs anymore and cannot get her feet into her shoes because of swelling.

A. What symptoms and signs of heart failure should you look for?
B. What tests do you want to order?
C. What treatment is indicated if she has an EF of 28% and moderate volume overload?

CASE 24–4. An 80-year-old man with a long history of hypertension presents with shortness of breath and exam reveals BP 180/95, JVP of 10 cm, an S_4 heart sound, lung crackles, and edema. ECG shows normal sinus rhythm at 90 with LVH without Q waves.

A. What is the most likely cause of his symptoms?
B. What tests should you order next?
C. What would be the best treatment for this man?

REFERENCES

Badgett RG, Lucey CR, Mulrow CD: Can the clinical examination diagnose left-sided heart failure in adults? JAMA 277:1712–1719, 1997.
Hunt SA, Baker DW, et al: ACC/AHA guidelines for the evaluation and management of chronic heart failure in the adult: Executive summary. J AM Coll Cardiol 38 (7):2101–2113, 2001.

USEFUL WEBSITE

ACC/AHA guidelines for the evaluation and management of chronic heart failure in the adult. *http://www.americanheart.org/presenter.jhtml?identifier=11841*

ISCHEMIC HEART DISEASE

▶ ETIOLOGY

What causes myocardial ischemia?

Myocardial ischemia occurs when myocardial oxygen demand exceeds oxygen delivery (Table 24–5). Ischemic heart disease is the leading cause of death and disability in the United States, and is most commonly caused by coronary atherosclerosis. While myocardial ischemia typically results in clinical syndromes of stable angina, unstable angina, or acute myocardial infarction, many patients with coronary artery disease (CAD) have episodes of ischemia that are atypical or even asymptomatic.

What is stable angina and what causes it?

Stable angina refers to ischemic chest pain that is reliably provoked by exertion and relieved by rest or nitroglycerin. Most patients with stable angina have one or more atherosclerotic plaques in their coronary arteries causing focal vessel narrowing. Blood supply may be adequate at rest but not with the increased demand of exertion.

What causes unstable angina and myocardial infarction?

Atherosclerotic plaques may destabilize and rupture. When this happens, platelets aggregate on the disrupted plaque causing subtotal or total occlusion of the coronary artery. Subtotal occlusion of a coronary artery results in unstable angina; this term

TABLE 24-5

Conditions That Exacerbate Cardiac Ischemia

Decreased Oxygen Supply	Increased Oxygen Demand
Cardiac	*Cardiac*
Coronary atherosclerosis	Cardiac hypertrophy
Coronary artery spasm	Tachyarrhythmia
Noncardiac	*Noncardiac*
Anemia	Exercise
Hypoxemia	Sinus tachycardia
Hypovolemia	Hyperadrenergic states (e.g., anxiety, cocaine)
Hemoglobinopathy	Hyperthyroidism
(e.g., sickle cell anemia)	

includes new onset angina, increasing angina, and rest angina. Plaque rupture with thrombus that totally occludes the coronary artery results in myocardial infarction (MI).

▶ EVALUATION

How do I diagnose stable angina?

The history and physical exam are the most important components of the initial evaluation of patients with chest pain. The history should focus on a thorough description of the chest pain and a review of the patient's CAD risk factors (Table 24–6 and Box 24–1). The physical exam should be directed at detecting the presence of the exacerbating factors (see Table 24–5). The likelihood of ischemia correlates with increasing patient age,

TABLE 24–6

Chest Pain Characteristics Predictive of Cardiac Ischemia

	Ischemia More Likely	Ischemia Less Likely
Quality	Squeezing/vise-like Pressure Heaviness Suffocating	Sharp Stabbing Knifelike
Location	Poorly localized Substernal Radiates to neck, jaw, teeth, shoulders, arms	Sharply demarcated
Duration	Minutes	Seconds only Hours to days
Provocation	Exertion	Position
Relief	Rest Nitroglycerin	Change in position

BOX 24–1

Coronary Artery Disease Risk Factors
Smoking
Hypertension
Hyperlipidemia
Diabetes mellitus
Family history of early CAD*

*First degree male relative with MI at less than 55 years or first degree female relative with MI at less than 65 years.

number of typical chest pain characteristics, and number of CAD risk factors. Upon completing your history and physical exam, you should be able to make a rough estimate of the likelihood that your patient's symptoms are caused by CAD. For example, a 60-year-old man with a history of hypertension and hyperlipidemia who complains of aching substernal chest discomfort that reliably begins about twenty minutes into his daily jog and clears within five minutes if he stops exercising has a high likelihood of CAD. A 50-year-old man with a history of tobacco who experiences sharp, substernal chest pain primarily when he uses his upper extremities has an intermediate likelihood of CAD as the cause of his symptoms.

When is a stress test indicated?

In patients with an intermediate likelihood of CAD, an exercise tolerance test (ETT) may aid diagnosis, with a positive test increasing the likelihood of CAD and a negative test decreasing its likelihood (Table 24–7). Both false-positive and false-negative tests are possible, so it is important to use clinical judgment in interpreting the results. You can see from the data presented in Table 24–7 that the ETT has little impact on your diagnostic certainty in patients with a high pretest likelihood of CAD. In these patients the ETT is still useful because it helps separate those patients who have a good prognosis from those at higher risk for progressing from stable angina to unstable angina or acute MI.

How do I diagnose unstable angina?

Unstable angina is characterized as ischemic chest pain that (a) is of new onset, (b) is of increasing severity, (c) occurs at rest, or (d) occurs post-MI or post-revascularization. The physical exam, ECG and cardiac enzyme levels may be normal in this setting and do not rule out unstable angina. When abnormal, however, they may alert you to patients who are at higher risk for progressing to myocardial infarction or sudden cardiac death (Table 24–8).

TABLE 24–7		
Predictive Ability of Exercise Treadmill Testing		
Pre-ETT Likelihood of CAD (Based on History)	**Post-ETT* Likelihood of CAD**	
	Positive Test (%)	*Negative Test (%)*
Low (5%)	21	3
Intermediate (50%)	83	36
High (95%)	98	83

*Assuming 50% sensitivity and 90% specificity.

TABLE 24-8

Risk Stratification of Patients with Unstable Angina

	Low Risk	Intermediate Risk	High Risk
History	New onset angina Worsening angina No ongoing pain	New onset angina, severe Rest pain, now resolved	Prolonged or ongoing angina
Exam	Normal	Hemodynamically stable	Hemodynamic instability, CHF
ECG	Normal	T-wave changes but no ST segment deviation	ST segment deviation New bundle branch block
Lab	Normal cardiac enzymes	Normal or minimally elevated cardiac enzymes	Elevated cardiac enzymes
Age	Younger		Older
MI Risk	3%–6%	9%	18%
Death Risk	0%	1.5%	6%

How do I diagnose acute myocardial infarction?

Acute MI needs to be diagnosed rapidly in order to optimize patient outcome. Early treatment decisions hinge on the ECG, so this should be obtained without delay in any patient with suspected MI. Most patients with acute MI present with chest pain. When chest pain radiates to the arms or shoulders and is associated with diaphoresis, MI is more likely. As many as 30% of patients with acute MI do not have chest pain at the time of presentation. These patients are more likely to be older, female, or diabetic and may instead present with fewer classic symptoms such as nausea, dyspnea, or palpitations. Other patients with acute MI have no symptoms at all and do not present for evaluation at the time of their MI. In these patients MI may be diagnosed months to years later based on ECG findings. The ECG is less sensitive than cardiac enzyme measurements for the detection of myocardial injury. Because of its virtually immediate availability, however, early treatment decisions depend on the ECG findings. Patients with new ST-segment elevations, new Q waves or a new conduction defect (e.g., left bundle branch block) in the setting of acute ischemic symptoms are assumed to have acute MI. When the initial ECG has normal or nonspecific findings and the patient has ongoing symptoms, repeat the ECG at ten-fifteen minute intervals. This may reveal evolving abnormalities that will allow the diagnosis of MI before cardiac enzyme levels become available.

What cardiac enzyme tests should be ordered?

While cardiac enzyme levels should be measured in all patients with acute coronary syndromes, they become critically important for diagnosing MI in patients whose symptoms and ECG findings are nonspecific. Creatine kinase (CK) and troponin I are the enzymes most frequently measured. Their serum levels begin to rise four to six hours after the onset of symptoms and thus initially may be normal in patients who seek care promptly. Serial measurements allow the detection of the rise and fall of these enzymes, which follow a typical time course when they are released from damaged myocardial cells (Table 24–9).

▶ TREATMENT

What are the goals of therapy for patients with stable angina?

The goals of therapy are to reduce symptoms, improve functional status, and prevent future myocardial infarction. Patients who achieve high levels of exercise without evidence of ischemia during exercise tolerance testing have a good prognosis. Less than 1% will die of their CAD within the next year.

Who can be treated medically for angina and what medicines can I use?   Aspirin + BB
                                                      Nitro PRN

Patients with stable angina and good exercise tolerance can be managed with medications. First line therapies are aspirin to prevent platelet aggregation and a β-blocker to decrease myocardial oxygen demand. Rapid acting nitroglycerin is used for episodes of angina that occur despite this therapy. Calcium channel blockers and long acting nitrates can be added to or substituted for β-blockers in those patients who do not completely respond, who are intolerant, or who have contraindications to β-blocker therapy. It is important to address each patient's CAD risk factors. Smoking cessation and treatment of hypertension and hyperlipidemia reduce the patient's risk for progressing to unstable angina or myocardial infarction.

Which patients with stable angina need referral to cardiology and what will happen to them?

Patients with chest pain or ECG findings at low exercise intensity on ETT have a poorer prognosis in that 5% or more of these

TABLE 24–9

Time Course for Cardiac Enzyme Elevations in Acute MI

	Onset	Peak	Duration
Troponin	4–6 hours	18–24 hours	Up to 10 days
Creatine kinase (CK)	4–6 hours	18–24 hours	36–48 hours

patients will die of their CAD in the next year. This group of patients should be referred to a cardiologist for further evaluation, which may include coronary catheterization and possibly revascularization, either by angioplasty, stenting, or coronary artery bypass surgery.

How do I treat patients with unstable angina?

Asprin, Nitrates, BB

The goals of initial management are to (1) rapidly relieve chest pain, (2) assess and reduce risk for acute MI and cardiac death, and (3) maintain stable hemodynamics. Admit patients with unstable angina to the hospital for continuous monitoring as hemodynamic instability can result from ischemia as well as its treatment. Initiate treatment with aspirin and intravenous heparin, which reduce mortality and the risk for progression to MI, possibly by preventing further clot development at the site of plaque rupture. If the patient is intolerant or hypersensitive to aspirin, clopidogrel or ticlopidine should be used. Nitrates and β-blockers reduce myocardial oxygen demand, may improve coronary blood flow, and are given to relieve chest pain or if cardiac enzymes are elevated. For ongoing ischemia despite these measures, or for planned angiography with stent/plasty, recent recommendations are to add a platelet GP IIb/IIIa receptor antagonist agent (eptifibatide or tirofiban).

Once the patient is pain free and hemodynamically stable, the patient's risk of dying or of having a nonfatal MI is formally assessed (see Table 24–8). Patients at high risk for progression to MI are referred for coronary catheterization while those at low risk may be managed with medications. Exercise treadmill testing is used to guide therapy in patients at intermediate risk. In general, those who do well on ETT testing may be managed medically while those who do poorly are referred for coronary catheterization.

TABLE 24–10		
Goals for Management of Acute Myocardial Infarction		
Immediate	**Subacute**	**Long-term**
Relieve pain	Identify patients with recurrent	Stop smoking
Restore hemodynamic stability	or ongoing ischemia	Control blood pressure
Initiate reperfusion within 30 min	Monitor for complications	Lower lipids
Prevent recurrent thrombosis		
Detect and treat arrhythmia		

How do I treat patients with acute MI?

The goals of treatment for patients with MI are listed in Table 24–10. As for patients with unstable angina, aspirin, nitrates, and β-blockers are the mainstays of early treatment. Attempts to reopen the occluded artery should begin as soon as possible. Thrombolytic medications and angioplasty are both effective and the decision about which approach to employ depends on individual patient characteristics and the availability of a cardiac catheterization facility. Depending on the technique used to re-establish perfusion in the affected artery, heparin or antiplatelet agents may be helpful in maintaining vessel patency. Angiotensin converting enzyme (ACE) inhibitors improve survival after acute MI but may cause hypotension and thus should be used with caution.

What are the complications of acute MI?

Patients should be monitored for complications of acute MI, which include atrial and ventricular arrhythmias, congestive heart failure, papillary muscle rupture leading to acute mitral regurgitation, and ventricular rupture. Patients with large anterior wall MI may develop clot in their left ventricle.

When is the patient ready for discharge?

Patients who have an uncomplicated post-MI course with no evidence of recurrent ischemia can undergo a low-level ETT within a few days of their MI. If the ETT is negative, they can be safely discharged from the hospital on medical management.

What medications should I prescribe when the patient is ready to leave the hospital?

First line therapies for patients following MI are similar to those for patients with stable angina. Unless there are specific contraindications to their use, aspirin and a β-blocker should be prescribed for all patients. Patients with reduced left ventricular function (ejection fraction less than 40%) benefit from the addition of an ACE inhibitor. Lipid-lowering therapy reduces the risk for recurrent MI; the target goal for LDL for patients with coronary artery disease is less than 100, so medication is recommended when low-density lipoprotein levels exceed 125 mg/dL. All these interventions offer a survival advantage.

K E Y   P O I N T S

▶ Myocardial ischemia occurs when myocardial oxygen consumption exceeds delivery.

▶ Atypical symptoms are common, particularly in women, the elderly, and in patients with diabetes.

▶ Treatment decisions are guided by risk for MI or cardiac death: refer high-risk patients for catheterization; manage low risk patients with medications.

▶ Time to reperfusion is critical to outcome in acute MI so make a diagnosis and begin treatment as quickly as possible.

▶ Aggressive management of CAD risk factors decreases the likelihood of disease progression in patients with CAD.

▶ Post-MI medications that offer a survival advantage include aspirin, β-blockers, ACE, and HMG CoA reductase inhibitors.

CASE 24–5. A 62-year-old woman with type II diabetes mellitus reports two weeks of nausea and heartburn each morning when she walks uphill to work. The symptoms resolve within a few minutes of arriving at work. Antacids have not helped. In your office, BP is 150/90. Her physical exam is otherwise normal. Resting ECG is shown in Figure 24–9.

   A. What is the most likely cause of her chest pain and what evidence supports this?
   B. Would you order any additional diagnostic tests at this time?
   C. How would you approach initial treatment?
   D. What additional information will help guide subsequent therapy?

CASE 24–6. A 72-year-old man with a history of CAD, hypertension, and hyperlipidemia comes to the ED with 30 minutes of dull substernal chest discomfort radiating to his jaw and both shoulders. He is nauseated

and vomited once on the way to the hospital. On exam he
is pale and diaphoretic. HR is 106 and BP is 96/50.
Cardiac exam reveals regular tachycardia without
murmur or gallop. Lungs are clear. His ECG is shown in
Figure 24–10.

  A. What is his diagnosis?
  B. What therapies are indicated at this time?

The patient undergoes balloon angioplasty of the left
anterior descending artery and subsequently does well
without recurrent chest pain or hemodynamic instability.
Four days later, he complains of sudden, sharp chest pain
and the nurse calls you because of a 12-beat run of
ventricular tachycardia. On exam the patient has a new
holosystolic murmur that can be heard across the
precordium and in his back.

  C. What is your differential diagnosis?

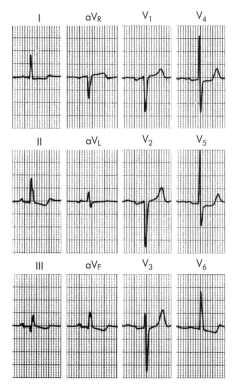

Figure 24–9. Electrocardiogram for patient in Case 24–5. (*From Davison
R: Electrocardiography in acute care medicine, St. Louis, 1995, Mosby.*)

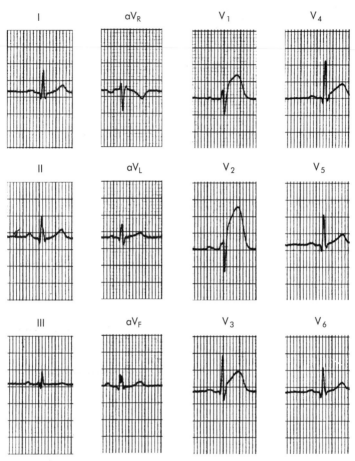

Figure 24–10. Electrocardiogram for patient in Case 24–6. (*From Davison R*: Electrocardiography in acute care medicine, *St. Louis, 1995, Mosby.*)

REFERENCES

Braunwald E, Antman EM, Beasley JW, et al: ACC/AHA guidelines for the management of patients with unstable angina and non–ST-elevation myocardial infarction. J Am Coll Cardiol 36:970, 2000.

Gibbons RJ, Chatterjee K, Daley J, et al: ACC/AHA/ACP–ASIM guidelines for the management of patients with chronic stable angina. J Am Coll Cardiol 33:2092, 1999.

Ryan TJ, Antman EM, Brooks NH, et al: ACC/AHA guidelines for the management of acute myocardial infarction. Circulation 100:1016, 1999.

USEFUL WEBSITE

American College of Cardiology site includes several recent cardiology guidelines. *www.acc.org*.

VALVULAR HEART DISEASE

▶ **ETIOLOGY**

Are all murmurs pathologic?

No. Many murmurs are "flow murmurs" without valvular pathology. These are benign, systolic, short murmurs heard in early systole that are 1-2/6 in intensity, are loudest at the upper sternal border, do not radiate to the neck and do not cause symptoms. Athletes and patients with anemia, fever or hyperthyroidism often have flow murmurs. Systolic murmurs are more likely pathologic if intensity is greater than 2/6, if they radiate to the carotids, are present in older people (older than age 55), or are accompanied by cardiac or pulmonary symptoms. A diastolic murmur, in contrast, is always pathologic.

What are common causes of systolic murmurs?

Flow murmurs, aortic stenosis (AS), and mitral regurgitation (MR) are common causes of systolic murmurs (Box 24–2). AS is most commonly due to calcification of a congenital bicuspid aortic valve in adults younger than 55, and degenerative valve change in adults older than 55. AS due to rheumatic heart disease occurs in people 40 to 60 years old, about 15 years after acute rheumatic fever. Aortic sclerosis is calcification of the aortic valve found in older individuals that can cause a murmur similar to AS. Aortic sclerosis can evolve into AS after time. Causes of MR are listed (see Box 24–2). A third cause of a systolic murmur is obstruction of the LV outflow tract with hypertrophic cardiomyopathy (HCM), a genetic disease that causes syncope with exertion. HCM has been the underlying cause of sudden death in some famous athletes and should be ruled-out in any sports physical.

What are the key causes of diastolic murmurs?

Aortic regurgitation (AR) and mitral stenosis (MS) are the most common causes. AR can occur with congenital bicuspid valves, rheumatic heart disease, endocarditis, ankylosing spondylitis, rheumatoid arthritis, and aortic root dilatation/dissection as with

---

BOX 24–2

Common Causes of Murmurs

Systolic Murmurs
Aortic stenosis (AS)
  congenital bicuspid valve (age less than 55)
  degenerative valvular disease (age greater than 55)
Flow murmur
  normal turbulence
  anemia, fever, hyperthyroidism
Hypertrophic cardiomyopathy (HCM)
Mitral regurgitation (MR)
  rheumatic heart disease
  mitral prolapse
  ischemic papillary muscle dysfunction

Diastolic Murmurs
Aortic regurgitation (AR)
  congenital bicuspid valve
  rheumatic heart disease
  endocarditis
  aortic root dissection
    Marfan's syndrome
    aortitis (syphilis, vasculitis)
Mitral stenosis (MS)
  rheumatic heart disease

Marfan's syndrome, vasculitis, or syphilitic aortitis. The predominant cause of MS is rheumatic heart disease.

▶ EVALUATION

My patient has a murmur. How should I proceed?

Place the murmur in systole or diastole by palpating pulse, grade the murmur on a scale of one to six (Table 24–11), and describe pitch, location, and sites of radiation (carotids, chest wall sites). For example, AR is described as an early diastolic, 2/6, high-pitched, decrescendo murmur heard best in the second right interspace radiating down the left sternal border.

How do I differentiate between the systolic murmurs of AS and MR?

Specific valvular abnormalities are often identifiable by the location and character of the murmur (Table 24–12, Figures 24–11 and 24–12). AS is diamond-shaped (crescendo-decrescendo in musi-

TABLE 24-11

Grading Cardiac Murmurs

Grade	Description
1	Cannot hear at first
2	Hear right away, not too loud
3	Loud but no palpable thrill
4	Loud and associated with palpable thrill
5	Heard with stethoscope angled on chest
6	Heard with stethoscope off chest

TABLE 24-12

Characteristics of Some Common Valvular Abnormalities

Lesion	Timing	Loudest Location	Radiation
AS	Systolic crescendo-decrescendo	2nd intercostal space	Carotid
MR	Pansystolic	Apex	Axilla, back
AR	Early diastole	Left sternal border	None
MS	Opening snap in early diastole, murmur in mid-diastole, with crescendo in late diastole	Apex, best to listen with bell in left lateral decubitus position	None

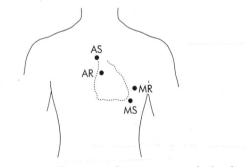

Figure 24–11. Location of murmurs from common valvular disorders.

cal terminology), heard best at the base, and radiates to the carotids. MR is holosystolic, heard at the apex, and radiates to the axilla. Severe AS damps and delays the carotid pulse (pulsus parvus et tardus). To differentiate between the murmurs of AS and MR from HCM, auscultate the heart while the patient abruptly stands from squatting or sitting, which decreases venous return.

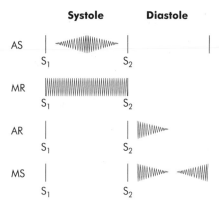

Figure 24–12. Visual representation of the sounds produced by common murmurs.

With this maneuver AS and MR murmurs *decrease* as stroke volume decreases the amount of blood rushing past the valves. However, in HCM the murmur intensity *increases* as the thickened outflow tract walls collapse toward one another with the stroke volume decrease.

How do the clinical presentations of the systolic murmur conditions differ?

For both aortic stenosis and mitral regurgitation, a long asymptomatic period may precede LV failure, which then causes fatigue, dyspnea on exertion, orthopnea. AS typically occurs in older patients and causes syncope and chest pain. Exertional syncope occurs due to fixed cardiac output in the setting of increased oxygen demand and vasodilation. Chest pain occurs due to poor coronary artery perfusion in diastole. MR may present acutely if myocardial infarction causes a ruptured papillary muscle. HCM usually occurs in younger patients with a family history of an autosomal dominant inheritance pattern of early cardiac problems, though incomplete penetrance may decrease the number of affected family members. Patients may have few symptoms before a sudden cardiac arrest/event. They may experience exercise intolerance, often masked by avoidance of exercise.

How can I differentiate between the diastolic murmurs of AR and MS?

The early diastolic, high-pitched decrescendo murmur of AR is heard maximally in the second right interspace with radiation down the left sternal border. It almost mimics a breath sound. A wide pulse pressure often accompanies a pulse with a rapid rise and fall. Use a diaphragm and have the patient lean forward with his or her breath held. In contrast, the MS murmur is low pitched, mid-diastolic, and heard at the apex. A presystolic crescendo is often heard as the atrial kick sends blood across the stenotic mitral valve. Use a lightly placed bell over the apex, or in the axilla, and ask the patient to lie in the left lateral decubitus position to best hear the murmur of MS.

How do the clinical presentations of the diastolic murmur conditions differ?

Both AR and MS can have long asymptomatic periods. AS eventually causes symptoms of left heart failure by way of increased LV work. The increased left atrial pressures from MS eventually can cause left atrial enlargement, atrial fibrillation, pulmonary congestion, and right heart failure. Occasionally, patients with MS present with hemoptysis.

Which patients need an echocardiogram or ECG?

Obtain both tests for murmurs with pathologic features: systolic murmur grade 3/6 or greater, age older than 55, any diastolic murmur, or concurrent cardiopulmonary symptoms.

▶ TREATMENT

How should I manage a patient with pathologic valvular disease?

All patients with pathologic valvular disease need close follow-up to detect onset of heart failure. Review cardiopulmonary symptoms and exam annually. Obtain an echocardiogram annually in patients with severe lesions, every two to five years in mild to moderate AS patients, or whenever patients report new or changing cardiopulmonary symptoms. Patients with AR benefit from afterload reducing agents (ACE inhibitors, hydralazine, and nifedipine) to increase cardiac output. These drugs can postpone or avoid surgery in asymptomatic patients with severe regurgitation. Atrial fibrillation is a common complication of atrial enlargement from MS or MR. Atrial fibrillation requires anticoagulation (warfarin), cardioversion, and/or heart rate control (β-blocker, calcium channel blocker, or digoxin). Refer asymptomatic patients for consideration of valve replacement when there are signs of LV dysfunction, an ejection fraction less than 55%–60%, or LV end systolic measurement greater than 45 mm for MR, and greater than 55 mm for AR. Refer all patients with cardiopulmonary symptoms. Acute AR and MR resulting from aortic dissection (AR), endocarditis (AR and MR), and myocardial infarction (MR) require urgent valve replacement to avoid LV failure.

Are there any special issues in managing patients with AS?

Avoid afterload reduction with ACE inhibitors or hydralazine in patients with AS because these agents worsen coronary artery perfusion. A pressure gradient greater than 80 mm Hg across the valve, a valve area less than 0.7 cm^2, and declining LV function are indications for valve replacement, but are controversial in asymptomatic patients.

Are there any special issues in managing patients with MS?

Diuretics can reduce pulmonary congestion. In patients with atrial fibrillation, rate control and/or cardioversion will markedly decrease symptoms. Systemic emboli can be a problem with MS and life-long warfarin is begun after any atrial fibrillation. Consider surgery for limiting dyspnea, uncontrollable pulmonary edema, recurrent systemic emboli on anticoagulation, and severe pulmonary hypertension with right ventricular hypertrophy and hemoptysis. Open mitral commissurotomy and percutaneous balloon valvuloplasty can be considered for nonregurgitant valves. Regurgitant or distorted valves require replacement.

How can I prevent endocarditis?

Give high-risk patients (those with prosthetic valves, damaged native valves) a single 2 gm oral dose of amoxicillin prior to dental, respiratory tract, or esophageal procedures, and ampicillin plus gentamicin for genitourinary or gastrointestinal procedures. Give moderate risk patients (e.g., acquired valvular dysfunction or mitral valve prolapse with regurgitation) amoxicillin for oral, pulmonary, GI, and GU procedures.

K E Y   P O I N T S

- ▶ All diastolic murmurs are pathologic.
- ▶ Monitor significant valvular disease by serial echoes and refer for valve replacement when there are symptoms or signs of LV dysfunction.
- ▶ Acute valvular regurgitation, such as MR with papillary muscle rupture and AR with endocarditis, requires urgent echocardiography and rapid intervention.
- ▶ Give endocarditis prophylaxis to all patients with valvular disease undergoing dental, respiratory, or GI or GU endoscopic procedures likely to result in bleeding.

CASE 24-7.

A 25-year-old man reports six months of low back pain. He is otherwise healthy. This pain is associated with morning stiffness and improves with exercise. In addition to reduced spine flexibility on Schober testing, you incidentally find a 3/6, high-pitched, diastolic decrescendo murmur that is present at the base and radiates down the left sternal border. In addition, there is a low-pitched rumble heard only at the apex.

A. What valvular lesion(s) is/are present?
B. What is the underlying disease process?
C. What diagnostic studies would you obtain?
D. Outline your management of the valvular lesion(s).
E. He is scheduled for a tooth extraction in two weeks. How will you prepare him for this?

CASE 24-8.

A 55-year-old male smoker complains of five weeks of exertional substernal heaviness. You detect a basal 4/6, diamond-shaped systolic murmur that radiates to the right carotid. The carotid pulse seems somewhat delayed. You diagnose aortic stenosis.

A. List as many physical exam features of severe aortic stenosis as you can.
B. Your assistant schedules an echocardiogram in two weeks. However, since there is an immediate opening in the exercise treadmill lab, your assistant schedules an appointment there for this afternoon. Is this plan acceptable?

REFERENCES

Etchells E, Bell C, Rob K: Does this patient have an abnormal systolic murmur? JAMA 277(7): 564–571, 1997.
Shipton B, Wahba H: Valvular heart disease: Review and update. Am Fam Physician 63(11):2201–2208, 2001.

USEFUL WEBSITE

http://www.wilkes.med.ucla.edu/intro.html

25

Dermatology

▶ ETIOLOGY

What are common causes of pruritus?

Xerosis (dry skin), scabies, and eczema are common causes of itching (pruritus). Less common causes include systemic diseases such as renal failure, cholestasis, polycythemia vera, or lymphoma.

▶ EVALUATION

How can I determine what is causing itching?

Xerosis (dry skin) usually causes diffuse pruritus and is common in the elderly and in patients who bathe frequently. The skin appears dry and may be cracked though there is usually no erythema. *Scabies* may be associated with burrows in the interdigital web spaces and a papular rash, especially in the axillae, around the waistline, on the male genitals, or on the buttocks. Red, itchy papules or nodules on the penis are pathognomonic for scabies infection. Sometimes a tiny scabies may be seen by looking at burrow scrapings under a microscope. Scabies burrows appear as white lines on the skin which are typically 1 mm wide and less than a half inch long. Patients with scabies may have affected family members and almost always suffer from intense pruritus, often worse at night. If a therapeutic trial for xerosis fails and scabies is not identified, consider work-up for a systemic illness with CBC and renal and liver function tests. Renal failure, cholestatic liver disease, and polycythemia vera are causes of pruritus that are screened with these tests.

▶ TREATMENT

What treatments are useful?

For dry skin, use moisturizers, minimize bathing, and avoid hot water and deodorant soaps. Use moisturizing soap sparingly and in essential areas only. Treat scabies with permethrin or lindane cream overnight to the whole body below the neck. Prescribe enough for the simultaneous treatment of all intimate contacts (don't use lindane in children), even if they are asymptomatic. Persistent egg capsules beneath the skin may cause itching to endure a week past the treatment of the infection. Repeated applications beyond once or twice may worsen skin irritation and pruritus due to irritation from the medication. In the morning, patients should wash their bedding and any clothes worn the previous two days. Itching may occur for one to two weeks after treatment but does not indicate treatment failure. A short course of prednisone may be indicated if the itching is very severe.

MACULOPAPULAR RASHES

▶ ETIOLOGY

What are the most common causes of erythematous macules or papules in adults?

Drug reactions and viral infections cause diffuse maculopapular rashes. A rash caused by a viral infection is referred to as a "viral exanthem." Scabies causes more localized papular eruptions and may cause diffuse pruritus.

▶ EVALUATION

How can I distinguish viral from drug-related rashes?

Because both drug reactions and viral exanthems cause a diffuse, truncal rash, history will best delineate the likely cause. If a new medication was recently started, particularly a sulfa antibiotic or penicillin, drug reaction is likely. If viral symptoms are present, a viral exanthem is more likely. Scabies also may cause papules, often intensely pruritic and crusted due to scratching. Although occasionally scabies is widespread, it is usually localized to the wrists, axillae, waist, or male genitals.

▶ TREATMENT

Viral exanthems resolve spontaneously. Drug reactions resolve with removal of the offending agent. See previous section for treatment of scabies.

SCALING RASHES

▶ ETIOLOGY

What are the most common scaling rashes in adults?

Psoriasis, eczema, seborrheic dermatitis, pityriasis rosea, and tinea infection are common causes of scaling rashes.

▶ EVALUATION

How can I tell these conditions apart?

The pattern of body sites involved is helpful (Figure 25–1). Besides distribution, the appearance of the border and scale are also useful. Psoriasis causes well-circumscribed, raised, salmon-colored plaques with adherent silvery scales. Eczema is often pruritic and frequently occurs in "atopic" individuals who are prone to allergies and asthma. Eczema rashes are often symmetrical and erythematous and may contain small vesicles or pustules. If eczema is long-standing, scaling and thickening (lichenification) can occur. Seborrhea is nonpruritic and has indistinct margins with fine, greasy, yellowish scales and mild erythema. Pityriasis rosea is a mysterious, self-limited rash with distinct, oval-shaped, hyperpigmented lesions, each with an inner scaling ring. These lesions are distributed in an evergreen tree pattern over the trunk. Tinea corporis causes distinct erythematous lesions with scaly borders that are usually not symmetrical. Tinea versicolor usually occurs on the chest, back, and arms. The lesions are pink to coffee colored

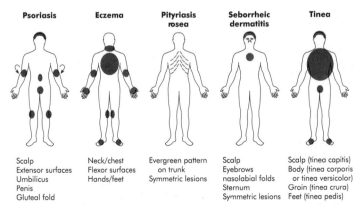

Psoriasis	Eczema	Pityriasis rosea	Seborrheic dermatitis	Tinea
Scalp	Neck/chest	Evergreen pattern on trunk	Scalp	Scalp (tinea capitis)
Extensor surfaces	Flexor surfaces	Symmetric lesions	Eyebrows	Body (tinea corporis or tinea versicolor)
Umbilicus	Hands/feet		nasolabial folds	Groin (tinea crura)
Penis			Sternum	Feet (tinea pedis)
Gluteal fold			Symmetric lesions	

Figure 25–1. Classic sites involved with common scaling rashes.

patches in patients who have had little sun exposure, and as hypopigmented spots in patients who are tan or of darker skin tone. Hyphae on a KOH prep of skin scrapings are diagnostic of tinea conditions.

▶ **TREATMENT**

What treatments are useful for scaling rashes?

Scaling rashes are generally treated with either topical steroids, antifungals, or both (Table 25–1). For eczema, further preventive measures include avoiding skin irritants, such as wool, newspaper ink, citrus peels, strong soaps, and household chemicals; minimizing scratching with antihistamines; keeping fingernails short; preventing skin dryness with nonlanolin moisturizers, decreased bathing, and hot water avoidance. If eczema is secondarily infected with bacteria (e.g., impetigo), treat with antibiotics.

SKIN CANCERS

▶ **ETIOLOGY**

What are the main types of skin cancer?

Melanoma is the most aggressive skin cancer. Associated with prior history of sunburns, it grows rapidly, metastasizes early, and can be deadly. Tissue depth of melanoma at the time of diagnosis determines prognosis. Basal and squamous cell skin cancers are slow-growing tumors associated with cumulative sun exposure, irrespective of whether patients experienced actual sunburns.

TABLE 25–1

Treatments for Scaling Rashes

Cause of Scaling Rash	Treatment
Psoriasis	Coal tar lotion or shampoo, topical steroids (high to very-high potency), sun exposure, UV light, methotrexate
Pityriasis rosea	Resolves without treatment after 2–8 weeks, antihistamines decrease itching
Seborrheic dermatitis	Selenium sulfide shampoo, steroid lotion (scalp), ketoconazole shampoo
Eczema	Topical steroids, moisturizer, irritant avoidance
Tinea	Antifungal cream

Although these skin cancers generally do not metastasize, they can invade and destroy local tissues if left untreated. Actinic keratoses are areas of mild atypia of the epidermis from chronic sun damage. They eventually can progress to squamous cell carcinoma, but the overall risk of progression is very small—less than 0.1% per year.

▶ EVALUATION

How do I recognize skin cancers?

Features that are concerning for melanoma are listed in Box 25-1. Basal cell carcinomas appear as shiny pink or pearly papules with telangiectasias. Squamous cell carcinoma is an indurated, yellowish plaque, often with scaling, erosions, or ulcerations. Actinic keratoses are usually more easily felt than seen: small patch of rough, adherent scale. While melanoma can occur anywhere, the other three types of lesions generally occur on sun-exposed areas, especially on the upper cheeks, below the eyes, on the ears, and around the nose.

How should a suspicious mole be evaluated?

If there is a low suspicion for melanoma, small lesions can be removed with a punch biopsy. If there is concern for melanoma, excisional biopsy is indicated. Never perform a shave biopsy on a pigmented lesion, since the depth of the lesion is critical to prognosis if the lesion is a melanoma.

▶ TREATMENT

Freeze actinic keratoses with liquid nitrogen. Be aware that the lesions are so superficial that a single ten-second freeze is usually sufficient. Refer to dermatology for wider excision of malignant lesions.

BOX 25-1

Features Concerning for Malignant Melanoma

A asymmetry, especially a notched border
B border irregularity, bleeding
C color variation
D diameter growing or >6 mm
E elevation irregularity, e.g., a raised area within a macule
F feeling changes, e.g., new itching or burning

VESICULAR LESIONS

▶ ETIOLOGY

What are common causes of vesicles?

Herpes zoster virus reactivating as shingles, herpes simplex infection, and contact dermatitis are common causes of vesicles.

▶ EVALUATION

How do I tell shingles from herpes simplex?

Shingles (or "zoster") is reactivation of dormant varicella zoster virus (the virus that causes chicken pox). Its dermatomal distribution, which typically does not cross the midline, clinches the diagnosis. Symptoms usually begin with painful burning along a single dermatome, followed by an outbreak of vesicles on an erythematous base in the same dermatome. Shingles occurs much more frequently in patients who are elderly or immunocompromised and is especially common in patients with HIV. Herpes simplex is usually sexually transmitted and causes vesicles and ulceration on the lips, in the mouth, or on the genitals; occasionally herpes affects the fingers with weepy ulcerations, called herpetic whitlow. To confirm the diagnosis of herpes simplex, obtain a sample of cells for viral culture from the base of an unroofed vesicle (rub firmly for an adequate sample).

What is post-herpetic neuralgia?

Post-herpetic neuralgia (PHN) is pain occurring after shingles resolves. It may last from a few weeks to a year or two in severe cases. The incidence and duration of PHN increases with age.

▶ TREATMENT

How do I treat herpes zoster and post-herpetic neuralgia?

Treat with seven days of acyclovir (800 mg 5x/day). Famciclovir (500 mg tid) and valacyclovir (1 gm tid) are equally effective but much more costly. These drugs shorten both the time to healing and the duration of PHN, but they do not affect the incidence of PHN. Prednisone may decrease the acute pain but has little to no effect on PHN, and so should be used only when the acute rash is severe. All patients with active zoster should avoid coming into contact with pregnant women and those who do not have a history of chicken pox or varicella vaccination. Patients who have lesions on the forehead, the nose, or around the eye, or those who have ocular symptoms should have urgent ophthalmologic evaluation to rule-out corneal involvement. Post-herpetic neuralgia may respond to tricyclic antidepressants, topical capsaicin cream, or to gabapentin.

How do I treat herpes simplex?

Outbreaks are self-limited but may be shortened by seven days of acyclovir (400 mg tid). Patients with frequent severe attacks can be given prophylactic acyclovir (400 mg bid). Lessen the risk of transmission by avoiding intimate contact with the involved area during outbreaks. Viral shedding occurs even without sores present, although the clinical impact is unclear.

K E Y P O I N T S

▶ Scabies causes pruritic papules on the wrists, axillae, waist, and genitalia.

▶ Scaling rashes respond to either steroids or antifungals, depending on the cause.

▶ Pityriasis rosea is a benign, self-limited rash that has a characteristic evergreen tree pattern.

▶ Seborrhea is a common scaling rash on the face that responds to low-potency steroids or ketoconazole.

▶ Psoriasis often responds to steroids, but if severe, may require referral for nontopical therapy.

▶ Eczema management consists primarily of skin moisturizing and topical steroids.

▶ Zoster should be treated with antivirals to speed healing and shorten the course of PHN.

▶ Basal and squamous cell carcinomas almost never metastasize; excision halts local spread.

CASE 25–1. A 28-year-old woman with allergic rhinitis and a history of childhood asthma reports an itchy rash on the flexor surfaces of her arms for four weeks. On exam she has symmetrical erythema on both antecubital fossae with significant excoriation, and one area of associated yellowish crust.

    A. What is the most likely diagnosis?
    B. What do you think of the yellowish crusting?
    C. What would you recommend for treatment?

CASE 25–2. A 62-year-old man has acute onset of facial pain followed by appearance of a rash on his forehead. His vision is normal. On exam, he has small, red vesicles on his left forehead.

    A. What is the most likely diagnosis?
    B. What would you recommend for acute treatment?
    C. Is any other evaluation needed?

CASE 25–3. A 52-year-old woman comes to clinic because her husband has noticed a mole on her back that has grown recently. On exam, there is a 5 mm pigmented, macular lesion just below the right scapula with a slightly irregular border.

    A. What other historical and physical exam features should be noted?
    B. What is the main diagnostic concern?
    C. What should be the next diagnostic step?

USEFUL WEBSITE

Indiana University interactive site with interesting cases with dermatology findings.
http://erl.pathology.iupui. edu/cases/dermcases/dermcases.cfm

26

Endocrinology

ADRENAL DISORDERS

▶ ETIOLOGY

What causes adrenal insufficiency?

Adrenal insufficiency has three forms: primary, secondary, and tertiary. *Primary insufficiency* also known as Addison's disease, is due to destruction of both adrenal glands. Greater than 90% of both glands must be destroyed before clinical signs of insufficiency appear. Worldwide, TB is the most common cause of primary adrenal gland destruction. In the U.S., autoimmune destruction is more common and is often part of a polyglandular deficiency syndrome type 1 (hypoparathyroidism and mucocutaneous candidiasis), or type 2 (autoimmune thyroiditis and type 1 diabetes mellitus). *Secondary adrenal insufficiency* is caused by decreased adrenocorticotropic hormone (ACTH) production due to disruption of pituitary function.

What is tertiary adrenal insufficiency?

The most common cause of adrenal insufficiency in the U.S. is *tertiary insufficiency* from exogenous steroid use, which suppresses but does not destroy the gland. Insufficiency can occur in the early weeks following steroid discontinuation if the steroid is not tapered appropriately and can also occur despite the patient's usual steroid dose if the body is under great stress and the suppressed adrenals are unable to respond. For example, a 65-year-old woman on chronic steroids for rheumatoid arthritis who develops pneumonia may present with hypotension and tachycardia. While she may be septic, this is also a common presentation for adrenal insufficiency. Uncommon causes are listed in Box 26–1.

What types of adrenal excess are there?

Adrenal hypertrophy, adenoma, or carcinoma can all produce excess aldosterone, cortisol (Cushing's syndrome), or cate-

---

BOX 26-1

Causes of Adrenal Insufficiency

Common causes
Autoimmune disease
Steroid use*
TB

Uncommon causes
Bilateral adrenal hemorrhage
Fungal infection
CMV adrenalitis (AIDS patients)
Lymphoma
Metastatic cancer
Pituitary failure[†]

---

*"tertiary adrenal insufficiency"
[†]"secondary adrenal insufficiency"

cholamines (pheochromocytoma). Cushing's syndrome is a state of chronic glucocorticoid excess from any source. Long-term steroid use is the most common cause. Cushing's disease is caused by a pituitary adenoma secreting ACTH and is the second most common cause of Cushing's syndrome. Less common causes are adrenal hyperplasia, adrenal adenoma, and ectopic ACTH production, usually from small cell lung cancer.

▶ EVALUATION

How does adrenal insufficiency present?

In the ambulatory setting, chronic adrenal insufficiency presents with nonspecific chronic complaints, particularly fatigue, arthralgias, myalgias, vague abdominal complaints, and episodes of volume depletion or hypotension. Acute adrenal insufficiency, or adrenal crisis, occurs with cardiovascular collapse mimicking sepsis (Table 26-1). These episodes are often precipitated by gastroenteritis, viral illness, bacterial infection, or some other systemic stress. With chronic primary adrenal gland failure, the compensating pituitary overproduces ACTH and a byproduct, melanocyte stimulating hormone (MSH), which results in diffuse hyperpigmentation accentuated in the palmar creases and gums. Secondary adrenal insufficiency due to pituitary failure usually presents with similar fatigue, arthralgias/myalgias, but the abdominal pain and hypotension are less prominent because mineralocorticoid production is preserved. Hypothyroidism and hypogonadism may also be present. Hyperpigmentation does not occur because the pituitary is producing neither ACTH nor MSH. Lab abnormalities are listed in Table 26-1.

TABLE 26–1

Presenting Signs and Symptoms of Adrenal Insufficiency and Cortisol Excess

	Adrenal Insufficiency	Cortisol Excess (Cushing's Syndrome)
Symptoms	Weakness/fatigue	Weakness/fatigue
	Dizziness	Easy bruising
	GI symptoms: anorexia, nausea, vomiting, abdominal pain, diarrhea	Acne
	Fever	Hirsutism
	Myalgias, arthralgias	Psychiatric symptoms
	Amenorrhea	
	Anxiety, irritability, confusion, depression, psychosis	
Signs	Hypotension/orthostasis*	Hypertension
	Weight loss	Central obesity with thin extremities
	Hyperpigmentation*	Edema
	Small heart on CXR	Facial plethora, moon face
		Abdominal striae
		Ecchymoses
		Osteoporosis
		Proximal muscle wasting
Laboratory test results	Hyperkalemia*	Hypokalemia
	Nongap metabolic acidosis	Metabolic alkalosis
	Hyponatremia	Hypernatremia
	Hypoglycemia	Hyperglycemia
	Eosinophilia, lymphocytosis, neutropenia	Leukocytosis, lymphocytopenia

*Occur with primary adrenal insufficiency, not in secondary adrenal insufficiency where mineralocorticoid levels are preserved.

How do I diagnose adrenal insufficiency?

A random cortisol greater than 20 µg/dL rules out adrenal insufficiency. In patients on chronic glucocorticoids, a random cortisol concentration does not reliably assess the adequacy of the adrenal response to stress. In these cases, stimulation tests are used to determine the adrenal response. The standard screening for patients with suspected pituitary insufficiency is with an ACTH stimulation test: a plasma cortisol of less than 20 µg/dL measured thirty–sixty minutes after supraphysiological concentrations of 250 µg synthetic ACTH (cosyntropin, given IV) indicates insufficiency. An ACTH level greater than 250 pg/mL then distinguishes adrenal from pituitary (ACTH less than 50 pg/mL) causes. This test has low sensitivity in patients with acute adrenal insufficiency. For such patients the low-dose (1 µg) ACTH test is used. A single cortisol concentration measured thirty minutes following ACTH administration reliably reflects adrenal function without false-positive results. Small adrenal glands on CT scan suggest autoimmune destruction; large adrenals suggest metastasis or early TB.

When should I suspect adrenal excess?

Poorly controlled hypertension can arise from excess aldosterone, cortisol, or catecholamine. Laboratory abnormalities of hypokalemia, hypernatremia, and metabolic alkalosis can occur with elevated aldosterone or cortisol. Screen for adrenal excess with careful history, exam, and electrolytes in very young hypertensive patients and in those with difficult-to-control hypertension. Clues to excess cortisol include a cushingoid appearance with facial plethora, central obesity, hirsutism, and proximal muscle wasting. Pheochromocytoma causes episodic severe hypertension, with associated sweating, flushing, and headaches. Some pheochromocytomas are associated with neurofibromatosis or medullary thyroid cancer.

How do patients with Cushing's syndrome present?

Patients rarely complain of symptoms that will suggest this diagnosis. It is diagnosed by an astute physician who thinks to look for it. Consider the diagnosis in patients who look "cushingoid," who present with hypertension and central obesity, hyperglycemia, or unexplained metabolic alkalosis. If one feature is present, look for others to confirm your suspicion (see Table 26–1).

How do I diagnose Cushing's syndrome?

Screen for cortisol excess by a twenty-four-hour urine cortisol (normal less than 100 µg/24 hours). Levels greater than 250 µg/day diagnose Cushing's syndrome, while levels less than 65 exclude the diagnosis. False-positive tests occur with depression, anorexia, stress, alcoholism, and oral contraceptive use.

How do I work-up patients for hyperaldosteronism or pheochromocytoma?

Some centers use a serum aldosterone-to-renin ratio for diagnosis of hyperaldosteronism, where aldosterone greater than 20 ng/dL and a ratio greater than 100 (with renin units in ng/ml/three hours) are highly specific for the diagnosis. If your center does not offer this test, a twenty-four-hour urine aldosterone greater than 20 µg in the setting of a low plasma renin less than 5 µg/dL makes the diagnosis. Suspect pheochromocytoma with presence of the 5 Hs (each usually episodic): Hypertension, Headache, Hyperhidrosis (sweating), Hypotension (orthostatic), and Hyperglycemia. Screen for pheochromocytoma by twenty-four-hour urine catecholamines, metanephrines, or vanillylmandelic acid. If screening is positive, obtain abdominal MRI to look for the source.

▶ TREATMENT

How do I treat adrenal insufficiency?

In patients with suspected primary adrenal insufficiency and hemo-dynamic instability, give dexamethasone 4 mg IV immediately, which will not interfere with subsequent urine testing, or hydro-cortisone 100 mg IV q eight hours. Search for precipitating infection or other physical source of stress. Maintenance therapy for chronic adrenal insufficiency includes dexamethasone 0.5 mg or prednisone 5 mg qhs. Alternatively, give hydrocortisone 15 mg qam and 5–10 mg in early afternoon. Mineralocorticoid replacement for patients with primary adrenal insufficiency is with fludro-cortisone 0.1 mg qd. Educate patients with primary and secondary adrenal insufficiency about the disease, how to manage minor and major stresses, and how to self-administer stress dose steroids. For patients with presumed tertiary insufficiency on long-term exogenous corticosteroids, there is sparse and mixed data regard-ing stress-dose steroids for surgery or acute illness. Current prac-tice includes hydrocortisone 100 mg IV on call to the OR, or 50–100 mg IV q8 h for twenty-four hours, then rapidly tapered when the patient stabilizes.

How do I treat adrenal excess syndromes?

When aldosterone, cortisol, or catecholamine excess is due to an adrenal tumor, surgical removal is indicated. This must be done carefully with pheochromocytoma. Prepare the patient preopera-tively with α- and β-blockade to avoid life-threatening cate-cholamine bolus. Aldosterone excess due to adrenal hyperplasia can be treated with surgical removal or lifelong spironolactone therapy. Cushing's disease due to pituitary or ectopic ACTH pro-duction requires surgical removal of the source of ACTH.

<table>
<tr><td>

K E Y   P O I N T S

</td></tr>
</table>

▶ Adrenal insufficiency is most commonly the tertiary form, due to steroid use.

▶ Patients who look septic might have adrenal insufficiency.

▶ If you suspect adrenal crisis, do not wait for test results—give hydrocortisone or dexamethasone immediately.

▶ Hyperpigmentation, hypotension, and hypokalemia occur with primary, but not secondary, adrenal insufficiency.

▶ Consider hyperaldosteronism, Cushing's syndrome, and pheochromocytoma in patients with poorly controlled hypertension.

▶ Suspect cortical excess in patients with hypertension, diabetes, central obesity, hypokalemia, and characteristic physical findings.

CASE 26–1. A 55-year-old man with severe COPD is markedly confused immediately following an elective cholecystectomy. T is 101.5°F, P is 130, BP is 76/42, and RR is 12. Staples are intact, abdomen is not distended but is tender, without guarding or rebound. Blood loss was minimal during the surgery and 2 L of fluid were administered.

   A. What is the most likely cause for his confusion and hypotension?
   B. What further work-up should be done?
   C. What treatment does he need?

CASE 26–2. A 40-year-old woman presents for evaluation of fatigue. Medical history is notable for morbid obesity (she weighs 200 lbs and is 5′5″ in height), recent onset of diabetes, and major depression. Her blood pressure is 190/100. On physical exam you note facial fullness, acne, and hirsutism.

   A. What is the most likely diagnosis?
   B. What tests would you order to evaluate for Cushing's syndrome?

REFERENCES

Boscaro M, Barzon L, Fallo F, Sonino N: Cushing's syndrome. Lancet 357:783–791, 2001.
Oelkers W: Adrenal insufficiency. N Engl J Med 335:1206–1212, 1996.

DIABETES

▶ ETIOLOGY

What is the difference between type 1 and type 2 diabetes?

Diabetes occurs when inadequate insulin results in a high blood sugar. Patients with type 1 diabetes stop making insulin. A combination of genetic predisposition and an environmental trigger (possibly a viral infection) causes autoimmune destruction of pancreatic islet β cells. These patients are generally young and slender. In type 2 diabetes, insulin secretion is not absent and in fact may be elevated, but is insufficient to overcome insulin resistance. Patients are usually obese and older than age 30.

What are the risk factors for diabetes?

The major risk factor for type 1 diabetes is an identical twin with type 1 diabetes. Risk factors for type 2 diabetes include prior gestational diabetes or newborn greater than 9 lb, overweight, inactivity, race (Native American, Hispanic, African American, Asian American, or Pacific Islander), hypertension, family history of type 2 diabetes, dyslipidemia, polycystic ovary syndrome, and history of glucose intolerance. Many drugs can exacerbate glucose intolerance including steroids, thiazide diuretics, niacin, protease inhibitors, glucosamine, and β-blockers.

What is diabetic ketoacidosis?

Diabetic ketoacidosis (DKA) occurs in type 1 diabetes when glucose cannot be utilized due to lack of insulin, causing accelerated starvation that forces the body to make ketones for fuel. Key features include hyperglycemia, elevated ketones, and anion-gap acidosis. Common precipitants include infection (50%), lack of insulin, and new diabetes.

What is hyperglycemic hyperosmolar nonketotic coma (HHNC)?

When patients with type 2 diabetes get extremely hyperglycemic, they become hyperosmolar. Ketoacidosis is uncommon because patients have enough insulin to prevent ketone production. High glucose draws free water out of cells and creates an osmotic diuresis, leading to dehydration and altered mental status. Many patients with HHNC are elderly and unable to drink enough fluids to compensate. Coma occurs in 10%; mortality is 10%–17%. Common precipitants include infection, heart attack, stroke, uremia, pancreatitis, and parenteral nutrition.

▶ EVALUATION

How do I diagnose diabetes?

Diagnose diabetes by a single plasma glucose greater than or equal to 200 mg/dL with symptoms such as polydipsia, polyuria, polyphagia, and weight loss, or a fasting plasma glucose greater than or equal to 126 mg/dL on two occasions. Glycosylated hemoglobin ($HgbA_{1c}$), called "A1C" is too insensitive to use for diagnosis. Oral glucose tolerance testing is used only to screen for gestational diabetes.

Who should be screened for diabetes?

Patients have type 2 diabetes on average 10–12 years prior to diagnosis. The American Diabetes Association recommends screening those with one or more risk factors beginning at age 30. Screening includes risk factor evaluation and fasting plasma glucose.

How do patients with diabetes present?

Patients under 20 years old with type 1 diabetes usually present abruptly, often in ketoacidosis precipitated by an acute stressor such as a bacterial infection. Ketoacidosis may be accompanied by coma (10%), Kussmaul breathing (rapid deep breaths in response to acidosis), fruity breath from elevated acetone, dehydration, hypotension, and tachycardia. Some patients with type 1 diabetes present with more gradual onset of malaise, weight loss, polydipsia, polyuria, or blurred vision. Patients with type 2 diabetes more commonly present without obvious symptoms, or within weeks to months of polyuria, polydipsia, weight loss, or symptoms of end-organ complications such as altered vision (retinopathy), peripheral edema (nephropathy), or sensory changes in the distal extremities (neuropathy). Patients with diabetes can also experience recurrent infections such as boils, carbuncles, and vaginal yeast infections. Elderly patients with new onset type 2 diabetes may be in life-threatening hyperosmolar coma.

Once I have made the diagnosis, what other evaluation is important?

Among patients with type 2 diabetes, 10%–15% have neuropathy, 37% have retinopathy, and 50% have coronary artery disease at diagnosis. Pertinent history and exam (Table 26–2) as well as lab monitoring should be aimed to detect complications (Table 26–3). $HgbA_{1c}$ estimates average blood glucose over the prior three months. Obtain a baseline $HgbA_{1c}$ and repeat every six months in patients who are stable at target, and every three months in patients above target or who are changing therapy. Because patients with type 1 diabetes may have autoimmune destruction of other endocrine glands, check TSH.

What tests are appropriate for patients with DKA or hyperosmolar coma?

Obtain electrolytes, renal function, arterial blood gas, complete blood count, and urinalysis. Look for a precipitating infection with

TABLE 26–2

Pertinent History and Physical in Patients with Diabetes

	History	Exam
New diagnosis of diabetes	<ul><li>duration of symptoms</li><li>polyuria, polydipsia</li><li>current diet and exercise pattern</li><li>cardiovascular symptoms</li><li>cardiovascular risk factors cigarette use cholesterol hypertension family history of CV disease</li><li>family history of diabetes</li><li>vision disturbance</li><li>sensory changes in the extremities</li><li>medications</li></ul>	<ul><li>blood pressure (assess CV risk)</li><li>weight and height for body mass index</li><li>funduscopic exam (for retinopathy)</li><li>thyroid exam (concurrent autoimmune disease)</li><li>carotid, femoral, abdominal renal artery bruits (for atherosclerotic disease)</li><li>sensory exam with monofilament (neuropathy)</li><li>extremities for edema, ulcers</li><li>skin (fungal infections may provide portal of entry for cellulitis)</li><li>acanthosis nigricans</li></ul>
Periodic follow-up	<ul><li>hyper- or hypoglycemia symptoms</li><li>glucose monitoring results</li><li>changes in vision</li><li>changes in foot sensation</li><li>daily self exam of feet</li><li>medication tolerance</li><li>diet and exercise habits</li></ul>	<ul><li>same as above</li></ul>

TABLE 26-3

Screening and Treatment for Complications of Diabetes

	Screening Test	Recommendation	Treatment
Retinopathy	Ophthalmology referral	• Type 1: yearly beginning 5 years after diagnosis: at diagnosis if age >30 • Type 2: yearly starting at diagnosis	• Laser therapy
Nephropathy	Urine protein/creatinine ratio or 24 hour urine (microalbuminuria =30–300 mg/24 hours)	• Type 1: yearly beginning 5 years after diagnosis • Type 2: yearly	• ACEI • Angiotensin receptor blocker • BP control
Neuropathy	Foot exam: deformity, lesions, and sensory testing with a 5.0 monofilament	• Daily patient self checks • Foot exam at every visit • Yearly sensory testing	• Tricyclic antidepressants • Gabapentin • Carbamazepine • Capsaicin cream
Heart disease	ECG at diagnosis in patients with type 2; pursue testing if chest or respiratory complaints	• Type 1: fasting lipids at diagnosis, then follow lipid screening guidelines • Type 2: fasting lipids yearly	• Lower lipids with statin to LDL <100 • β-Blockers post-MI
Gastroparesis	Ask about symptoms of early satiety, nausea, emesis	• Upper GI series or nuclear medicine gastric emptying study	• Metoclopramide • Erythromycin

blood and urine cultures as well as CXR, even if the patient is afebrile. An elevated WBC (12–15), glucose greater than 250 mg/dL, elevated potassium due to cellular shifts, and anion gap acidosis with compensatory respiratory alkalosis are expected. Serum osmolarity greater than 330 can cause altered mental status. If the serum osmolarity is less than 330 with altered mental status, or if mental status does not reverse after several hours of treatment, consider head CT and lumbar puncture.

▶ **TREATMENT**

What are the goals of treatment?

In the Diabetes Control and Complications Trial (DCCT), type 1 patients treated with intensive therapy were 50%–75% less likely to have progression of retinopathy, nephropathy, and neuropathy than those treated with conventional therapy. The goal of such intensive treatment for type 1 diabetes is an HgbA$_{1c}$ less than or equal to 6.5% (normal 4%–6%), with fasting glucose less than 110 mg/dL, and two hour postprandial glucose less than 140 mg/dL. Similar goals are reasonable for type 2, though fewer outcome data exist.

How do I start treatment in patients with newly diagnosed diabetes?

Diet, exercise, and self-monitoring of blood glucose (SMBG) are the foundation of treatment. Aggressively lower coronary artery disease risk with smoking cessation and treatment for elevated blood pressure and hyperlipidemia. Glucose is best checked two–four times daily, before meals or before bed. Type 1 patients require insulin; type 2 patients may require oral medications or insulin. When starting medications, educate patients about sweating, shaking, hunger, and confusion as signs of hypoglycemia and about averting a reaction with candy or juice. Careful glucose monitoring should accompany any change in regimen.

How do I choose a starting dose of insulin?

Patients with type 1 diabetes need multiple daily subcutaneous insulin injections: short-acting to cover meals (prandial) and long-acting for basal requirements. A number of preparations are available (Table 26–4). Estimate total daily insulin dose by weight, starting at 0.5–1.0 U/kg/day. Type 1 patients and patients who have type 2 DM with little insulin resistance need less insulin. Basal (glargine)/prandial (lispro) combination regimens give half of insulin as basal and the other half prior to meals as lispro based on pre-meal glucose level and the anticipated amount to be eaten. For less intensive therapy with two shots per day, use neutral protamine Hagedorn (NPH) and regular or lispro insulin, giving two thirds of

TABLE 26-4

Selected Human Insulin Formulations and Pharmacokinetics

Insulin	Action	Onset (=lag time*)	Peak (hours)	Duration (hours)
Lispro (Humalog)	Immediate	5–15 min	0.5–1.5	≤5
Regular (Humulin R)	Rapid	30–60 min	1–5	5–7
NPH (Humulin N)	Intermediate	3–4 hours	6–12	18–28
Ultralente (Humulin U)	Prolonged	4–6 hours	12–24	36
70/30 (Humulin, 70%N/30%R)†	Mix of intermediate and rapid	30–60 min 3–4 hours (N)	6–15	22–28
Glargine (Lantus)	Prolonged	2 hours	No peak	24

*Lag time refers to the amount of time between an insulin injection and when a patient should eat. Lag time is approximately equal to onset of action (e.g., 30 minutes for regular insulin; little or no lag time with Lispro).
†Humulin 75/25, 75% N and 25% Lispro, is available and may be better for people with high carbohydrate diets.

the dose in the AM 2/3 NPH, 1/3 regular), and one third in the evening (split 1/2 NPH, 1/2 regular). If nighttime hypoglycemia is a problem, give NPH at bedtime instead of with dinner so the peak effect occurs later when early AM growth hormone and cortisol levels naturally increase blood sugar. Alternatively substitute glargine for NPH since glargine provides twenty-four hours of basal insulin and is peakless and less likely to cause hypoglycemia.

When are medications necessary in patients with type 2 diabetes?

Asymptomatic patients near ideal body weight, with no complications, or with a fasting glucose level less than 200 mg/dL may do well with diet and exercise alone. For patients who are symptomatic, have complications, or have a fasting glucose greater than 300 mg/dL, diet and oral agents are usually not enough, so insulin is appropriate initial therapy. Most patients with type 2 diabetes require diet and an oral agent. About a third of type 2 patients eventually need insulin; many patients feel better and achieve better glycemic control on insulin.

Which oral agent should I use?

Multiple oral agents are available (Table 26–5). Nonobese patients who need more than dietary treatment should start with a sulfonylurea to stimulate pancreatic insulin secretion and decrease insulin resistance. Patients who are overweight or have high triglyc-

TABLE 26-5

Common Oral Agents Used To Treat Patients with Type 2 Diabetes

Drug Example	Primary Action	Major Side Effects	Can be Used in Combination	Dose
Sulfonylureas Glyburide	Increase pancreatic insulin secretion	hypoglycemia weight gain	metformin insulin	1.25–10 mg/d
Biguanides Metformin	Decrease gluconeogenesis	GI intolerance lactic acidosis	sulfonylurea	1000–2550 mg/d divide bid-tid
Meglitinides* Repaglinide	Increase pancreatic insulin secretion	Hypoglycemia, weight gain	metformin	0.5–4 mg before each meal
Thiazolidinediones Pioglitazone Rosiglitazone	Increase uptake at the muscle	edema, weight gain, CHF, possibly liver toxicity	sulfonylurea metformin insulin	15–45 mg/d 2–8 mg/d
Alpha glucosidase inhibitors Acarbose	Slows down absorption	intestinal gas abdominal pain	sulfonylurea metformin	50–100 mg tid

*Repaglinide has shorter half life, can be given with meals and skipped when meals are skipped. Possibly less hypoglycemia, but more expensive than sulfonylureas.

erides do well on metformin, which lowers lipids and doesn't cause the weight gain common with sulfonylureas and insulin. Metformin is contraindicated in patients older than age 80, and those with CHF, liver disease, excessive alcohol use, or creatinine greater than 1.4 mg/dL because of the risk of lactic acidosis. Metformin should also be stopped temporarily in patients with sepsis, hypoxia, or dehydration, and in patients undergoing surgery or procedures requiring intravenous contrast dye. Increase doses of oral medications weekly as needed. Oral agents lower the HgbA$_{1c}$ 1%–2% except acarbose (0.5% reduction).

What should I do if one oral agent is not enough?

Many patients require combination therapy, either with a sulfonyl-urea plus metformin or an oral agent plus insulin. The combina-tion of metformin and glyburide lowers the A1C about 3%. Intermediate or long-acting insulin (0.1 u/kg) can be added at bed-time. Bedtime insulin decreases fasting glucose and causes less weight gain. Acute illness or medications such as prednisone can exacerbate hyperglycemia, necessitating short-term insulin use.

How can I prevent nephropathy and renal failure?

Slow the progression of nephropathy by controlling hypertension aggressively to BP less than 130/85 (goal approximately less than 120/85). Use angiotensin converting enzyme inhibitors (ACEI) when urine microalbumin is greater than 30 mg/L. ACEIs cannot be used in pregnancy, or when they cause hyperkalemia or angioedema. Elevated creatinine alone should not prevent ACEI use, as even patients with creatinines of three-four may benefit. Patients with higher creatinines are at increased risk for hyper-kalemia. Monitor their electrolytes and keep them volume replete. Be sure the patients do not take potassium supplements. β-Blockers and thiazide diuretics are strong choices for hyperten-sion despite mild adverse effects on glycemic control and lipids, and patients with coronary artery disease gain greater benefit than harm from β-blockers.

How do I adjust therapy when patients can't eat?

When patients are ill or fasting for a procedure, adjust therapy to avoid hypoglycemia. Patients with type 2 diabetes can hold or decrease sulfonylurea doses and monitor chemsticks. Patients on metformin should stop this medication prior to procedures or sur-gery because of the small risk of lactic acidosis; restart after forty-eight hours if creatinine is stable.

Patients with type 1 diabetes always need insulin, regardless of food intake, to prevent ketoacidosis. Since hepatic production accounts for about half of the serum glucose, give patients half their usual insulin in long-acting form, and monitor frequently. Alternatively, you may use an insulin drip.

How do I treat hypoglycemia?

Hypoglycemia is the most common endocrine emergency. Intensive therapy and decreased renal clearance of insulin or sulfonylureas are risk factors. Low serum glucose alters mental status and induces a catecholamine response (sweating, shakiness, weakness, nausea, and anxiety). β-Blockers blunt hypoglycemic symptoms except for sweating. Give oral glucose to conscious patients, and intravenous glucose and glucagon to unconscious patients. Hospitalize if the patient does not respond rapidly or if decreased renal clearance may cause recurrent symptoms.

When do I need to hospitalize patients with diabetes?

DKA, hyperosmolar coma, severe infections, severe nausea and vomiting, and cardiac ischemia are common reasons to hospitalize patients with diabetes. Cellulitis and foot ulcers often require intravenous antibiotics. Malignant otitis externa is an uncommon but life-threatening pseudomonal infection of the external ear canal which requires intravenous antibiotics. Other life-threatening infections seen with diabetes include rhinocerebral mucormycosis, emphysematous cholecystitis (*E. coli* or *Clostridium*), emphysematous pyelonephritis (*E. coli* or other gram-negative rods) and necrotizing fasciitis (mixed anaerobes and aerobes).

A patient with diabetes is hospitalized for cellulitis. How should I manage the glucose?

Patients can be given their usual regimen if glucose is less than 200 mg/dL. "Supplemental" insulin (additional insulin before meals for high glucose measurements) may be appropriate. "Sliding scale" insulin given for a high glucose without anticipating caloric intake is unacceptable because of the risk of hypoglycemia. If the patient's glucose cannot be easily controlled by insulin injections, use an insulin drip, and add glucose if the patient is not eating.

How do I treat patients with DKA?

Patients with DKA usually require intensive care for aggressive hydration with normal saline, intravenous insulin, and electrolyte monitoring and replacement. Give regular insulin, 10 U/IV bolus, followed by an insulin drip for at least twelve–twenty-four hours, with hourly glucose checks; adjust as needed. Check potassium and phosphate as these are often depleted. Serum potassium levels may not reflect total body depletion because acidosis causes a shift from cells to plasma. When the serum glucose drops to 250, intravenous fluid can be changed to D51/2NS to prevent hypoglycemia and provide calories and free water. Insulin can be changed to the outpatient regimen when bicarbonate normalizes and the patient can eat. Continue the insulin drip at least one hour after the first subcutaneous injection to prevent recurrent ketone production. Give DVT prophylaxis to comatose patients. Look carefully for a precipitating infection and use antibiotics when indicated.

How do I treat patients with hyperosmolar coma?

Hydration with isotonic saline is the mainstay of therapy. Insulin may be needed in lower doses than for DKA (5–10 U/IV bolus and 0.1 U/kg/h). As with DKA, look for and treat any precipitating infection.

K E Y   P O I N T S

▶ Type 1 diabetes is caused by lack of insulin.

▶ Type 2 diabetes results from insulin resistance.

▶ Diagnose diabetes by two fasting glucose values greater than 126, or a random glucose greater than 200 in addition to symptoms.

▶ Patients with type 1 diabetes require insulin to avoid DKA; intensive therapy reduces complications.

▶ Therapy for type 2 diabetes begins with diet and exercise; oral agents or insulin may be required to optimize glucose levels and prevent complications.

CASE 26–3. A 32-year-old woman reports thirst, frequent urination, and a 30 lb weight loss over eight weeks. She has felt markedly anorexic in the last week. She has no significant medical history and takes no medications. She is adopted and works at a sedentary job. Her weight is 220 lb, height 5'7". Vital signs and exam are normal. Her glucose is 780 and her urine is positive for glucose, and 1+ ketones.

  A. Does she have type 1 or type 2 diabetes and what evidence do you need to decide?
  B. Assuming she needs insulin, and needed 100 U/IV insulin in the first twenty-four hours in the hospital, design a regimen of basal/bolus insulin.
  C. What screening for complications does she need now?

CASE 26-4. A 58-year-old woman presents for an annual exam, having not been seen for four years. Random glucose on screening is 190 mg/dL. Review of symptoms shows nocturia. Her BMI is 31 (obese).

A. What else do you need to know at this time?

B. Her A1C comes back at 8.8%. How does the A1C correlate with her average glucose and how often should you check the A1C?

C. What therapy do you recommend?

D. BP is 140/90 and cholesterol is 240: LDL 145, HDL 45, TG 250. What interventions are warranted?

REFERENCE

The Expert Committee on the Diagnosis and Classification of Diabetes Mellitus. Report of the expert committee on the diagnosis and classification of diabetes mellitus. Diabetes Care, 20:1183, 1997.

USEFUL WEBSITE

American Diabetes Association web site:
http://www.diabetes.org/main/application/commercewf

HYPERLIPIDEMIA

▶ ETIOLOGY

Why are lipids important?

Hyperlipidemia is associated with an increased risk for coronary artery disease (CAD), the leading cause of morbidity and mortality in the United States. In particular, treating high levels of low density lipoprotein (LDL) has been shown to reduce the risk of future CAD events. Depressed high density lipoprotein cholesterol (HDL) and elevated triglyceride (TG) levels are also independently associated with increased risk of CAD events, although treatment of these isolated conditions has not been shown definitively to decrease the risk of future events. Very high triglyceride levels (greater than 1000 mg/dL) can also cause life-threatening pancreatitis.

What causes hyperlipidemia?

While some lipid abnormalities are caused by known, inborn errors of lipid metabolism, the majority of lipid disorders arise from a combination of dietary factors, lack of exercise, and some degree of genetic susceptibility. Coexisting conditions and medications may also affect lipid levels (Box 26–2).

▶ **EVALUATION**

Whom should I test for hyperlipidemia?

Anyone with known cardiovascular disease should be tested for hyperlipidemia. Controversy exists about when to screen persons without known cardiovascular disease. The National Cholesterol Education Program (NCEP) currently recommends screening every five years in all adults older than age 20. The U.S. Preventive Services Task Force, which uses stricter requirements for the evidence on which they base their guidelines, recommends screening men ages 35 to 65 and women ages 45 to 65. A reasonable approach would be to begin screening at age 35, and earlier only if the patient has significant cardiovascular risk factors (Box 26–3) or a family history of hyperlipidemia. Whether or not to screen asymptomatic patients after the age of 65 is unclear, but lipid testing is important at any age in the setting of known CAD.

What tests are available?

A complete lipid panel provides direct measurement of total cholesterol (TC), HDL, and TG and is measured after a 12-hour fast, usually in the morning before breakfast. LDL is calculated based on the formula LDL = (TC) – (HDL) – (TG÷5). You may also order isolated TC, TG, or HDL levels.

BOX 26–2

Secondary Causes of Hyperlipidemia

Poorly controlled diabetes mellitus
Hypothyroidism
Obstructive liver disease
Nephrotic syndrome
Chronic renal failure
Smoking
Drugs
    Corticosteroids
    Anabolic steroids
    Progestins
    Protease inhibitors

BOX 26–3

Cardiovascular Risk Factors, per NCEP* Guidelines, besides Elevated LDL Cholesterol

Age (men ≥ 45 years or women ≥ 55 years)
Cigarette smoking
Diabetes mellitus
Family history of premature CAD:
    CAD event in a first-degree male relative < 55 years
    CAD event in a first-degree female relative < 65 years
HDL < 40 mg/dL
Hypertension (≥ 140/90 or on medication)
Note: HDL ≥ 60 counts as a negative risk factor

---

*National Cholesterol Education Program

What test should I use?

For screening purposes, measure nonfasting levels of TC and HDL for convenience and decreased expense. If the TC is greater than or equal to 200 mg/dL or the HDL is less than 40 mg/dL, a complete fasting lipid panel is indicated. For any patient in whom treatment is possible or currently under way, obtain a fasting lipid panel to guide therapeutic decisions. When looking for causes of pancreatitis, an isolated TG level may be useful.

What happens when the lab can't calculate the LDL level?

If the patient's TG level is greater than 400, the LDL cannot be accurately calculated. This is problematic, as treatment guidelines are generally based on LDL levels. To circumvent this problem, you can assume the TG to be 400. This provides a conservative (high) estimate of your LDL (LDL = TC – HDL – 400÷5, i.e., 80) because a TG level higher than 400 would actually subtract more from the LDL figure.

▶ **TREATMENT**

How do I decide whom to treat?

Treatment decisions are usually based on an estimation of your patient's overall risk of future CAD events and the LDL level. Aggressive treatment is indicated for anyone with known CAD, other atherosclerotic disease, or diabetes mellitus. The NCEP extends those guidelines to anyone with a calculated ten-year risk of CAD events greater than or equal to 20%. For patients with less risk, treatment is less aggressive (Table 26–6). The ten-year risk

TABLE 26-6

NCEP Guidelines (Simplified) for Treatment of Hypercholesterolemia

Patient's Cardiovascular Risk Factor Profile	Goal LDL (by diet or drugs)	Threshold LDL for Starting Drug Therapy
CAD, other atherosclerotic disease, diabetes mellitus, or 10-year risk >20%	<100 mg/dL	≥130 mg/dL
2+ risk factors, and 10-year risk 10%–20%	<130 mg/dL	≥130 mg/dL
2+ risk factors, and 10-year risk < 10%	<130 mg/dL	≥160 mg/dL
0–1 risk factors	<160 mg/dL	≥190 mg/dL

of events can be calculated using a point system or computerized risk model. One example of such a risk calculator, based on the Framingham study, is provided on the National Heart, Lung, and Blood Institute website (see website reference later).

Are diet, exercise, and other lifestyle modifications helpful?

Diet, Weight loss, Exercise, ETOH restriction is first line therapy

A regular exercise program can lower LDL and TG levels and increase HDL levels. Eating a diet low in total fat (25%–35% of total calories) and saturated fats (less than 7% of total calories) and high in soluble fiber and plant stanols/sterols can decrease cholesterol levels. Although dietary interventions have not been clearly shown to reduce future CAD events, both diet and exercise are recommended in all persons with hyperlipidemia. Before starting medications, a six to twelve week trial of lifestyle modification, with or without referral to a dietitian, is often appropriate and can be sufficient to treat mild hyperlipidemia. Diet, exercise, weight loss, and alcohol restriction are first line therapy for hypertriglyceridemia.

What medications are used to treat hyperlipidemia?

Statin First line drugs

Decreasing the risk of future cardiovascular events has been most clearly documented with HMG CoA reductase inhibitors ("statins"), and these should be considered first line therapy in patients with known CAD and elevated LDL. Some consideration may be given to cost, differing effects on the lipid profile, and side effects (Table 26–7) when choosing between other available agents; however, treatment is focused on reducing LDL level. This is done most efficiently with statins. Side effects of statins include rare myopathy and generally insignificant liver enzyme elevations. For patients without known CAD who have high LDL and low HDL levels, niacin is a low-cost alternative. The flushing and headache associated with niacin can be attenuated by pretreatment with aspirin and slow upward dose titration. Older extended-release niacin preparations were associated

TABLE 26-7

Lipid-Lowering Medications

Drug	Cost	Action	Side Effects
HMG CoA reductase inhibitors "statins"	$$$	LDL ↓ ↓ TG ↓ HDL ↑	Myopathy Elevated liver enzymes GI distress Headache, Insomnia
Nicotinic acid niacin	$	LDL ↓ TG ↓ ↓ HDL ↑	Flushing, headache, tachycardia, pruritus Hyperuricemia Hyperglycemia Hepatotoxicity
Fibric acid gemfibrozil clofibrate	$	LDL ↓ TG ↓ ↓ HDL ↑ ↑	Myopathy, small ↑'d risk with statins, ↑ ↑ ↑'d with cyclosporine, erythromycin, and ketoconazole Gallstones Hepatotoxicity GI malignancy Nausea
Bile-acid sequestrants colestipol cholestyramine	$$	LDL ↓ TG ↑ HDL ↔	↓'d absorption of many other medications GI distress, constipation

[handwritten annotations in margin: "Best for Pt c̄ CAD" next to HMG CoA reductase inhibitors; "Best for s̄ CAD" next to Nicotinic acid]

with hepatotoxicity; newer preparations appear to be safer. In some patients who have very elevated TG, or low HDL levels in the absence of elevated LDL, a fibric acid derivative such as gemfibrozil may be indicated. Bile acid sequestrants may also be used, usually in combination with another agent, to further lower LDL levels. Both these agents commonly cause some gastrointestinal upset.

Is hormone replacement therapy a reasonable alternative for treatment of hyperlipidemia in postmenopausal women?

While estrogen has been shown to decrease LDL and TG levels and to increase HDL levels, evidence from randomized clinical trials casts doubt on the protective effects of estrogen against CAD seen in observational studies. Estrogen, with or without progestin, should not be used for the treatment of hyperlipidemia, although it may be indicated for other reasons.

Are there other alternatives to cholesterol-lowering medications?

Increasing dietary omega-3 fatty acids by consuming fish and fish oil (30 gm/day or two fish meals weekly) has been shown to reduce total cholesterol, triglycerides, raise HDL, and lower mortality. Soluble dietary fiber, found in legumes, oat bran, fruit, and psyllium, has also been associated with significant lowering of cholesterol levels. Mild-to-moderate consumption of alcohol (less than 1 oz/day = 2 oz whiskey = 8 oz wine = 24 oz of beer) is associated with increased HDL levels and reduced incidence of CAD. The potential harmful effects of excess alcohol ingestion preclude routine recommendations for its use in preventing CAD. Vitamin E and beta-carotene are antioxidants that have been shown to reduce the oxidation of lipids, but clinical trials to date have shown no benefit in clinical outcomes.

Are there any other ways to decrease the risk of future CAD events?

Yes. Assess and treat any other cardiovascular risk factors. Counsel patients to quit smoking, and aggressively treat hypertension and diabetes mellitus. These are well-established, effective ways of preventing CAD events.

K E Y   P O I N T S

▶ Screen otherwise healthy patients with nonfasting total cholesterol and HDL.

▶ Treatment goals should be commensurate with estimated future risk of CHD events.

▶ Statins prevent death and cardiovascular events in patients with known CAD.

CASE 26–5. For each of the following cases, decide whether to test for hyperlipidemia and choose which test you would order:

A. 50-year-old man with hypertension and diabetes
B. 25-year-old woman whose father had a heart attack at age 60
C. 45-year-old woman with pancreatitis and no history of alcoholism or gallstones
D. 36-year-old man presenting for a history and physical
E. 60-year-old woman with hypertension presenting 6 weeks after attempting diet and exercise therapy for a total cholesterol level of 220

CASE 26-6. A 50-year-old obese man with hypertension gets a complete fasting lipid panel: TC 240, HDL 40, TG 500, LDL "cannot be calculated."

A. Calculate the LDL level assuming the TG level is 400. Is the actual LDL level higher or lower than this estimate?

B. What therapy, if any, would you recommend to this man?

CASE 26-7. A 57-year-old postmenopausal woman has persistent hypercholesterolemia after six months of diet therapy. Her only other risk factor is hypertension. Total cholesterol = 293, TG = 159, LDL = 215, HDL = 46, glucose = 90, and TSH = 9.3 (high).

A. What is her goal cholesterol?

B. Would you start a medication now and, if so, which medication would you choose?

REFERENCES

Executive Summary of the Third Report of the National Cholesterol Education Program (NCEP) Expert Panel on Detection, Evaluation, and Treatment of High Blood Cholesterol in Adults (Adult Treatment Panel III). JAMA 285(19):2486–2497, 2001.

Screening and Treating Adults for Lipid Disorders: Recommendations and Rationale. U.S. Preventive Services Task Force. Am J Prev Med 20(3S):73–76, 2001.

USEFUL WEBSITE

National Heart, Lung, and Blood Institute website risk calculator: *http://hin.nhlbi.nih.gov/atpiii/calculator.asp? usertype*=prof

MALE HYPOGONADISM

▶ ETIOLOGY

What is male hypogonadism?

Male hypogonadism is a syndrome of low serum androgen levels associated with gynecomastia, sarcopenia (loss of muscle mass), weakness, osteopenia, sexual dysfunction, and loss of sense of well-being. Sometimes, hypogonadism is diagnosed in men whose serum testosterone levels are in the low-normal range at the time of diagnosis. These men may benefit from treatment because their serum testosterone level is below their normal baseline level. The male gonads have two important functions: production of sex steroid hormones and spermatogenesis. Men with deficient testosterone production inevitably have decreased or absent spermatogenesis and diminished fertility. Technically, an isolated defect in spermatogenesis is a form of male hypogonadism, but the term "hypogonadism" is normally used to connote testosterone deficiency.

What are the types of male hypogonadism?

Primary hypogonadism is defined as testosterone deficiency due to a testicular defect. Secondary hypogonadism occurs when pituitary or hypothalamic dysfunction results in decreased secretion of the gonadotropins, follicle stimulating hormone (FSH), and luteinizing hormone (LH).

What causes hypogonadism?

The most common cause of primary hypogonadism is Klinefelter's syndrome, a syndrome associated with an XXY karyotype. Other causes of primary hypogonadism include postpubertal orchitis (mumps), bilateral orchidectomy, and testicular trauma (Table 26–8). Common causes of secondary hypogonadism include large pituitary tumors (macroadenomas) and hemochromatosis. Hypogonadism is often the first sign of these diseases. Supraphysiological (endogenous or exogenous) corticosteroids also suppress gonadotropin secretion and cause secondary hypogonadism. A rare (1 in 10,000 male births) congenital cause of secondary hypogonadism is Kallmann's syndrome, which is associated with inadequate secretion of gonadotropin-releasing hormone from the hypothalamus to the pituitary. Any severe chronic systemic illness, such as uremia and HIV, may also cause secondary hypogonadism. Many of these patients will benefit from androgen replacement therapy. Men who are hospitalized with any

TABLE 26–8	

Common Causes of Primary and Secondary Hypogonadism

Cause	Distinguishing Features
Primary hypogonadism	
Klinefelter's syndrome	Very small testes, XXY karyotype
Postpubertal mumps orchitis	Soft testes, normal size
Orchidectomy	No testes
Trauma	Soft testes, normal size
Secondary hypogonadism	
Pituitary macroadenoma	Headaches, visual complaints
Cushing's syndrome	Easy bruisability, thin skin
Hemochromatosis	Advanced disease: hyperpigmented skin liver failure

severe acute disease might have transient suppression of circulating gonadotropins and testosterone levels that normalize with resolution of the acute disease. Older men (more than 60 years) often have low or low-normal serum testosterone levels. It is controversial whether these men have hypogonadism that will benefit from androgen replacement therapy.

▶ DIAGNOSIS

When should I suspect male hypogonadism?

Male hypogonadism is a very common disorder that is often undiagnosed for years after the onset because the symptoms and signs are often vague and nonspecific (Box 26–4). Hypogonadism

BOX 26–4	

Common Manifestations of Male Hypogonadism

Symptoms
 Decreased sexual function (diminished libido)
 Decreased energy
 Diminished sense of well-being
 Weakness
 Tender gynecomastia
 Infertility

Signs
 Decreased rate of facial hair growth
 Gynecomastia extending beyond areola
 Small or soft testes (<3.5 cm in longest axis)
 Atraumatic/osteoporotic fracture

should be suspected in men who complain of gynecomastia, weakness, or sexual dysfunction. Sexual dysfunction due to hypogonadism usually manifests as decreased libido and sexual pleasure. Hypogonadism is seldom the sole cause of erectile dysfunction. All men with osteopenia should be evaluated for hypogonadism. It should also be suspected in men with unexplained hypoproliferative anemia.

What tests should I order to make the diagnosis of hypogonadism?

When male hypogonadism is suspected, order serum total testosterone, FSH, and LH levels. Although there are commercial assays for free (unbound) bioactive serum testosterone, these assays are fraught with problems, tend to underestimate the true free testosterone levels, and lead to the over-diagnosis of hypogonadism. In the next few years, it is likely that useful assays of serum bioavailable or calculated free testosterone will become available. FSH and LH levels are helpful in determining the etiology of the hypogonadism and can help to confirm hypogonadism in men with low-normal serum testosterone levels. In primary hypogonadism, serum FSH and LH levels are elevated even in those men with low-normal serum testosterone levels. No further evaluation is necessary, although a serum karyotype may be done to look for Klinefelter's syndrome. In secondary hypogonadism, serum testosterone levels are low, and serum FSH and LH levels are inappropriately normal or low. If secondary hypogonadism is diagnosed, order head MRI to exclude a pituitary macroadenoma and ferritin or transferrin saturation to exclude hemochromatosis. A careful H & P for evidence of thin skin (easy bruisability and violaceous striae) and proximal muscle weakness is generally an adequate evaluation for Cushing's syndrome as the cause of secondary hypogonadism.

▶ TREATMENT

How do I treat male hypogonadism?

Treatment should address both androgen replacement and fertility restoration. Androgen replacement should be considered for all hypogonadal men, but therapy to restore fertility is expensive and should be reserved for men with secondary hypogonadism who are attempting to conceive within the next year. Men with primary hypogonadism are generally infertile and will not respond to medical therapy to improve fertility. Men with secondary hypogonadism might have improved fertility after normalization of FSH and LH levels by appropriate treatment with gonadotropin-releasing hormone or gonadotropin replacement therapy.

What are the options available for androgen replacement therapy?

Androgen replacement therapy may be safely and effectively accomplished with transdermal (a patch system or a gel) testosterone or intramuscular testosterone injections (Table 26–9). Transdermal testosterone provides hormone levels that mimic normal circadian rhythm—highest in the morning with an evening nadir. Intramuscular administration peaks at twenty-four to forty-eight hours and gradually decreases without the diurnal variation until the next dose. At normal intramuscular replacement doses, the peak testosterone level may be supraphysiological. Although the clinical significance of this is unknown, some men have difficulty with cyclic acne and moodiness around the time of the peak level.

What are the risks and benefits of androgen replacement therapy?

Androgen replacement therapy has been shown to increase strength, bone mass, sexual function, and sense of well-being in hypogonadal men. The most common side effect of androgen replacement therapy is erythrocytosis, and an HCT must be checked periodically (at least annually). Overall, the data suggest

TABLE 26–9

Forms of Androgen Replacement Therapy Available in the U.S.

Route	Frequency	Advantages	Disadvantages
Scrotal patch	Daily	Provides physiological testosterone levels	Expensive Requires scrotal shaving Patch often falls off Difficult to adjust dosage May not provide enough testosterone
Nonscrotal patch	Daily	Provides physiological testosterone levels	Expensive Often causes dermatitis Difficult to adjust dosage May not provide enough testosterone
Transdermal gel	Daily	Provides physiological testosterone levels Easy to adjust dosage	Very expensive
Intramuscular injection	Every 7–14 days	Inexpensive if self-injected (or injected by friend) Relatively easy to adjust dosage	Does not provide physiological testosterone level Requires injections

that there is a neutral effect or a small benefit to cardiovascular risk factors when hypogonadal men take androgen replacement therapy. There is no evidence that androgen replacement therapy increases the risk of prostate disease, but hypogonadal men should be offered counseling and screening for prostate disease just as you would for age-matched eugonadal men.

K E Y   P O I N T S

▶ Hypogonadism should be excluded in all men with sexual dysfunction, osteoporosis, unexplained weakness, unexplained anemia, or symptomatic gynecomastia.

▶ It is important to distinguish between primary hypogonadism (with elevated serum gonadotropins) and secondary hypogonadism (with low or inappropriately normal serum gonadotropins).

▶ A pituitary macroadenoma, hemochromatosis, and Cushing's syndrome are the most common causes of secondary hypogonadism.

CASE 26–8. A 32-year-old man reports painful, enlarged breast tissue. He and his wife have had difficulty conceiving. His physical examination is unremarkable except that he has tender gynecomastia that extends beyond both areolas, and he has small testes. His serum testosterone level is low and his serum gonadotropins are elevated.

     A. What type of hypogonadism does he have?
     B. What is the most likely diagnosis?
     C. What is the treatment?

CASE 26–9. A 42-year-old man reports fatigue, decreased energy, and diminished sex drive. He has recently started taking a β-blocker for treatment of hypertension. His serum testosterone level is low, and his gonadotropin levels are normal.

     A. What is the differential diagnosis of his syndrome?
     B. What further diagnostic studies should be done?

REFERENCES

Anawalt BD, Merriam GR: Neuroendocrine aging in men: Andropause and somatopause. Endocrinol Metab Clin of North Am 30:647–671, 2001.
Nehra A: Treatment of endocrinologic male sexual dysfunction. Mayo Clin Proc 75:540–545, 2000.

THYROID DISEASE

▶ ETIOLOGY

What are the most likely causes of hyperthyroidism?

Graves' disease is commonly seen in young women and is due to an antibody that turns on the TSH receptor. *Toxic multinodular goiter* is seen in the elderly and occurs when one or more clones of cells grow into nontender, autonomously functioning nodules. *Subacute thyroiditis* follows viral respiratory infection and causes a painful enlarged thyroid gland, elevated ESR, and transient hyperthyroidism followed by transient hypothyroidism. *Silent thyroiditis*, occurring postpartum, may be a nonpainful variant of subacute thyroiditis. There may be no preceding viral infection or elevated ESR.

What causes hypothyroidism?

In over 95% of patients, hypothyroidism is due to thyroid gland failure or removal. *Iatrogenic* hypothyroidism from ablation or removal of the thyroid gland is the most common cause in developed nations. *Iodine insufficiency* is the most common cause of hypothyroidism worldwide and causes diffuse thyroid enlargement or goiter. With iodine plentiful and the thyroid intact, *Hashimoto's thyroiditis* is the next most common condition, an autoimmune disease associated with antimicrosomal antibodies against thyroid peroxidase. Hashimoto's thyroiditis may coexist with other autoimmune disorders, including Sjögren's disease, diabetes, pernicious anemia, or lupus, and can be complicated by lymphoma, especially in the few men with Hashimoto's. Less than 5% of hypothyroidism is secondary, usually due to *pituitary failure*. This diagnosis is important to make since thyroid replacement in panhypopituitarism can precipitate fatal adrenal insufficiency if no mineralocorticoids or glucocorticoids are given.

What causes thyroid nodules?

Though thyroid nodules are recognized in only 5% of cases, autopsies show 50% prevalence. Approximately 5%–10% of solitary thyroid nodules are malignant, the majority of which are papillary or follicular carcinomas—well-differentiated, slow-growing, and curable by resection when found early. Medullary thyroid carcinoma is uncommon and may be sporadic or inherited as part of a multiple endocrine neoplasia syndrome, MEN-2. Lymphoma rarely complicates Hashimoto's thyroiditis. Anaplastic thyroid carcinoma is rare but aggressive with average survival less than one year.

▶ EVALUATION

What questions are pertinent if I suspect hyperthyroidism?

Ask about weight loss despite a healthy appetite, nervousness, emotional lability, excessive sweating, tremor, palpitations, heat intolerance, frequent bowel movements, diarrhea, altered menses (usually amennorrhea), and insomnia. Elderly patients may present less typically, with "apathetic" hyperthyroidism manifesting as anorexia, weakness, blunted affect, depression, or slowed mentation. CHF, angina, or arrhythmias may be precipitated or worsened by thyroid disease, so do a good cardiopulmonary review of systems (Box 26–5).

How does thyroid storm present?

Thyroid storm is a life-threatening presentation of extreme hyperthyroidism. Decompensation in one or more organ systems occurs with fever as high as 106°F, delirium or even frank psychosis, seizures, tachyarrhythmia, angina, high output cardiac failure, or

BOX 26–5

Symptoms and Signs of Hyperthyroidism

Symptoms
Weight loss
Fatigue, insomnia
Palpitations
Tremor
Weakness
Sweating, heat intolerance
Nervousness, irritability
Diarrhea, frequent stools
Menstrual irregularities (usually amenorrhea)

Signs
Tachycardia, atrial fibrillation, CHF, hypertension
Abnormal thyroid gland exam
Proximal muscle weakness
Lid lag (all causes)
Proptosis (Graves' only)
Pretibial myxedema (Graves' only)

cardiogenic shock. Precipitants include infection, surgery, iodine in contrast dyes, ablative therapy, amiodarone, and trauma.

What should I look for on exam when I suspect hyperthyroidism?

Observe for agitation, fine tremor, nail clubbing, and onycholysis (fingernail separation from the nail bed). Feel for velvety moist skin from excess sweating. Palpate the thyroid. Multiple nodules suggest multinodular goiter; diffuse enlargement is consistent with Graves' disease; and a tender, hard gland suggests viral thyroiditis. Ask patients to rise from a chair with arms crossed to detect proximal muscle weakness. Check for signs of sympathetic overstimulation: tachycardia, arrhythmias, hyperreflexia, lid lag on oculomotor testing (white sclera visible above the iris with downward gaze), and widened palpebral fissures causing a frightened stare. These reverse with therapy for the hyperthyroid state. Check for exophthalmos (protrusion of the eyeballs) due to infiltration of the eye muscles in Graves' disease. Unlike lid lag, exophthalmos does not reverse with treatment. Look for pretibial myxedema, an infiltrative dermopathy seen on the anterior shins due to Graves' disease.

What history and exam suggests hypothyroidism?

Onset is often insidious and may be overlooked by patients and physicians because hypothyroidism can mimic normal aging. Hypothyroid patients are often fatigued (although most fatigued patients do not have hypothyroidism). Ask about dry skin, slowed speech, hoarseness, cold intolerance, myalgias, weakness, muscle cramps, depression, constipation, altered menses (usually menorrhagia), and weight gain. Paradoxical weight loss may occur from poor bowel motility and anorexia, especially in the elderly. On exam, look for hypothermia, bradycardia, pale cool doughy skin, pitting edema in the lower extremities, periorbital edema, coarse skin and hair, macroglossia, pleural effusion, and distant heart sounds suggesting a pericardial effusion. Neurologic manifestations can include impaired mentation, dementia, ataxia, psychosis, deafness, carpal tunnel syndrome, "hung-up" reflexes with a delayed relaxation phase, and bradykinesia. Severe hypothyroidism may cause cardiac failure or coma (Box 26–6).

What studies do I order if I suspect thyroid disease?

Order a TSH. If the TSH is low, then check a free T4. Other lab abnormalities that may accompany hypothyroidism include anemia, hypercholesterolemia, hyponatremia, elevated SGOT, LDH, and CPK. CXR may reveal cardiomegaly in hypothyroid patients due to pericardial effusion. ECG may show bradycardia or decreased voltage, if pericardial effusion is present, with hypothy-

---

BOX 26–6

Symptoms and Signs of Hypothyroidism

Symptoms
Weight gain
Fatigue, hypersomnolence
Weakness, myalgias, muscle cramps
Hoarseness
Cold intolerance
Impaired mentation, depressed mood
Peripheral and periorbital edema
Dry skin
Coarse hair
Constipation
Menstrual irregularities (usually menorrhagia)

Signs
Altered mental status, coma, depression, psychosis
Bradycardia, hypotension, CHF
Edema
Pleural effusion
Pericardial effusion
Reflexes with a delayed relaxation phase

---

roidism. Sinus tachycardia or possibly atrial fibrillation may accompany hyperthyroidism. Consider bone density testing in patients with prolonged hyperthyroidism to assess for bone loss.

What does it mean if my patient has a high TSH?

TSH cannot be interpreted alone. The most common cause of a high TSH is an underactive thyroid gland (primary hypothyroidism). A concomitant low free T4 confirms this. Since TSH is very sensitive to small changes in T4, it may rise before a drop in T4 is detected. This situation is called subclinical hypothyroidism because patients are usually asymptomatic. In rare cases, both free T4 and TSH are high, implicating a TSH-producing pituitary or GYN tumor. TSH takes four to six weeks to reflect changes in thyroid hormone replacement.

Does a low TSH imply primary hyperthyroidism?

Yes, usually. This is confirmed by the clinical picture and a high free T4. In the rare instance where both TSH and free T4 are low with hypothyroid symptoms, secondary hypothyroidism from pituitary failure is likely.

When do I need to check a free T3?

T4 is the inactive form of hormone produced in the thyroid and converted to active T3 in the periphery. Elevated T3 can be missed if not specifically measured. If TSH is low in the setting of hyper-thyroid symptoms but free T4 is normal or low, obtain free T3 to look for T3 toxicosis.

When do I need to check antithyroid antibodies?

Most Hashimoto's and many Graves' disease patients have antimi-crosomal and/or antithyroglobulin antibodies. Graves' patients may also have antithyroid receptor antibodies. Occasionally, Graves' ophthalmopathy causes proptosis without hyperthyroidism. The presence of thyroid antibodies obviates the need for further work-up for retro-orbital mass or vascular lesion. Patients with other autoimmune disorders can be checked for antithyroid antibodies to determine if frequent TSH monitoring is warranted.

How do I tell the difference between a malignant and benign thyroid nodule?

The strongest risk factor for thyroid malignancy is prior head and neck irradiation: one third of nodules are malignant in these high-risk patients. Other risk factors include male gender, family his-tory, childhood onset, rapid growth, hard fixed nontender nodules larger than 4 cm, hoarseness, local compressive symptoms, and ipsilateral adenopathy or a Delphian node in the midline just above the thyroid isthmus. *Fine needle aspiration* (FNA), the initial nod-ule evaluation of choice, yields a benign diagnosis in 70%–80% of patients and a malignant diagnosis in 5%. The remaining 10%–20% are nondiagnostic and require further work-up, usually by surgical removal. Although ultrasound distinguishes solid from cystic lesions, this is not useful as either of these lesions could be malignant. Radioactive iodine scan identifies the 10% of nod-ules that are "hot" nodules (take up radiolabeled iodine) and there-fore are unlikely to be malignant. Of the remaining 90% of nondiagnostic-FNA nodules, surgical exploration is mandatory as two of ten are malignant.

▶ TREATMENT

What are the options for treatment of hyperthyroid patients?

Hyperthyroidism causes unpleasant and potentially dangerous symptoms in the short-term, and long-term may cause osteo-porosis, cardiac arrthymias, and CHF. Medications for symptom management include *propranolol* to block sympathetic stimulation and thereby decrease tremor, palpitations, and tachycardia. The negative inotropy may worsen CHF, however. In acute thyroiditis, *glucocorticoids* shorten the course and decrease thyroid pain but are rarely needed. Antithyroid medications *propylthiouracil* (PTU) and *methimazole* decrease thyroid hormone production and release. PTU also blocks peripheral conversion of T4 to active T3. Although most patients achieve a euthyroid state by six weeks on these medications, 35%–40% experience relapse. Because these antithyroid drugs rarely cause agranulocytosis, CBC monitoring is important especially in older patients. *Radioiodine ablation* is effective for both Graves' disease and multinodular goiter but leads to iatrogenic hypothyroidism in 75% of the cases. Check TSH periodically after ablation. *Surgical removal* of the thyroid gland is reserved for local compressive symptoms, failure to respond to other therapies, or possible malignancy.

How do I treat hypothyroid patients?

Asymptomatic patients with subclinical hypothyroidism (normal free T4 and mildly elevated TSH) can be followed without therapy, although patients may feel better if treated with low-dose thyroxine. Start clearly hypothyroid patients on oral thyroxine at around 100 µg/day. Start more gingerly at 25 µg/day in elderly patients and those with known coronary artery disease; this avoids precipitating angina or MI. Intravenous thyroxine is reserved for life-threatening coma.

When should I hospitalize a patient for thyroid disease?

Hypothyroid myxedema coma is an endocrine emergency with stupor, hypothermia, bradycardia, and hypoventilation. It may be associated with hypoglycemia, anemia, hyponatremia, or adrenal insufficiency. Treat the patient in the hospital with parenteral levothyroxine, high dose glucocorticoids to prevent adrenal crisis, and intensive supportive therapy. Myxedema coma may develop insidiously or may be precipitated by infection, cold exposure, sedative drugs, or failure to take thyroid replacement. Life-

---

K E Y   P O I N T S

▶ TSH is very sensitive: small changes in T4 cause large changes in TSH.

▶ When TSH and free T4 are abnormal at opposite levels, there is a primary thyroid problem.

▶ TSH levels lag behind dosage changes by about four to six weeks.

▶ In the elderly or in those with coronary artery disease, start with low-dose replacement.

▶ The procedure of choice for the initial work-up of a thyroid nodule is FNA.

threatening hyperthyroidism, or thyroid storm, also requires hospitalization for monitoring and initiating antithyroid drugs, iodine to inhibit hormone release, and β-blockers to decrease adrenergic effects and block peripheral conversion of T4 to T3. Glucocorticoids may have a role. Iopanoic acid or ipodate (radiographic contrast agents) can be added to block hormone release and decrease peripheral T4 to T3 conversion.

CASE 26–10. A 75-year-old man is brought to your office by his daughter because he seems depressed and weak. He has been losing weight with a poor appetite, has become much less interactive, and is now unable to climb the three stairs to his room without assistance. On exam he is a slender, elderly man in no acute distress with a mild tremor, an irregular pulse of 100, a lumpy, nontender thyroid, and clear lung sounds.

  A. What is your differential diagnosis?
  B. TSH is less than 0.1, free T4 is elevated. What thyroid condition is most likely?
  C. What treatment do you want to offer him?

CASE 26–11. A 63-year-old woman is brought to the ED. Her landlord found her slumped in her easy chair after he noticed that she hadn't paid her rent. On exam, she moans to painful stimuli, T is 34, P is 45, BP is 110/80, RR is 6. Skin is cool, dry, and doughy; tongue is large. Heart sounds are inaudible; lungs reveal diffuse rales; rectal vault contains hardened pellets of stool; CXR reveals a massive heart, pleural fluid, and pulmonary vascular cephalization.

  A. What is your differential diagnosis for her altered mental status?
  B. TSH is very high at 95, free T4 is low. Name your diagnosis and seven features of her presentation to support it.
  C. How will you manage this patient?
  D. What other labs are likely to be abnormal?
  E. What are likely causes of the hypothyroidism?

REFERENCES

Helfand M, Redfern CC: Clinical guideline, part 2. Screening for thyroid disease: An update. American College of Physicians. Ann Intern Med 129:144, 1998.

Mulder JE: Thyroid disease in women. Med Clin North Am 82:103, 1998.

27

Gastroenterology

▶ ETIOLOGY

What are causes of biliary tract disease?

Blockage of the bile ducts leads to cholecystitis or cholangitis. Blockage is usually due to gallstones, but rarely is caused by cholangiocarcinoma, primary sclerosing cholangitis, or extrinsic compression by tumor or adenopathy. Cholecystitis is inflammation or infection of the gallbladder from obstruction of the cystic duct, usually by a gallstone. Cholangitis is a deadly infection arising in the common bile duct due to ductal obstruction. The gallbladder is usually uninvolved. Primary sclerosing cholangitis (PSC) causes inflammation and scarring from unclear cause. PSC leaves the biliary ducts thickened and irregularly narrowed and eventually causes cirrhosis and hepatic failure. Patients with ulcerative colitis are at risk for PSC.

▶ EVALUATION

What is a pertinent history?

The classic patient with gallstones is "fat, fertile, forty, and female," a derogatory but accurate characterization of the risk factors. Cystic duct occlusion occurs as postprandial right upper quadrant pain, worse with fatty food ingestion, as much as three to four hours after eating. It commonly occurs at night between 10 PM and 2 AM. It can be intermittent or progressive. If blockage persists, pain becomes steady, often radiating to the right shoulder. High fever is rare. In contrast, cholangitis is a gastrointestinal emergency, the patient presenting with a triad of high spiking fevers with rigors, jaundice, and right upper quadrant pain. If tumor is obstructing the common bile duct, painless jaundice may develop gradually over weeks prior to onset of infection. When bile flow to the intestine is completely obstructed, urine is dark (bilirubinuria) and stools are light. More than 30% of patients with cholangitis have concomitant pancreatitis, with pain radiating to the back. With PSC, patients have intermittent flares of jaundice, pruritus, right upper quadrant pain, and sometimes frank cholangitis.

What do I look for on physical exam?

Fever, tachycardia, hypotension, right upper quadrant pain, and guarding can occur with both cholecystitis and cholangitis. Peritoneal signs are usually absent. Jaundice is a feature of cholangitis, but is absent in cholecystitis. Fifty percent of patients with cholecystitis have a palpably enlarged gallbladder. The classic exam finding is Murphy's sign. Palpate the liver edge deeply at the midclavicular line and ask the patient to inhale. When the inflamed gallbladder meets the hand, the patient abruptly stops breathing in. Unfortunately, sensitivity and specificity are low for this maneuver.

What labs and studies should I order?

When either cholecystitis or cholangitis is suspected, order CBC, blood cultures, liver function tests, amylase, and imaging. The hallmarks of ductal blockage are elevated alkaline phosphatase, GGT, and bilirubin. A thickened, edematous gallbladder wall on ultrasound or CT suggests cholecystitis. Common bile duct dilation suggests cholangitis. If cholecystitis is suspected but ultrasound is normal, an HIDA scan can confirm cholecystitis by absence of tracer uptake in the gallbladder. ERCP confirms PSC by the beaded appearance of the bile ducts or cholangiocarcinoma by biopsy.

▶ TREATMENT

What treatment steps are appropriate for patients with cholecystitis or cholangitis?

For cholecystitis or cholangitis, start broad-spectrum intravenous antibiotics to cover gram-negative enterics, gram-positives (*Clostridium*, enterococcus), and anaerobes (*Bacteroides*). Volume resuscitate as needed. Patients with cholecystitis may respond to antibiotics alone and warrant eventual elective cholecystectomy. Asymptomatic patients with gallstones do not require their removal. Worsening fever or leukocytosis does warrant urgent cholecystectomy. For cholangitis, consult GI immediately for emergent ERCP with sphincterotomy to decompress the common bile duct.

Do most patients get better from cholecystitis and cholangitis?

At least 25% of patients with cholecystitis require urgent surgery. Complications of cholecystitis include empyema, gangrene, or gallbladder perforation with a mortality, 30%. Cholangitis is fatal if untreated.

K E Y   P O I N T S

▶ Right upper quadrant pain, high fever, and jaundice prove cholangitis until shown otherwise.

▶ Cholangitis is a GI emergency and warrants urgent imaging and GI consultation.

CASE 27-1. A 49-year-old woman with obesity, diabetes, and hypertension reports several hours of severe, steady abdominal pain with an episode of emesis. T is 102°F, P is 120, BP is 100/80, and RR is 28. Her abdomen is obese with right upper quadrant tenderness.

A. What information do you need to narrow your differential diagnosis?
B. Which of the diseases on your list of possibilities is most worrisome? Most likely?
C. Where do you want to take care of her?
D. What intervention is likely most important right now?

REFERENCES

Kalloo AN: Gallstones and biliary disease. Primary Care; Clinics in Office Practice 28(3):591–606, 2001.
Lee YM, Kaplan M: Medical progress: Primary sclerosing cholangitis. N Engl J Med 332:924–933, 1995.

LIVER DISEASE

▶ ETIOLOGY

How is liver disease categorized?

Liver disease is categorized by whether it affects the biliary tree or the parenchymal cells. Biliary tree disorders generally elevate alkaline phosphatase and bilirubin. Hepatocellular injury elevates liver transaminases (ALT, AST) more dramatically than bilirubin or alkaline phosphatase. This chapter focuses on causes of hepatocellular/parenchymal injury.

What are the causes of elevated transaminases?

Transaminases greater than 2000 mg/dL are caused by viral hepatitis, drug-induced hepatitis, or ischemic hepatitis such as with shock. Other causes of hepatocellular injury that raise transminases more modestly include alcohol, passive liver congestion from right-sided heart failure, autoimmune disorders, inherited storage disorders, tumors, and non-alcoholic steatohepatitis.

What epidemiologic features distinguish the major causes of viral hepatitis?

Viral hepatitis epidemiology is summarized in Table 27–1. Hepatitis A and E are passed by the fecal-oral route, while hepatitis B, C, and D are acquired parenterally, usually through sexual contact, transfusion, or injection-drug use. *Hepatitis A virus* (HAV) is endemic in developing countries where it causes approximately 35% of cases of acute viral hepatitis. Infection with *hepatitis B virus* (HBV) is often asymptomatic. Less than 5% of individuals who are infected as adults develop chronic infection; by contrast, 90% of perinatally acquired hepatitis B infections become chronic. *Hepatitis C virus* (HCV) is the most common chronic blood-borne infection in the U.S., with 60% of transmission due to injection-drug use. Unlike hepatitis B, most individuals develop chronic infection with hepatitis C.

TABLE 27–1

Epidemiologic Features of Viral Hepatitis				
Virus	Transmission	Risk factors	% Who become chronic carriers	Incubation period (days)
A	Fecal–oral	Travel in developing countries	None	15–60
B	Parenteral	IDU, male-male sex, health care worker, unprotected sex, tattoos	10% (90% if perinatal)	45–160
C	Parenteral	Same as HBV, intranasal cocaine use	80%	14–180
D	Parenteral	IDU, coinfection with HBV, unprotected sex	2–70%	42–180
E	Fecal–oral	No cases seen in U.S.	None*	15–60

*Hepatitis E infection carries a 30% mortality if acquired in the 3rd trimester of pregnancy.

The course of infection is insidious, and most patients do not notice any symptoms during the first two decades of infection. *Hepatitis D virus* (HDV) requires coinfection with HBV in order to replicate. Seroprevalence is low in the U.S. except in injection-drug users and recipients of multiple transfusions. *Hepatitis E virus* (HEV) infection is usually inconsequential and self-limited, although mortality rates greater than 30% have been seen in women infected during the third trimester of pregnancy.

What are the most important causes of chronic liver disease?

Chronic liver disease is any condition that causes hepatic inflammation for longer than six months. Chronic liver disease from all causes is the tenth leading cause of death among U.S. adults. The most common causes include chronic viral hepatitis from HBV and HCV. Other etiologies include alcohol, autoimmune disease, drugs, hemochromatosis, Wilson's disease, and α1-antitrypsin deficiency. Each of these disorders can lead to cirrhosis, with alcohol abuse as the leading cause. Alcohol is also a common co-contributor to cirrhosis in the other conditions, particularly hepatitis C.

How does alcohol cause liver damage?

The pathogenesis is unknown. The spectrum of disease includes fatty liver infiltration, alcoholic hepatitis, and cirrhosis. Cirrhosis occurs more frequently in individuals who have a history of alcoholic hepatitis and continue to drink.

What drugs cause hepatocellular injury?

Methyldopa, acetaminophen, trazodone, phenytoin, nitrofurantoin, isoniazid, antilipid agents (statins and fibrates), and sulfonamides are associated with drug-induced hepatitis.

What is autoimmune hepatitis?

Autoimmune hepatitis causes liver inflammation. Although autoantibodies are often found, they do not directly cause the hepatitis. Type 1 is responsible for 80% of adult cases in the U.S. Most of type 1 occurs in young women, whereas type 2 is more common in children.

What are some of the inherited causes of liver disease?

Autosomal recessive causes of liver disease include hemochromatosis, Wilson's disease, and α1-antitrypsin deficiency. Hemochromatosis results from abnormally increased intestinal iron absorption and iron deposition in a variety of organs including the liver, heart, pancreas, and pituitary. In Wilson's disease, impaired copper excretion into the bile results in accumulation of copper in the liver and other tissues resulting in cirrhosis and/or neuropsychiatric abnormalities. A new diagnosis of Wilson's disease is extremely rare in patients older than 35 years of age. The α1-antitrypsin deficiency causes emphysema, chronic hepatitis, and eventual cirrhosis.

▶ EVALUATION

When should I suspect liver disease?

Acute hepatitis is often obvious, occurring with right upper quadrant pain and jaundice. Nausea, anorexia, and malaise are often also present. If hepatic failure has occurred, encephalopathy and coagulopathy are likely as well. Chronic hepatitis, in contrast, is often insidious and nonspecific with fatigue, anorexia, and/or pruritis. You must use your H & P to detect risk factors and subtle signs (see later).

What components of the clinical history are pertinent?

Assess risk factors for viral hepatitis (e.g., intravenous drug use, prior transfusion, tattoos, cocaine use, occupational exposure, sexual behavior, travel history, birthplace in an endemic area). Ask about toxin exposure, including alcohol and medication. Family history of liver or autoimmune disease is also pertinent.

What clues to liver disease should I look for on physical exam?

Scleral icterus is visible when bilirubin level is above 3 mg/dL. Most patients with chronic liver disease remain anicteric until acute exacerbation or end-stage disease occurs. Other signs of chronic liver disease result from cirrhosis and include spider angiomata, palmar erythema, Terry's nails (dark red distal nail, pale proximal nail), gynecomastia, and jaundice. Advanced disease occurs with postnecrotic cirrhosis and advanced hepatic fibrosis. Portal hypertension develops and, beyond a critical threshold, results in ascites, seen as bulging flanks, or detected as shifting dullness. To look for shifting dullness, percuss to find a point where tympany turns to dullness on the side of the abdomen. Shift the patient to lie in the lateral decubitus position with that side down, and percuss again. The point shifts toward the umbilicus if fluid is present but remains the same if there is no ascites. Other manifestations of portal hypertension include caput medusa (engorged vessels around the umbilicus), bleeding esophageal varices, severe hemorrhoids, muscle wasting, encephalopathy, and peripheral edema. Patients with hemochromatosis may have bronze skin color. Patients with either alcohol-induced liver disease or hemochromatosis may have testicular atrophy, although this is not seen in patients with other causes of liver disease. Patients with α1-antitrypsin deficiency may present with early emphysema in the lung bases.

What laboratory tests should I order when I suspect liver disease?

Liver enzymes (transaminases or aminotransferases) are sensitive indicators of liver injury. These include alanine aminotransferase (ALT) and aspartate aminotransferase (AST). The ALT is more specific for liver injury, whereas the AST may be elevated owing to skeletal, cardiac, and liver muscle injury or injury to the brain and kidney. Transaminases are elevated with all causes of hepatitis. The degree of elevation is usually higher in acute than in chronic injury and correlates with the severity of liver injury only in acute, but not chronic, hepatitis. Acute viral hepatitis can cause transaminase elevations up to 100 times normal. In contrast, alcohol-induced hepatitis usually elevates transaminases to about two to three times normal, with a characteristic AST/ALT ratio of 2:1.

In advanced cirrhosis, enzymes may be normal despite ongoing damage because nearly all the normal hepatocytes have been destroyed. Once you detect liver disease, continue work-up with viral hepatitis antibody screening. If viral serology results are negative, look further for storage or autoimmune disorders (see later). For patients with alcohol use that is mild, or who deny a previously applied diagnosis of alcohol-induced liver disease, have a low threshold for ruling out other treatable causes of liver disease.

What labs can I use to assess the severity of liver disease?

Unlike acute hepatitis, aminotransferase levels do not correlate well with the degree of accumulated injury in patients with chronic hepatitis. Albumin and prothrombin time are more sensitive markers of hepatic biosynthetic function in patients with chronic liver disease. Albumin less than 3 g/dL or an increased prothrombin time (above eleven to sixteen seconds) indicates significantly reduced hepatic synthetic function.

How do I interpret hepatitis serologic profiles?

Some general rules are helpful: antigen is present with active infection, either acute or chronic; IgM antibodies signal early response to acute infection; and IgG antibodies develop later in infection and persist with chronic infection or resolution (Table 27–2). In hepatitis

TABLE 27-2

Interpretation of Serologic Tests for Viral Hepatitis

Test	Interpretation
Hepatitis A	
IgM antibody	acute infection
IgG antibody	past infection
Hepatitis B	
Surface antigen (HBsAg)	acute or chronic infection
Envelope antigen (HBeAg)	correlates with higher infectivity
IgM antibody against core protein (HBcIgM)	acute infection
IgG antibody against core protein (HBcIgG)	prior infection or vaccination
Hepatitis C	
IgG antibody	infection, likely chronic
Viral load	active infection

C infection, the likelihood of becoming a chronic carrier is so high, positive antibody tests are usually presumed to indicate chronic infection. Active HCV infection can be confirmed by testing for HCV RNA by PCR.

When should I screen for hemochromatosis?

Screen all 1st-degree relatives of affected patients for iron overload with serum iron, ferritin, transferrin saturation, and consider testing for the hemochromatosis gene, if present in the affected relative. Screen patients with chronic liver disease and negative viral serology findings. Elevated ferritin, or a transferrin saturation greater than 55%, is suggestive, but not specific, for hemochromatosis. Liver biopsy is required to confirm the iron overload. Be aware that other causes of chronic liver disease may also elevate these results, making interpretation challenging. Some physicians advocate screening the general white population over age 30, given the high prevalence of heterozygotes (7%) and the therapeutic efficacy of early phlebotomy in preventing cirrhosis. This is currently not an established standard, but is under review.

What labs suggest autoimmune hepatitis?

Type 1 autoimmune hepatitis is characterized by hypergamma-globulinemia, antinuclear antibody (ANA), and antismooth muscle antibody (ASMA). Type 2 is characterized by antibody to liver/kidney microsome type 1 (anti-LKM1) without ANA and ASMA. Either type may be accompanied by other autoimmune diseases, although this is more common with type 2.

What lab tests do I use to diagnose Wilson's disease?

Wilson's disease lowers the serum ceruloplasmin to less than 20 mg/dL and increases urinary copper excretion. Up to 20% of patients with Wilson's disease have normal ceruloplasmin. An elevated twenty-four-hour urine copper excretion suggests the diagnosis, and liver biopsy with quantitative copper measurement confirms the diagnosis. Kayser-Fleisher rings, a single brownish line on the outer edge of the cornea seen using a slit lamp exam, are pathognomonic but not always present.

What are the complications of cirrhosis that I should recognize?

Cirrhosis leads to fibrosis of the liver parenchyma with increased vascular resistance in the hepatic sinusoids, resulting in increased resistance to portal blood flow. This is referred to as portal hypertension. Associated clinical features with portal hypertension may include esophageal varices, as blood detours around the liver through small vessels in the esophagus; massive GI bleeding if these varices rupture; and ascites due to leakage of fluid from the portal system with risk of associated spontaneous bacterial peritonitis. Cirrhosis may also result in hepatic encephalopathy, hepatorenal syndrome, and hepatocellular cancer.

Should I screen for hepatocellular carcinoma in patients with chronic liver disease?

Serum α-fetoprotein and imaging studies, such as ultrasound and CT, are used to detect hepatocellular carcinoma. No evidence exists that screening increases the rate of detecting potentially curable tumors, however, despite the fact that cirrhosis of any etiology is associated with the development of hepatocellular carcinoma. In areas where hepatitis B is endemic, one half of patients with hepatocellular carcinoma are HBsAg positive. A similar risk pattern is seen with HCV infection.

When should a patient be referred for liver biopsy?

Use liver biopsy to confirm hemochromatosis and Wilson's disease and to determine eligibility for antiviral therapy in hepatitis B or C. Biopsy is also a prognostic tool. Patients with evidence of portal or mild periportal hepatitis tend to have a benign course. Those with bridging or multilobular necrosis or cirrhosis are at a high risk for progressive disease.

▶ TREATMENT

What treatments are available for chronic viral hepatitis?

The treatment of chronic viral hepatitis is a rapidly evolving field. The goals of therapy for hepatitis B and C differ. Hepatitis B treatment is directed at halting viral replication and sustaining seroconversion as evidenced by the development of anti-HBeAg antibody. Hepatitis C treatment is directed at eliminating the virus. α-Interferon is FDA-approved for the treatment of both hepatitis B and C. This treatment is expensive and has multiple side effects, including flulike symptoms, fatigue, bone marrow suppression, and neuropsychiatric effects. With hepatitis B, treatment is reserved for those with active viral replication and elevated aminotransferases. Thirty to forty percent of treated individuals respond to therapy as evidenced by loss of HBeAg and return of the serum ALT to normal. Lamivudine is a second-line therapy for chronic hepatitis B infection with fewer side effects but half the overall sustained virologic response due to development of viral resistance to the drug. In patients treated with lamivudine, long-term maintenance therapy may be required to prevent viral recurrence and return of hepatic inflammation.

Interferon is recommended for chronic hepatitis C in patients at the greatest risk for the progression to cirrhosis, as evidenced by elevated ALT levels, detectable HCV RNA, and liver biopsy findings of either portal or bridging fibrosis. Fifty percent of treated individuals have normalization of ALT levels and 33% have loss of detectable HCV RNA. Unfortunately, 50% experience relapse when therapy is stopped, leaving only 15%–25% with a sustained response. Studies in patients with chronic hepatitis C show better sustained response (up to 40%) with the use of combination therapy, including both interferon and ribavirin for 24 weeks in patients with genotype 2 and 3 or 48 weeks for those with genotype 1 or high viral load. Future treatments are under investigation, so refer patients to a hepatologist for consideration of inclusion in clinical trials. Advise patients with chronic hepatitis of any type to abstain from all alcohol ingestion to prevent accelerated progression to cirrhosis.

What treatments are available for drug-induced or autoimmune hepatitis?

Stop the drug and watch to make sure liver function tests and clinical symptoms improve. For autoimmune disease, steroids prolong survival and may be augmented with azathioprine.

What is the treatment for alcoholic liver disease?

By stopping the use of alcohol there may be reversal of liver damage.

How do I treat the complications of cirrhosis?

Treat *ascites* with sodium restriction to less than 2g/day. A loop diuretic such as furosemide and/or an aldosterone antagonist such as spironolactone can be added. Use large volume paricentesis for tense ascites in symptomatic patients in whom diuretics fail or are contraindicated. *Esophageal variceal hemorrhage* is treated with endoscopic variceal banding (preferred) or sclerotherapy. Transjugular intrahepatic portal systemic shunt (TIPS) decompresses portal hypertension and thereby reduces recurrent variceal bleeding and refractory ascites. β-Blockers, with or without oral nitrates, are effective at reducing both first time esophageal hemorrhage and recurrent esophageal hemorrhage. The mainstay of treatment for *hepatic encephalopathy* is lactulose, which facilitates the removal of ammonium ion.

Hepatorenal syndrome with oliguria and poor renal perfusion causing a renal sodium concentration less than 10 mEq/L is a grave prognostic sign. There is no treatment other than temporizing with dialysis while awaiting liver transplantation. *Hepatocellular tumors* can be resected if they involve only one lobe of the liver. Otherwise, elective palliative therapy involves angiographic embolization of affected areas.

How do I treat hemochromatosis?

Treat hemochromatosis with phlebotomy, removing 500 mL one to two times/month to a goal hemoglobin less than 11 gm/dL and ferritin less than 100 ng/mL. This prevents iron overload and cirrhosis.

Who should be referred for liver transplantation?

Patients with end-stage liver disease or fulminant hepatic failure should be referred early to centers for consideration of liver transplantation. Waiting lists are long, and patients must fulfill specific criteria including mental stability, psychosocial support, survival probability, and funding. Contraindications are based on outcome data and include alcohol intake over the preceding six months, other substance abuse, AIDS, infection outside the hepatobiliary system, metastatic liver disease, hepatic carcinoma, and uncorrectable coagulopathies.

How can I prevent hepatitis?

Vaccines are available for both hepatitis A and B. The hepatitis A vaccine is given in two doses six to twelve months apart and is recommended for travelers to endemic areas, military personnel, people with chronic liver disease, and people engaging in high-risk sexual activity. Hepatitis B vaccine is given in three doses, spaced by one and six months. It is recommended in infants, people at occupational risk, sexually active young adults, injection-drug users, inmates of correctional facilities, hemodialysis patients, international travelers, and populations where HBV is endemic.

K E Y   P O I N T S

▶ The most common presenting symptoms of chronic liver disease are fatigue, anorexia, and pruritus.

▶ Hepatitis B rarely progresses to chronic infection and cirrhosis unless acquired perinatally.

▶ Hepatitis C is the most common chronic blood-borne infection in the U.S., with the majority unaware that they are infected.

▶ Prothrombin time and albumin reflect the extent of irreversible liver injury in patients with chronic liver disease.

CASE 27–2. A 70-year-old man comes to clinic ten days after hospital discharge, concerned that he has been looking yellow for the last week. He reports feeling quite tired and is particularly bothered by generalized itching. His stool is light in color, and he thinks that his urine looks brown. He hasn't been eating due to loss of appetite.

   A. What is your differential diagnosis?
   B. What laboratory tests would be useful in determining the etiology of his illness?
   C. What other information would be useful?

CASE 27–3. A 50-year-old man is diagnosed with hepatitis C. He believes that he initially was infected on his 40th birthday when he injected IV drugs for the first and only time. He has had no subsequent care and is referred to a hepatologist for further evaluation.

   A. Which diagnostic studies will be useful in determining the extent of his disease?
   B. What factors would lead you to treat him?
   C. What advice would you offer to prevent accelerated progression to cirrhosis?

REFERENCES

Gordon SC: Treatment of viral hepatitis—2001. Ann Med 33: 385–390, 2001.

Lauer GM, Walker BD: Medical progress: Hepatitis C virus infection. N Engl J Med 345:41–52, 2001.

Maddrey WC: Alcohol-induced liver disease. Clin Liver Dis 4(1):115–131, 2000.

Walsh K, Alexander GJ: Update on chronic viral hepatitis. Postgrad Med J 77(910):498–505, 2001.

PANCREATITIS

▶ ETIOLOGY

Causes of acute pancreatitis are listed in Table 27–3 with no cause identified in 15%–20% of cases. Pancreatitis can become chronic if the underlying cause is not treated.

▶ EVALUATION

How do patients with pancreatitis present?

Patients report severe steady epigastric pain, often radiating to the back, worse lying down, and relieved sitting up. Nausea and vomiting are common and are exacerbated by eating. If pancreatic edema or gallstones occlude the common bile duct, jaundice ensues.

What do I look for on physical exam?

Look for tachycardia, hypotension, volume depletion due to third spacing of fluids, or low-grade fever due to inflammation or infec-

TABLE 27–3

Causes of Pancreatitis	
Common	**Uncommon**
Alcohol	Drugs (ddI, ddC, d4T, sulfonamides, tetracycline, thiazides, pentamidine,
Gallstones	azathioprine, estrogen, valproate)
	Viral
	Triglycerides >1000
	Idiopathic
	Trauma
	Hypercalcemia

tion. The abdomen is usually diffusely tender. Retroperitoneal pancreatic hemorrhage may manifest as bruising around the umbilicus (Cullen's sign) or flank (Turner's sign), although both these signs are rarely seen.

What tests should I order?

Order complete blood count, amylase or lipase, chemistry panel, calcium, liver function, LDH, glucose, triglycerides, x-rays of the abdomen and chest. Pancreatic calcifications on x-ray are pathognomonic of chronic pancreatitis. CXR may show pleural effusion. Abdominal CT scan may show necrotic pancreatic tissue, an indication for antibiotic prophylaxis. If patients are refractory to therapy, repeat abdominal CT scan may show developing complications such as pancreatic pseudocyst or abscess. Follow CBC, calcium, BUN, PaO_2, and base deficit from the arterial blood gas to assess for worsening prognosis by Ranson criteria (Box 27–1).

▶ TREATMENT

Treatment is mostly supportive, such as resting the bowel, allowing inflammation to subside, and treating complications. Use bowel rest (nothing to eat) and IV fluids (normal saline) as needed for resuscitation and then maintenance (D5 1/4 normal saline). Place a nasogastric tube to low-intermittent suction if vomiting is present. ERCP relieves an obstructing gallstone, but may worsen pancreatic inflammation. Manage pain with patient-controlled intravenous narcotics. Watch for complications of pseudocyst, abscess, sepsis, and adult respiratory distress syndrome (ARDS). Severely ill patients and those with necrotic pancreatic tissue on CT scan may benefit from prophylaxis with broad-spectrum antibiotics (imipenem or cefuroxime). Follow daily amylase, liver function tests, and CBC until they return to normal to track resolution of inflammation. Refer for elective cholecystectomy when the pancreatitis resolves if stones were the cause. Mortality is 10% overall in patients hospitalized with pancreatitis.

BOX 27–1

Ranson Criteria Predict Mortality Rates

Initial evaluation	Changes in the first 48 hours
Age >55	HCT drop >10%
WBC >16,000	BUN rise >5 mg/dL
SGOT >250	Ca <8
LDH >350	PaO_2 <60
Glucose >200	Base deficit >4

Mortality is 2% with 0–2 criteria, 40% with 5–6 criteria, nearly 100% with >7 criteria

---

K E Y   P O I N T S

▶ Pancreatitis radiates to the back, while cholecystitis radiates to the right shoulder.

▶ Gallstone disease and alcohol abuse are the two main causes of pancreatitis.

CASE 27–4. A 45-year-old man has several hours of severe abdominal pain radiating to the back with emesis worsened by eating. He smokes half a pack of cigarettes and drinks at least six-pack of beer daily: P 90, BP 145/90, T 99°, RR 20. Upper midabdomen is very tender, and you cannot find any costovertebral angle or point tenderness on his back.

     A. Name three possible causes of abdominal pain that are associated with back pain.
     B. Which of the three diagnoses you named is most likely for this patient and why?
     C. What will help you confirm your diagnosis and assess his prognosis? Amylase = 500 (normal 20–90), WBC = 19, SGOT = 300, glucose = 160.
     D. He has several more episodes of emesis. What treatment is warranted now?

REFERENCE

Cartmell MT, Kingsnorth AN: Acute pancreatitis. Hosp Med 61(6):382–385, 2000.

28

Geriatrics

► ETIOLOGY

What causes benign prostatic hyperplasia (BPH)?

BPH, a nonmalignant enlargement of the prostate, is due to excessive cellular growth of both glandular and stromal elements of the prostate. Increasing evidence suggests that BPH is an endocrinopathy related to dihydrotestosterone (DHT, the chief intracellular androgen) and aging.

► EVALUATION

How do I make the diagnosis of BPH?

The diagnosis of BPH is suggested by symptoms that reflect bladder irritation (urinary frequency, urgency, nocturia) and obstruction (hesitancy, straining, weak stream, dribbling, retention). Rule out other conditions causing these symptoms (e.g., prostatitis, urethral stricture, infection, prostate, bladder cancer) by history, rectal examination, and urinalysis.

How can I gauge the severity of my patient's BPH?

The American Urological Association (AUA) Symptom Index is a valid and reliable indicator of symptom severity using seven questions regarding specific symptoms (Table 28–1). Peak urine flow (normal greater than 15 mL/sec) and postvoid residual (normal less than 100 mL) are useful to gauge disease severity. Prostate size does not correlate well with symptom severity or the degree of obstruction.

Besides symptoms, are there any other serious problems associated with BPH?

Longstanding BPH can infrequently cause urinary retention, renal insufficiency, urinary tract infections, gross hematuria,

TABLE 28–1		
The American Urological Association Symptom Index for Patients with BPH		
Over the Past Month, How Often Have You...	**Answer Score**	
1. Had the sensation of not emptying your bladder completely? 2. Had to urinate again within 2 hours of last void (frequency)? 3. Stopped and started again several times while urinating? 4. Found it difficult to postpone urination (urge)? 5. Had a weak urinary stream? 6. Had to push or strain to begin urination? 7. Had to get up to urinate after going to bed?	0 = not at all 1 = less than 1 time in 5 2 = less than half the time 3 = half the time 4 = more than half the time 5 = almost always One point for each time	

Symptom score (sum of answers): mild (0–7), moderate (8–19), or severe (20–35)

and/or bladder stones. If these occur, surgery is generally indicated.

▶ TREATMENT

How do I decide when and how to treat BPH?

BPH is a disease that primarily affects quality of life. Thus, patient perception of symptom severity (AUA Symptom Score) is a major determinant in making treatment decisions. Treatment options range from watchful waiting to surgery (Figure 28–1).

What medications are used to manage BPH?

Two classes of medication and one herbal remedy improve BPH symptoms. α-*Adrenergic blockers* such as doxazosin, terazosin, and tamsulosin work fairly rapidly (within several weeks) via blocking α_1-adrenergic receptors in the bladder neck and prostate that constrict outflow. Side effects in 5%–10% of patients include orthostatic hypotension and weakness. Tamsulosin selectively blocks prostatic α-receptors and causes less asthenia, dizziness, and hypotension but can cause more retrograde ejaculation. The second class of medication includes *finasteride*, which works by decreasing prostatic DHT and shrinking prostate size by about 20%. Over six to twelve months, finasteride reduces urinary retention symptoms and need for surgery. Finasteride has fewer side effects (decreased libido, impotence in 3%–4%) than α-blockers. The natural product *saw palmetto* appears to be at least as effective as finasteride in relieving the symptoms of prostate obstruction with minimal side effects. The mechanism of action of saw palmetto is debated. *Invasive or surgical interventions* offer benefit for

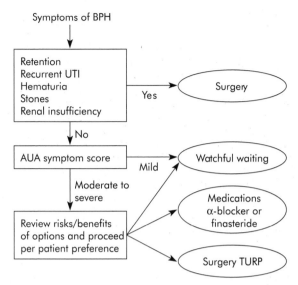

Figure 28–1. Treatment algorithm for benign prostatic hyperplasia.

patients in whom medical therapy fails, but risks include impotence, incontinence, blood loss requiring transfusion, and infection. The most common surgical procedure is transurethral resection of the prostate (TURP).

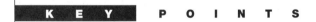

K E Y   P O I N T S

▶ Use history and directed evaluations to detect and assess severity of BPH.

▶ Patient symptoms and preferences should guide interventions for BPH.

DEMENTIA

▶ ETIOLOGY

What are the three most common causes of dementia in older adults?

Alzheimer's disease accounts for about two thirds of dementia cases. Traditionally, multi-infarct dementia is cited as the next most common cause of dementia, at 15%–25%. Studies suggest that vascular dementia may be over-diagnosed and that a previously under-diagnosed entity, Lewy body dementia, may account for up to 10%–20% of cases. Alcohol, at 10%, is the third most common cause of dementia in some case series.

What are the most common causes of "reversible dementia"?

Drugs and depression ("pseudodementia") are by far the most common reversible causes. After drugs and depression, only 5% of remaining cases are potentially treatable; 1% or less are truly fully reversible. The most common potentially reversible causes of cognitive impairment are B_{12} deficiency, hypothyroidism, and normal pressure hydrocephalus. Dementia is often only partially reversed with treatment of these conditions (perhaps because they often coexist with Alzheimer's disease).

▶ EVALUATION

How does one establish the diagnosis of dementia?

Although a hallmark sign, memory deficits alone are not sufficient to diagnose dementia. Impairments must exist in at least one other cognitive area (e.g., language, motor skills, personality), at a level severe enough to interfere with usual function. The mini-mental state examination (MMSE) is a useful 30-item instrument to objectively measure and document cognitive impairment.

What is the appropriate work-up for a patient suspected of having dementia?

Perform a thorough history and examination with focus on neurologic and mental status. Obtain CBC, electrolytes, BUN, creatinine, liver function tests, vitamin B_{12}, thyroid screen, and syphilis serology. Most experts recommend a noncontrast head CT to rule out tumor, subdural hematoma, or hydrocephalus, and brain imaging is absolutely indicated for patients with focal neurologic signs, headache, or other atypical features. Lumbar puncture and EEG are not routinely required.

What red flags increase the likelihood of a diagnosis other than Alzheimer's disease?

Sudden onset or onset at a younger age (especially age younger than 60), history of rapid cognitive decline over weeks to months rather than years, or presence of focal neurologic signs or symptoms increases the chance of a diagnosis other than Alzheimer's disease.

▶ TREATMENT

What are the basic management approaches to patients with dementia?

Review and discontinue drugs likely to impair cognition. Consider depression; begin a trial of selective serotonin reuptake inhibitor (SSRI) therapy. Diagnose and treat coexisting medical conditions that, although not the cause of cognitive impairment, can affect mood and function. Use nonpharmacologic approaches to improve patient function and behavior, along with caregiver education, support, and respite.

What pharmacologic treatments are available to patients with Alzheimer's dementia?

Three cholinesterase inhibitors (donezepil, rivastigmine, and galantamine) are currently available to treat Alzheimer's disease. These agents can significantly improve cognition, behavior, and overall function, but their main effect appears to be to slow rates of decline. Vitamin E and ginkgo biloba have also been shown to slow the rate of decline in Alzheimer's disease but data on these agents have not been as strong or consistent as studies with the cholinesterase inhibitors. Although estrogen, anti-inflammatory agents, and statin lipid-lowering drugs have been associated with lower prevalence rates of Alzheimer's disease, estrogen failed to slow progression of Alzheimer's disease in one randomized trial, and further study is needed before these drugs should be considered for prevention or treatment of Alzheimer's disease.

How about managing common behavioral problems such as agitation and sleep problems?

Nonpharmacologic strategies may work as well as, if not better than, medications. Seek out and address medication side effects, infection,

---

K E Y   P O I N T S

▶ Most dementia is not reversible; Alzheimer's disease is the most common cause.

▶ Drugs and depression are the most common potentially reversible causes of dementia.

▶ Function and behavior are optimized through excellent general medical care, nonpharmacologic intervention, and judicious use of drugs.

injury or pain, exacerbation of preexisting illness, or inconsistency in the environment that may be causing agitation. Low dose neuroleptics (e.g., haloperidol 0.5 mg, risperidone 0.5 mg, olanzapine 2.5 mg) may be helpful for severe agitation, persistent hallucinations, or delusions. Trazodone may be useful for sleep problems.

CASE 28–1. A 68-year-old woman is concerned about her memory. She is an accountant and reports increased difficulty doing her work and difficulty concentrating. These problems started a few months ago and seem to be steadily worsening. She has had trouble sleeping and has been taking Tylenol PM for insomnia. She admits to increased stress at work and a lack of energy but denies depressed mood. Her other medical problems include longstanding hypertension treated with atenolol and recently diagnosed diabetes newly treated with glipizide. On examination she appears somewhat anxious, S_4 gallop is present, neurologic examination is nonfocal, and Mini-Mental State Examination (MMSE) score is 24/30, with the patient stating that she could not do serial calculations after getting the first calculation correct, and forgetting two of three memory recall items.

A. Does this patient have dementia?
B. What is the most likely cause of her cognitive difficulties?
C. What other factors could be contributing to her symptoms?
D. What diagnostic work-up is warranted?
E. What interventions should you consider?

POLYPHARMACY

▶ ETIOLOGY

Why do older adults have more adverse drug effects than younger patients?

Most studies on the efficacy and safety of medications exclude the very old (older than age 75) and those with multiple medical problems. As a result the benefits, risks, and dosages of drugs seen in younger, healthier populations may not apply to older patients. Older adults are at higher risk for adverse effects because they take more medications (30% take at least four drugs) and have more underlying disease. Older adults also have altered pharmacokinetics (e.g., reduced renal clearance not accurately reflected by serum creatinine) and pharmacodynamics (e.g., more sensitive to warfarin and psychoactive drugs). Polypharmacy decreases compliance, with its own adverse effects.

▶ EVALUATION

When should I suspect an adverse effect from drugs/polypharmacy?

Always suspect drugs as a cause of new symptoms. Adverse consequences are often nonspecific, such as dizziness, falls, confusion, or altered bowel and bladder function. Particularly scrutinize hospitalized patients because up to 25% of admissions of older adults are for drug-related problems—most often resulting from adverse effects rather than patient error or noncompliance.

Are particular medications more commonly associated with adverse effects in the elderly?

Problematic drugs include antihypertensives, NSAIDs, H_2-blockers, tricyclic antidepressants, narcotics, and sedatives. These agents are often clearly medically indicated; they are mentioned here to increase vigilance rather than prohibit their use. Review over-the-counter agents as well.

▶ TREATMENT

How can I best avoid polypharmacy and adverse drug events in elderly patients?

Regardless of age, the risk for adverse reactions increases with each added medication. Thus, be particularly judicious when initiating drugs in the elderly. Try to limit patients to, at most, four drugs, which is often difficult in patients with multiple chronic conditions. Start at the lowest recommended dose. Carefully assess for drug interactions and for dosage changes necessitated by altered metabolism. Calculate creatinine clearance rather than relying on serum creatinine to assess renal function. Use Medisets (a box with compartments for each day to hold pills), simple regimens, and patient education to reduce patient errors.

How can I safely withdraw medications in older adults?

Although some drugs (i.e., steroids or drugs that interact with receptors such as β-blockers, benzodiazepines, antidepressants) require slow tapering to avoid physiologic withdrawal, do not be reluctant to carefully withdraw drugs whenever problematic polypharmacy is suspected. In one study of drug reduction among older adults, about one in four medications were stopped and 74% of drug discontinuations occurred without incident. No deaths were associated with the infrequent disease exacerbations that did occur when medications were stopped.

K E Y   P O I N T S

▶ **The biggest risk factor for adverse drug events is number of medications prescribed.**

▶ **Compliance decreases as the number of drugs that an individual takes increases.**

▶ **With careful monitoring, many medications can be safely stopped in older adults.**

URINARY INCONTINENCE

▶ ETIOLOGY

What are the basic categories of urinary incontinence?

Keeping in mind that mixed etiologies are common, there are four basic categories, each with characteristic symptoms and risk factors (Table 28–2).

What are the common causes of acute incontinence?

Remember reversible causes with the mnemonic DRIP (Box 28–1). These often occur suddenly and are usually treatable. Frequently implicated drugs include diuretics, anticholinergic

---

BOX 28–1

Common Reversible Causes of Acute Incontinence, by the Mnemonic "DRIP"

D Drugs, delirium
R Restricted mobility, retention
I Infection, fecal impaction
P Polyuric states, such as CHF, diabetes

TABLE 28–2

Mechanisms, Symptoms, and Treatment of the Four Types of Urinary Incontinence

Incontinence Type	Mechanisms and Risk Factors	Characteristic Symptoms	Treatment

Overflow	Outlet obstruction BPH, stricture
	↓ Bladder contractility
	Diabetic neuropathy
		Hesitancy, dribbling
		Small-volume leakage
			Avoid anticholinergic agents
			For BPH
			  α-blockers
			  finasteride
			  saw palmetto
			  TURP
			For stricture
			  urethral dilation

Stress	Weak sphincter Altered pelvic muscle strength Multiple childbirth Vaginal atrophy	Exacerbated by cough, laugh, bending Small-volume leakage	Pelvic muscle exercises Pessary Periurethral collagen injections Surgery α-agonists* Imipramine Estrogen**

Urge	Detrusor hyperreflexia
	
	↓ CNS inhibition
	Parkinson's, stroke
	Detrusor overactivity
	↑ Bladder contraction
	UTI, renal stone
	Outlet obstruction
		Sudden urge
		
		Large-volume leakage
			Avoid irritants (caffeine, alcohol)
			Scheduled voiding
			Anticholinergic agents
			  oxybutynin
			  imipramine
			Antispasmodic agents
			  dicyclomine,
			  propantheline

Functional	Physical impairment Cognitive impairment	Inability to get to toilet Large-volume leakage	Adapt environment Commode, urinal, condom catheter Scheduled voiding

*α-agonist, phenylpropanolamine no longer available; imipramine effective by its α-agonist effect
**Estrogen has been used historically, but recent data show little or no benefit.

agents that impair bladder contractility, and narcotics. Isolated nocturnal incontinence is often caused by volume overload states (CHF, lower extremity edema) due to the diuresis that occurs with recumbence.

▶ EVALUATION

What is the best way to discern the cause of my patient's incontinence?

Inquire about timing and volume of urine loss and about specific symptoms related to urge or stress incontinence, outlet obstruction, and functional problems. If incontinence is new or suddenly worse, consider DRIP causes. Because the bladder control reflex arc is located at S2-S4, focus the examination on relevant neurologic evaluation of sacral dermatomes and lower extremity function. Perform rectal exam (impaction, prostate, sphincter tone, anal wink) and pelvic exam (atrophy, vaginitis, prolapse). Assess for volume-overload state, cognitive impairment and/or physical impairment. Obtain urinalysis, glucose, BUN/creatinine, and calcium. Obtain postvoid residual (PVR)—greater than 100 mL is likely overflow, whereas less than 100 mL is likely urge or stress incontinence.

▶ TREATMENT

What are common nonpharmacologic treatment approaches to incontinence?

More than 50% of patients are cured and most others are markedly improved with standard therapies. Nonpharmacologic interventions include scheduled voids, bladder training (Kegel exercises to strengthen pelvic muscles as well as biofeedback and imagery to decrease urges), addressing mobility issues, and adult protective garments. Sometimes surgery is helpful (Table 28–2 and Figure 28–2). Refer to urology for hematuria, PVR greater than 100 mL, prostate nodule, uterine prolapse, or unclear diagnosis after initial evaluation and/or empiric therapy fails.

What medicines work to improve urinary incontinence?

Medications for incontinence act at cholinergic receptors, which cause bladder contraction (overactive in those with urge and underactive for those with overflow incontinence), and α-receptors, which cause sphincter contraction (underactive in those with stress incontinence). For urge incontinence, anticholinergics oxybutynin and tolteridine block stimulation of the bladder muscle and have the best efficacy. Anticholinergic side effects (dry mouth, confusion) may limit its use, especially in elderly patients. Other agents to try include dicyclomine, propantheline, and imipramine. Imipramine may also improve sphincter tone (by its α-agonist effect) in patients with stress incontinence and is a reasonable agent to try for mixed stress and urge incontinence. There are no medications that help overflow incontinence. Avoid anticholinergic medications that may decrease bladder tone and worsen obstruction.

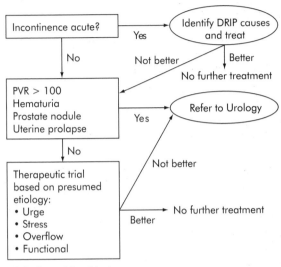

PVR, Postvoid residual.

Figure 28–2. Algorithm for the management of urinary incontinence.

K E Y   P O I N T S

▶ Most urinary incontinence can be cured or markedly improved using combined nonpharmacologic and pharmacologic interventions.

▶ History and directed exam are the keys to determining the causes of incontinence.

CASE 28–2. A 76-year-old man reports several months of worsening urinary incontinence of small volumes of urine, worsened by bending over. For many years he has had mild bladder symptoms of hesitation, slightly decreased force of stream, and nocturia two to three times per night, but he never has had continence problems until the past few months. He has noted a

Continued

CASE 28.2 *continued*

marked worsening in his hesitancy and in his diminished force of stream in the past few weeks. His other medical problems are hypertension treated with amlodipine, and seasonal allergies that he treats with over-the-counter (Dimetapp). On exam he is afebrile, has no flank tenderness, no abdominal masses, and his prostate is soft, enlarged, and nontender. Sphincter tone is normal.

A. What type of incontinence do you think he has and how can you confirm this diagnosis?
B. What factors are likely contributing to his difficulty in emptying his bladder?
C. What treatment options should be considered?

REFERENCE

Geriatrics At Your Fingertips, 2001 Edition. Published by the American Geriatrics Society, this is a concise guide to the evaluation and management of diseases and disorders that most commonly affect older persons. Available for under $10 through Kendall/Hunt Publishing Company 1-800-338-8290.

USEFUL WEBSITE

The American Geriatrics Society website has many cross-references to clinical guidelines and updates regarding health problems of older adults. *http://www.americangeriatrics.org/*

29

Hematology and Oncology

BLEEDING DISORDERS

▶ ETIOLOGY

What general processes cause abnormal hemostasis?

Hemostasis requires a dynamic balance between factors that promote clot formation and factors that promote anticoagulation. The tendency to bleed or to clot can be inherited or acquired. The types of bleeding problems you encounter in the outpatient setting are likely to be quite different from those you might see in hospitalized patients.

What are the most common causes of abnormal bleeding?

Common causes are summarized in Table 29–1. *Von Willebrand disease* (vWD) is the most likely inherited cause, due to a lack of the protein that links platelets to damaged endothelium. The most common acquired cause is *nonsteroidal anti-inflammatory drugs* (NSAIDs and aspirin), with bleeding in up to 10% of patients on these agents. *Immune thrombocytopenic purpura* (ITP) is an acquired disease caused by autoantibodies that bind to the surface of platelets and shorten their life span. These antibodies may be associated with a variety of systemic illnesses such as lupus, HIV infection, or lymphoproliferative disorders. ITP is usually an outpatient diagnosis. Hospitalized patients with thrombocytopenia should be evaluated for alternate causes.

What are some of the most likely causes of bleeding in a hospitalized patient?

The leading diagnosis depends on how sick your patient is, and what underlying medical problems are present. In the ICU setting, for example, *disseminated intravascular coagulation* (DIC) is a fairly common cause of abnormal bleeding. This is a final com-

TABLE 29-1

Prevalence of Common Inherited and Acquired Bleeding
Disorders

Bleeding Disorder	Prevalence	Factors Involved
Inherited disorders		
vWD	1/100	von Willebrand factor deficiency
Hemophilia A	1/5,-10,000*	VIII deficiency
Hemophilia B	1/30,-50,000*	IX deficiency ("Christmas disease")
Acquired disorders		
NSAIDs	1/10	Platelet dysfunction
ITP	1/10,000	Platelet antibodies
DIC		Platelet and factor consumption
End stage liver disease		Vit K-dependent factor deficiency (II, VII, IX, X)
Warfarin	1/100/year	Vit K-dependent factor deficiency (II, VII, IX, X)

*Prevalence among live male births only, as these are X-chromosome-linked conditions

mon pathway of many conditions including sepsis, massive trauma
and transfusion, acute head injury, acute promyelocytic leukemia,
and adenocarcinoma. *Liver disease,* acute or chronic, with its
associated vitamin K dependent factor deficiencies (II, VII, IX, X)
is common in the patient who is bleeding briskly enough to be
hospitalized. Unfortunately, over-anticoagulation is a common
cause of bleeding necessitating hospitalization. Of the several million patients in the U.S. on *warfarin* for CHF or atrial fibrillation,
about 1% per year have significant bleeding complications.

What is hemophilia?

Hemophilia A and B are X-linked deficiencies of factors VIII and
IX, respectively (see Table 29–1). Although we expect a pedigree
like that of the royal families of Victorian Europe, about 30% of
hemophilia patients have a spontaneous, de novo mutation.

▶ EVALUATION

How do I gauge if prior bleeding is "excessive"?

Although prior excessive bleeding is your clue to a true bleeding
disorder, it is often over-reported. Quantify the blood loss. Did epistaxis require cautery, packing, or transfusion? Was transfusion
required after a minor surgical procedure (dental extraction, tonsillectomy, circumcision)? Have menses been heavy for longer than
three days or prolonged for more than six to seven days? Has
there been anemia or iron therapy in the past, especially in men.

How do I distinguish between hereditary and acquired disorders?

A careful history reveals helpful clues. Ask about lifelong problems with hemostasis to uncover inherited problems: at birth, circumcision, tonsillectomy, tooth extractions requiring wound packing or suturing, postpartum bleeding, nosebleeds. The one exception to this rule is vWD because severity is variable and may worsen later in life. Ask about medications, especially the recent addition of an anti-inflammatory or anticoagulant, which might suggest an acquired cause. Acute bleeding in a hospitalized patient who has a history of excellent hemostasis is almost always from an acquired condition.

Does the type of bleeding help me generate a differential diagnosis?

Yes (Table 29–2). Hematochezia, melena, hematemesis, hemoptysis, and hematuria are almost never caused by a bleeding disorder, so evaluate these patients for an anatomic cause of blood loss.

What lab tests do I order if I suspect a bleeding problem?

Common tests ordered are listed in Table 29–3. CBC determines if bleeding has caused anemia. Platelet count identifies altered platelet numbers, but tells you nothing about platelet function. Bleeding time assesses platelet function (primary hemostasis). Prothrombin time (PT) assesses activity of the extrinsic and common pathways in the coagulation cascade and is elevated with

TABLE 29–2

Type of Bleeding Suggested by Particular History and Exam Clues

Clinical Symptom	Likely Bleeding Problem
Bruising	Connective tissue disorder (Ehlers-Danlos, scurvy), vitamin K deficiency (liver failure)
Bruises on extremity extensor surfaces	Physical abuse
Delayed (hours-days) postsurgical bleeding	Hemophilia, vitamin K deficiency, factor deficiency (secondary hemostasis problem)
Joint or deep muscle bleed	Hemophilia
Oozing catheter sites in hospitalized patient	DIC
Palpable purpura	Vasculitis, cryoglubulinemia, endocarditis
Petechiae, mucosal hemorrhage, bruises from minor trauma	Decreased or dysfunctional platelets (primary hemostasis problem)

TABLE 29-3

Key Features of Lab Abnormalities Seen with Specific Bleeding Disorders

Condition	BT	Plts	PT	PTT	TT	FDP	F	Other tests
ASA or NSAIDs	↑↑							
vWD	↑	↓ in IIB						Platelet aggregation ↓ only with ristocetin
Hemophilia A or B				↑				Factor levels*
Warfarin			↑↑↑	↑↑				LFTs
Liver disease		↓	↑↑	↑↑	↑			Exam, LFTs
DIC	↑↑	↓↓	↑	↑	↑↑	↑↑↑	↓↓	

Key: BT = bleeding time, F = fibrinogen, Plts = platelets, PT = prothrombin time, PTT = partial thromboplastin time, TT = thrombin time, FDP = fibrin degradation products, F = fibrinogen.

*Factor VIII levels may be low in vWD as well as hemophilia A because von Willebrand factor complexes with factor VIII and prolongs its half-life in the circulation.

warfarin, vitamin K deficiency, liver disease, and DIC. Partial thromboplastin time (PTT) measures intrinsic pathway activity and is prolonged with DIC and heparin use, but not LMWH. Prolonged PTT can also occur with deficiency of a clotting factor or presence of a lupus inhibitor. To tell which one, mix some normal serum in with the patient's sample (a "1:1 mix") and repeat the assay. Factor deficiencies correct, whereas inhibitors continue to prolong, the PTT. Fibrin degradation products appear with thromboembolism or DIC.

▶ TREATMENT

How do I use blood products?

Supply the missing components needed for adequate hemostasis (Table 29-4). If the problem is DIC, the key to your patient's survival is to quickly correct the underlying disorder. Mortality in DIC attributed to shock and sepsis exceeds 50%.

If the diagnosis is most likely ITP, do I give platelets?

No. Transfused platelets will be destroyed about as fast as they are infused. Use high dose prednisone (1 mg/kg/day) to block the immune process responsible for destroying platelets for two to seven days, or until the platelet count rises above 30,000/μl. Then taper prednisone slowly over three to four weeks. If bleeding is severe, or if the initial platelet count is below 10,000/μl, give IV immunoglobulin (IVIG) (1 gm/kg/day) for two days. The response to IVIG is quicker than to prednisone, such that the platelet count

TABLE 29-4

Use of Blood and Other Products for Bleeding Disorders

Product	Contents	When to use
Fresh frozen plasma (FFP)	All clotting factors, no platelets	Multifactor deficiency, vitamin K deficiency, warfarin excess, liver disease with bleeding
Vitamin K		Same as for FFP
Cryoprecipitate (from FFP)	Fibrinogen, VIII, vWF, XIII	PTT prolonged, heparin excess, severe vWD, fibrinogen depletion, DIC, factor VIII deficiency
Protamine sulfate		PTT prolonged from regular heparin (NOT low molecular weight)
Platelets		Bleeding time prolonged, NSAIDs, aspirin, DIC, massive bleeding or transfusion
Rho (D) immunoglobulin		ITP in HIV infection, Rh+ patients
Specific factor concentrates	VIII or IX	Hemophilia chronic maintenance
Desmopressin (DDAVP)*		Preoperatively for mild vWD

*Do not use DDAVP in patients with type IIB vWD as it will exacerbate associated thrombocytopenia and may worsen hemostasis.

usually rises within twenty-four hours. About two thirds of patients with chronic ITP require splenectomy. Immunize these patients with the hemophilus, polyvalent pneumococcal, and meningococcal vaccines several weeks before splenectomy. Platelet count greater than 30,000 in ITP is sufficient for adequate hemostasis.

K E Y   P O I N T S

► Ask about prior dental procedures, surgeries, and menses to uncover excessive bleeding.

► Mucosal and catheter site oozing in hospitalized patients suggests DIC; petechiae suggest a platelet problem; palpable purpura suggests vasculitis or immune complex deposition; delayed bleeding suggests factor deficiency.

► Bleeding from the bowel, bladder, or lungs is generally NOT caused by a bleeding disorder and requires rapid evaluation to find the cause.

► Give fresh frozen plasma to stop bleeding in patients with liver disease or warfarin excess.

► Give prednisone or IVIG, not platelets, to patients with ITP.

CASE 29–1. A 37-year-old woman with a history of rheumatoid arthritis presents with a new rash around her ankles and multiple dime- to quarter-sized bruises on her arms after working in her garden. She denies any recent illness or problems with bleeding or bruising and takes no medications. On exam, there are palatal petechiae. There are several purpuric lesions on each of her forearms, all less than 1.5 cm in diameter, and most less than a week old (i.e., little change in color to green or yellow). There is no adenopathy or organomegaly. The rash around her ankles consists of nearly confluent, nonblanching, pinpoint erythematous lesions.

　　A. What is the most likely diagnosis and how is her history of rheumatoid arthritis relevant?
　　B. What laboratory studies would you order to investigate this?
　　C. What do you recommend for therapy?

REFERENCE

Cobas M: Preoperative assessment of coagulation disorders. Int Anesthesiol Clin 39(1):1–15, 2001.

CLOTTING DISORDERS

▶ ETIOLOGY

What are heritable causes of hypercoagulability?

The list of possible heritable causes is growing steadily; all causes listed subsequently are autosomal dominant. Deficiencies of the physiologic anticoagulant proteins C, S, and antithrombin III are detected in 5%–15% of patients younger than age 45 with deep venous thrombosis (DVT). Activated protein C resistance, also called factor V Leiden mutation, may be diagnosed in up to 50% of patients with DVT. This is extremely common in women who develop blood clots while taking oral contraceptives. The prevalence of this mutation is estimated at 3%–5% in whites, although is less common in Asian- and African-Americans. A prothrombin (G20210A) polymorphism has been identified as associated with an increased risk of thromboembolism and MI in young patients (3% prevalence in whites). Hyperhomocystinemia is associated with arterial and venous clots. Thromboembolism remains idiopathic in 25% of cases.

What are the risk factors for thrombosis?

Risk factors for arterial thrombosis (MI, stroke) include hypertension, hyperlipidemia, elevated lipoprotein(a), diabetes, smoking, and vasculitis. Risk factors for venous clotting include immobilization, anesthesia, surgery, pregnancy, estrogen use, malignancy (typically mucin-secreting adenocarcinomas), nephrotic syndrome, CHF, age older than 50, and prior thrombosis.

What is a lupus anticoagulant?

Lupus anticoagulants are acquired IgG or IgM antibodies, also called antiphospholipid or anticardiolipin antibodies, that artifactually prolong the PTT assay. The term is a misnomer, because these antibodies are not uniformly associated with lupus, and they cause clotting rather than bleeding. Presence of a lupus anticoagulant is also called antiphospholipid antibody syndrome (APAS) and is an acquired hypercoagulable state associated with lupus and other autoimmune disorders. It is typically seen in young women with recurrent spontaneous abortions and thrombocytopenia. Up to 35% of patients with APAS suffer venous and/or arterial thromboembolism; the risk of thrombosis approaches 70% with APAS and concurrent lupus.

▶ EVALUATION

Whom do I screen for the presence of an underlying hypercoagulable state?

The British Society for Hematology has recommended screening in the following situations:

- Thrombosis younger than age 45 without risk factors even with the first event

- Recurrent thrombosis or thrombosis at an unusual site (cerebral- or visceral-vein thrombosis)

- Arterial thrombosis before the age of 30

- Family history of venous thrombosis

- Stillbirth OR three or more unexplained spontaneous abortions

How do I screen for a hypercoagulable state?

Obtain protein C and S levels before starting warfarin, but remember these may be artifactually low owing to consumption of factors in the acute thrombosis. Obtain antithrombin III before starting heparin. Activated protein C resistance (by PCR), the presence of antiphospholipid antibodies, and homocysteine levels can be assayed while patients are on either anticoagulant. The prothrombin procoagulable polymorphism can be detected on DNA/PCR screening, Although this test may not yet be widely available.

▶ TREATMENT

How do I anticoagulate a patient with a DVT?

Start with an IV heparin bolus of 80 u/kg (ideal body weight) followed by a continuous infusion at 18 u/kg/hour. As this is a rough estimate, adjust infusion rate to maintain PTT at 1.8–2.5 times control. PTT can be followed to monitor heparin therapy every six hours until stable, then less often. Twice-daily subcutaneous low molecular weight heparin can be given instead. It is more expensive per dose, but total cost may be less. LMWH does not alter PTT so it does not require monitoring and can be used in outpatients. Begin oral warfarin twenty-four to forty-eight hours after initiating heparin. Physicians vary widely in how aggressively they "load" the warfarin therapy, starting with 5–10 mg for the first few days, then adjusting based on the PT INR. Continue heparin until patient is therapeutic on warfarin (INR greater than 2). Some hematologists continue heparin two days beyond the time a therapeutic INR has been reached to prevent warfarin-associated skin necrosis, especially a risk in patients with protein C or S deficiency. Warfarin necrosis occurs because of rapid loss of short half-life clotting factors during the initiation of warfarin, causing a transient imbalance in the clotting cascade toward thromboembolism. Generally, the target INR is 2–3. Patients with APAS routinely fail less intense therapy and are at high risk of recurrence (greater than 70%), so their target INR is higher at 3–4.

My patient with a postsurgical DVT has been on a therapeutic level of heparin for five days, but his platelet count is dropping and by duplex ultrasound, his DVT is enlarging. What's going on?

Yours is one of about 2% of patients who develop heparin-induced thrombocytopenia (HIT). HIT is suspected when platelets drop below normal or decline more than 50% from baseline. Unfortunately, extension of the DVT despite adequate anticoagulation means your patient is also one of the 0.2%–0.6% who develop HIT-associated thrombosis (HITT). A heparin-dependent antibody, usually IgG, that activates platelet aggregation causes HITT. The clotting events associated with HITT may be venous or arterial and are life-threatening. STOP all heparin, including catheter flushes. Remove all heparin-bonded catheters. Post a sign above the patient's bed explicitly stating, "NO HEPARIN FLUSHES." Call a hematologist to assist with options for replacing heparin. Lepirudin is the leading choice, but requires continuous IV infusion and careful monitoring. Danaparoid, a heparinoid, and LMW heparin are NOT options because they worsen the problem 10% and 80% of the time, respectively. If an arterial thrombosis develops, directed thrombolytic therapy may be necessary to save a limb. HIT and HITT are the reason careful platelet monitoring must accompany all heparin use.

How long do I continue warfarin therapy?

Warfarin is usually given for three to six months after an initial event when a reversible cause was present such as pregnancy, surgery, or trauma. Consider indefinite warfarin therapy if the hypercoagulable state is a persistent risk (APAS, CHF, paroxysmal nocturnal hemoglobinuria, nephrotic syndrome, active malignancy). Lifelong anticoagulation is recommended in those with a history of multiple events, multiple genetic risk factors, a strong family history, regardless of the results of the ~$3000 work-up, or an initial event in an unusual site. Although it is tempting to hinge the length of warfarin therapy on the severity of the initial event, this has no real bearing on the patient's subsequent risk for recurrence. Of patients who develop a diagnosed lower extremity DVT, 40%–50% will suffer a pulmonary embolism. Overall, the risk of a significant bleeding complication caused by warfarin therapy is about 1% per year. Avoid warfarin in women planning pregnancy and through the 1st trimester.

When should I consider prophylactic anticoagulation?

Give prophylactic subcutaneous heparin during immobility (e.g., postop) to any patient with a prior clot (i.e., with surgery) or with an identified genetic risk, even in the absence of a history of thrombosis. Women with factor V Leiden mutation who become pregnant are at a much greater risk for DVT (odds ratio, 16.3, 95% confidence interval, 4.8 to 54.9). There is evidence supporting prophylaxis in this population unless there is a history of DVT.

Is there a role for aspirin in the hypercoagulable patient?

Aspirin and NSAIDs are antiplatelet agents and are useful in preventing arterial thrombosis, such as in MI and stroke. A patient with APAS who has a history of predominately arterial thromboses is often treated with the combination of warfarin and aspirin, with very close monitoring of the INR and clinical status. In all other patients taking warfarin for venous thrombosis, aspirin and NSAIDs are discouraged as the risk of bleeding complications increases with the use of these agents.

K E Y	P O I N T S

▶ Factor V Leiden accounts for 50% of clotting disorders.

▶ Overlap heparin and warfarin use in patients with DVT to prevent warfarin-induced clotting.

▶ Screen for hypercoagulable state in patients with recurrent thromboses, recurrent fetal loss, unusual or arterial sites of clotting, a family history of frequent blood clots, or those patients younger than age 45 with DVT and no risk factors.

▶ Monitor platelets in patients prior to and during heparin use to look for heparin-induced thrombocytopenia.

CASE 29–2. A 27-year-old woman of Irish descent is admitted to the medical floor with a left iliofemoral DVT four weeks postpartum. She is G4P3SAB1 (4 pregnancies, 3 live births, and one spontaneous abortion). She denies any prior thrombosis. Her family history is significant for a maternal grandmother who died of a pulmonary embolism at the age of 63 as well as a maternal uncle who developed a DVT following a transpolar flight to London from Seattle.

A. What are the two most likely diagnoses?
B. What laboratory studies would you perform, and how would anticoagulation therapy affect the accuracy of the evaluation?
C. What do you recommend for therapy?
D. How would you approach diagnostic screening of the extended family?

REFERENCES

Thomas RH: Hypercoagulability syndromes. Arch Intern Med 161: 2433–2439, 2001.

Whiteman T, Hassouna HI: Hypercoagulable states. Hematol Oncol Clin North Am 14(2):355–377, 2000.

USEFUL WEBSITE

American Society of Hematology Education Book has the best overview of thrombophilia (clotting). Search table of contents under either thrombosis or bleeding, and there are two chapters of interest. *www.asheducationbook.org*

BREAST CANCER

See section on Breast Health.

COLON CANCER

▶ **ETIOLOGY**

Who gets colon cancer?

In the U.S., 56,000 people die from colon cancer each year, making it the second deadliest malignancy after lung cancer. As with breast cancer, most victims have no risk factors other than age. Lifetime incidence of colon cancer is 5% overall. Lack of physical activity, consumption of red meat, obesity, alcohol and cigarette use are associated with higher rates of colon cancer. Certain uncommon conditions impart a particularly high risk. A family history of colon cancer in a 1st degree relative raises risk two- to threefold. Ulcerative colitis raises risk 20-fold after ten years of active disease. Hereditary nonpolyposis colorectal cancer (HNPCC), an autosomal dominant condition, accounts for 2%–5% of colon cancer, with early onset of cancer of the colon and other organs, and multiple affected relatives. Patients with HNPCC have a 70%–90% chance of developing colon cancer. Familial adenomatous polyposis (FAP), also autosomal dominant, accounts for less than 1% of colon cancer. The colon becomes studded with polyps at an early age, with a colon cancer diagnosis on average by age 16, and 100% diagnosed with colon cancer by age 50. HNPCC and FAP should be considered in families with early onset colon cancer, other associated malignancies, and multiple affected relatives.

▶ **EVALUATION**

What screening is recommended?

Starting at age 50, screen for polyps with sigmoidoscopy every three to five years in addition to annual occult blood stool testing, or colonoscopy every decade. People at higher risk need earlier and more frequent screening. For patients with a 1st degree relative with colon cancer, begin screening at ten years younger than when the relative developed the disease. Digital rectal exams may detect rectal cancers but have not been shown to improve outcome.

What symptoms might my patient with colon cancer develop?

Distal colon cancers tend to obstruct, producing cramps, thin stools, bloating, or perforation. Stool in the proximal colon is more liquid, so cancers there cause symptoms by ulcerating and bleeding. Every adult with unexplained iron-deficiency anemia needs a colonoscopy. Dyspnea may be the chief complaint of your patient with a cecal carcinoma and a low HCT. Unfortunately, many patients present with an abdominal mass or liver metastases from advanced disease.

How do I stage colon cancer?

The Dukes' classification is a simple staging system that guides treatment and prognosis (Table 29–5).

▶ TREATMENT

How do I treat colon cancer?

Stage A, B, and C tumors are resected. Stage C tumors are also treated with chemotherapy, usually 5-fluorouracil with leucovorin. Stage D tumors receive chemotherapy or irradiation. Small isolated liver metastases can be resected. Studies of adjuvant chemotherapy for stage B tumors have shown little or no benefit.

How do I catch recurrences early?

Once treated, perform regular exams, labs, and colonoscopy. Measure the carcinoembryonic antigen (CEA) level before excision. A persistently elevated or rising level predicts recurrence.

K E Y   P O I N T S

- ▶ Common risk factors are age greater than 50, family history, and ulcerative colitis.
- ▶ Screen people older than age 50, or earlier if there are risk factors.
- ▶ Elevated CEA levels after excision predict recurrence but require a preop level for comparison.

TABLE 29-5

Dukes' Classification of Colon Cancer

Stage	Definition	Treatment	Five year Survival (%)
A	Limited to mucosa and submucosa	Excision	95
B	Local extension to subserosa or beyond	Excision	75
C	Regional lymph node involvement	Excision, plus 5-fluorouracil and leukovorin	50
D	Metastases (liver first; then lung, bone, CNS)	Chemotherapy or irradiation, excision of 1-3 liver metastases	5

LEUKEMIA

► ETIOLOGY

What causes leukemia?

Leukemias are the neoplastic, clonal proliferation of blood cells or their precursors. Leukemias are classified according to the stage of maturation (blast or mature-appearing cells) and type of cell involved (lymphoid or myeloid). Thus, there are four common leukemias: chronic lymphocytic leukemia (CLL), chronic myelogenous leukemia (CML), acute lymphocytic leukemia (ALL), and acute myeloid leukemia (AML). CLL and AML are diseases of the elderly, with average presentation at ages 60 and 65, respectively. CML is a disease of middle age, with an average age of 42 at presentation. ALL incidence peaks in young children, but is seen in adults. Almost all patients with CML have a translocation between chromosomes 9 and 22, called the Philadelphia chromosome. AML is associated with the myelodysplastic syndrome. Certain genetic conditions, exposure to radiation, benzene, and chemotherapy are all associated with the development of acute leukemias, but the majority of cases have no identifiable risk factors.

► EVALUATION

What are common symptoms of leukemia?

Patients may describe fatigue, night sweats, or low grade fever. Infiltration of tissues may result in enlarged nodes, liver and spleen, or masses in the gingiva, skin (leukemia cutis), or soft tissue (chloroma). When the WBC is over 150k, vascular sludging, or leukostasis, may result in stroke, headache, tinnitus, blindness, priapism, or myocardial injury. Infiltration of normal bone marrow causes pancytopenia (neutropenia, anemia, and thrombocytopenia), resulting in infection, dyspnea, fatigue, bleeding especially from the nose or gums, and bruising.

What will I see on a peripheral blood smear?

If you see more than 15,000 mature lymphocytes in the blood of an elderly person, they likely have CLL. In CML, there are 30–300k WBCs, mostly myeloid cells in later stages of maturation with fewer than 5% blast forms. When blast forms exceed 30%, the CML has progressed to a more acute blast phase. Leukemoid reactions, or reactive elevations of white cells caused by certain infections, such as TB, may look similar. Leukemoid reactions can be differentiated from leukemias by their high serum leukocyte alkaline phosphatase (LAP). Pancytopenia is the hallmark of acute leukemia, usually with circulating blasts of either myeloid (AML) or lymphocytic (ALL) lineage. It is important to note that leukemia can present with a low, high, or numerically normal WBC. Auer rods are pathognomonic for AML; they look like red cigars in the myeloid blast cell cytoplasm.

What other tests are used to diagnose leukemias?

Bone marrow biopsy and aspiration are helpful: greater than 30% mature B lymphocytes are present in CLL; mature cells predominate in CML; blasts predominate in AML and ALL. Flow cytometry of bone marrow aspirate specimens identify membrane antigens that differentiate the blast forms seen with acute leukemias. Cytogenetics can be performed on bone marrow or serum specimens to identify genetic rearrangements in malignant cells, which provide diagnostic and prognostic information, as well as aid in choosing therapy. The Philadelphia chromosome is pathognomonic for CML.

What special complications should I watch for?

In CLL, clonal lymphocytes produce monoclonal immunoglobulins and depress the synthesis of normal immunoglobulins. The resulting hypogammaglobulinemia impairs humoral immunity, causing infections by *Staphylococcus aureus*, *Streptococcus pneumoniae*, and *Haemophilus influenzae*. Fifteen percent of patients have antibodies against erythrocytes or platelets, conditions known as autoimmune hemolytic anemia or thrombocytopenia. In AML/ALL, bone marrow failure at presentation is the rule, often with sepsis, DIC, or renal failure. Cranial nerve palsies and leukemic meningitis are common in ALL, especially in children.

▶ TREATMENT

Do I need to treat the "chronic" leukemias?

Neither CLL nor CML requires urgent treatment in chronic, asymptomatic phases. CLL may not cause symptoms for many years, and it typically affects older people who often die of other diseases first. Indications for treatment include worsening fatigue, anemia, thrombocytopenia, or worsening lymphadenopathy. Chlorambucil orally every three weeks for six months was formerly the only treatment option. Fludarabine is now used for its higher response rate and more sustained effect, but requires intravenous infusion five days each month for four to six months. Newer options combining chemotherapy with antibodies against CLL cell antigens are currently being tested. Associated autoimmune hemolytic anemia or thrombocytopenia may require prednisone or splenectomy. For CML, chemotherapy agents effective at lowering white cell counts include hydroxyurea and α-interferon. Emergent leukapheresis can reduce cell counts rapidly when sludging causes end-organ damage. A new agent was approved, STI–571 (Gleevec), which specifically inhibits the tyrosine kinase up-regulated by the bcr/abl oncogene of CML, and appears to give excellent control of the disease at two years with few serious side effects or toxicity. Allogeneic bone marrow transplant is offered to patients younger than 60 years of age, which occurs more often with CML than with CLL. Transplant is most successful early in the chronic phase of disease. After several years, patients with CML develop a blast crisis, such as AML, that responds poorly to chemotherapy and is usually lethal.

How do I treat the acute leukemias?

ALL and AML are treated with combination chemotherapy (two or more drugs) in stages: induction, consolidation, and maintenance. Induction chemotherapy is the initial, often successful, attempt to induce a complete remission (CR). Recurrence within a year is the rule, unless monthly consolidation chemotherapy is given. The actual agents used depend on the leukemia cell type and patient age, but may include antimetabolites such as cytarabine or 6-thioguanine, anthracyclines such as daunorubicin or idarubicin, or etoposide. Patients with ALL require CNS chemotherapy to prevent CNS sequestration of leukemia cells. They also may require years of low-dose maintenance therapy. Autologous or allogeneic bone marrow transplants are sometimes used, especially for patients with poor response to chemotherapy or poor prognosis as predicted by cytogenetics. Long term disease-free survival is 15%–20% for AML, and up to 40% for ALL. (It is much better in children.)

What is the role of bone marrow transplant?

Hematopoietic stem cell transplantation (HSCT) is used to treat a variety of hematologic malignancies including AML, ALL, and CML. Otherwise lethal doses of chemotherapy and radiation are given, and the patient is "rescued" by an infusion of their own (autologous) or a donor's (allogeneic) stem cells. In the case of allogeneic transplantation, an immunologic "graft vs. leukemia" effect helps to control the underlying malignant clone. Because of the high degree of toxicity associated with transplantation, these therapies have traditionally been used in patients younger than age 60.

What are the potential complications of treatments for leukemia?

Hydroxyurea can cause bone marrow suppression. Interferon causes unpleasant flulike symptoms and can precipitate or exacerbate depression. STI–571 can cause capillary leakage (pulmonary edema, ascites, pleural effusions, edema), GI symptoms, cytopenias, and can be hepatotoxic, but is generally very well tolerated. Bone marrow transplantation purposefully ablates native bone marrow, leaving patients transiently susceptible to many serious infections and dependent upon red blood and platelet transfusions until the transplant repopulates the bone marrow. Treatment that rapidly lyses large numbers of tumor cells, such as induction chemotherapy for acute leukemia, can cause renal failure or tumor lysis syndrome, in which purine metabolites released from leukemic cells raise uric acid and potassium. Cytarabine and etoposide cause alopecia, mucositis, nausea, vomiting, neuropathy, and bone marrow suppression with a nadir around fourteen to eighteen days after administration. Daunorubicin is known to cause arrhythmias, heart failure even years after administration, secondary leukemias, and infertility in addition to the usual myelosuppression, GI effects, and alopecia seen with other chemotherapy agents.

K E Y   P O I N T S

▶ Symptoms of leukemia are caused by infiltration of organs, infiltration of bone marrow, alterations in immunity, and the large burden of clonal cells in the blood.

▶ Leukemia is diagnosed by peripheral smear, bone marrow biopsy, immunologic markers (flow cytometry), and cytogenetics.

▶ CLL may never need treatment; CML always becomes acute over time, and early transplant is the only hope of cure.

> ▶ Acute leukemias must be treated urgently with combination chemotherapy.

LUNG CANCER

▶ ETIOLOGY

Who gets lung cancer?

Lung cancer killed 160,000 people in the U.S. in 2000—more than any other cancer. Because of rising smoking rates among women, lung cancer mortality has surpassed that of breast cancer among American women. Ninety percent of patients who die of lung cancer are smokers, and many of the nonsmokers die from passive exposure. Workers exposed to asbestos (plumbers, shipbuilders) have up to four times the risk of nonsmokers. Smoking is synergistic with asbestos, and together they increase the risk of lung cancer 100 times. Although in theory screening for such a common fatal disease makes sense, trials of screening with sputum cytology and/or CXR have not shown a decrease in mortality, so are not recommended. Screening with chest CT has a higher sensitivity for smaller and potentially more curable lesions. Many noncancerous lesions are discovered that must be investigated, exposing the patient to potential harm and cost. At this time, there are no data from randomized clinical trials indicating decreased mortality with this procedure.

What types of lung cancer are there?

Multiple histologic types of lung cancer are classified into one of two groups based on natural history and response to therapy (Table 29–6). Think of *small cell lung cancer* (SCLC) as a "systemic" disease—it spreads very early to the mediastinum, nodes, liver, bone, and CNS. Coincidentally, "systemic" therapy, chemotherapy, is relatively effective in the short term, extending survival from weeks to months. Squamous cell, adenocarcinoma, and large-cell cancer, subtypes "giant-cell" and "clear-cell," are grouped as *non-small cell lung cancer* (NSCLC) because surgery may be curative for localized disease.

▶ EVALUATION

How might my patient present with lung cancer?

A lung mass may bleed or obstruct an airway, producing hemoptysis, dyspnea, cough, or postobstructive pneumonia. Local

TABLE 29-6

Classification of Lung Cancers

Stage	Involvement	Treatment	Five Year Survival (%)
Small Cell Lung Cancer			
Limited	1 lung, regional nodes (hilum, supraclavicular)	Chemotherapy + radiotherapy +/– prophylactic cranial irradiation rarely, surgical resection for limited disease	5-10
Extensive	More than "limited"	Chemotherapy +/– prophylactic cranial irradiation	<1
Non-Small Cell Lung Cancer			
1	No nodes or metastases	Surgical resection	40-60
2	Ipsilateral bronchial or hilar nodes only	Surgical resection	22-40
3	Distal nodes or local extension	Chemotherapy and/or radiotherapy	5-13
4	Distant metastases	Palliative radiotherapy or chemotherapy	1

extension to the mediastinum, pleura, and chest wall may result in pleural and pericardial effusions, compression of the superior vena cava, or paralysis of mediastinal nerves. Metastases may cause bone pain, liver failure, adrenal insufficiency, or neurologic symptoms. There are many paraneoplastic syndromes associated with particular lung cancers. For example, the syndrome of inappropriate antidiuretic hormone secretion (SIADH) occurs in about 10% of people with SCLC and causes hyponatremia. SCLC can also release ACTH and cause Cushing's syndrome. Humorally mediated hypercalcemia is common in squamous cell carcinoma. These tumors increase serum calcium by secreting parathyroid hormone analogues. Bone metastases are rarely a cause of hypercalcemia in lung cancer.

How do I evaluate a single nodule on a CXR?

Many diseases may cause nodules, such as benign tumors (hamartomas, lipomas), AV malformations, infections (TB, abscesses, fungal diseases), rheumatologic disease (Wegener's granulomatosis, rheumatoid arthritis), infarction, hemorrhage, primary lung or metastatic cancers. Thus, an H & P is important. Certain features of the nodule suggest cancer, including irregular borders and eccentric calcification. Nodules that are unchanged after two years are unlikely to be cancer, so old CXRs may be helpful. A CT scan might rule out cancer, but suspect lesions require biopsy.

► TREATMENT

What is the approach to treatment?

Limited SCLC, found in less than 10% of patients, may be cured with chemotherapy and radiotherapy. Your patient may need a bone marrow biopsy, brain imaging, and bone scan to ensure that the disease is limited. Up to 40% of patients with SCLC will have CNS metastasis requiring cranial radiation therapy. For NSCLC, the essential task is to determine which tumors can be resected for cure. Imaging with CT and/or PET scans, bone scans, and even mediastinoscopy may be necessary. For late-stage SCLC or NSCLC, treatment is palliative with chemotherapy or radiation to shrink, but not eliminate, bulky tumor masses impinging on crucial structures (see Table 29–6).

KEY POINTS

- ► SCLC is treated with chemotherapy; surgery cures a few early cases.
- ► NSCLC is best treated by surgery, but you must look carefully to prove that the tumor is resectable.
- ► Talk to smokers about quitting every time you see them.
- ► Hyponatremia due to SIADH and hypercortisolism due to tumor ACTH release can occur with small cell lung cancer.

NON-HODGKIN'S LYMPHOMA

► ETIOLOGY

What causes non-Hodgkin's lymphoma (NHL)?

Non-Hodgkin's lymphomas are a diverse group of lymphoid tumors of unknown etiology. They cause about 12,000 deaths each year, mostly in middle-aged people. NHL can be a complication of HIV infection. Other associations include human T cell leukemia virus (HTLV) infection, *H. pylori* infection, prior chemotherapy or radiation therapy, and autoimmune disease. Because of the relatively low prevalence, screening is not recommended.

What are the different types of non-Hodgkin's lymphoma?

Most lymphomas are caused by clonal proliferation of B-lympho-cytes residing in lymph nodes. Primary CNS lymphomas are usu-ally seen in immunocompromised patients, such as those with HIV infection. GI lymphomas have been associated with *Helicobacter pylori* infection, Crohn's disease, and celiac sprue. Hairy-cell lym-phoma is associated with prior Epstein-Barr virus infection. T cell lymphomas are less common, and the patient may present with cutaneous malignancy (mycosis fungoides) or in association with HTLV infection seen predominantly in southern Japan, parts of Africa and the Caribbean, and in IV drug users in the United States. Lymphomas are also classified as indolent, aggressive, or highly aggressive based on their rapidity of progression. In gen-eral, indolent lymphomas are not very responsive to therapy but impart prolonged survival. Aggressive and highly aggressive lym-phomas are very responsive to treatment, but are rapidly fatal if not treated.

▶ EVALUATION

How does NHL appear?

About two thirds of patients present with enlarged nodes. Indolent lymphomas may exist for years before the patient notices waxing and waning painless adenopathy. Sometimes, patients report abdominal fullness or early satiety due to hepatosplenomegaly. Aggressive lymphomas may act like acute leukemias, with rapid, progressive enlargement of lymph nodes. Any lymphoma may occur with generalized "B" symptoms: fever, night sweats, and 10% or greater weight loss over the previous six months. B symptoms more often accompany aggressive lym-phomas and portend a worse prognosis. Patients may report fatigue, pruritus, or GI symptoms. Physical exam should focus on presence of lymph nodes (including the neck, axillae, epitrochlear areas, groin, occiput, preauricular areas, tonsils, tongue, and nasopharynx), abdominal exam for organomegaly, as well as known sites of extranodal involvement such as the salivary glands, thyroid, breast, ovary, prostate, testicles, neuro-logic sites, and skin.

What work-up is necessary?

Lymphomas can involve any lymphoid tissue and the CNS, so a complete H & P is critical, with special focus as noted. You will also want a lymph node biopsy of an entire node to evaluate nodal architecture and adequately diagnose the type of lymphoma. Once lymphoma has been suggested by node biopsy, you will need bone marrow biopsy, lumbar puncture, and head and body imaging for staging the tumor. Basic labs should be drawn to identify complications including CBC, renal function, electrolytes, calcium, uric acid, and liver function tests. Serum β-2 microglobulin and LDH may reflect prognosis and disease activity in patients with NHL and help monitor response to therapy. Serum protein electrophoresis (SPEP) may reveal circulating paraproteins or hypogammaglobulinemia. Cytogenetics, cell surface immunophenotyping (flow cytometry), and cytochemistry may further characterize the malignant cells for diagnostic and treatment decisions.

What defines the stages of NHL?

The stages are I–IV, as follows: I—single site, II—several sites on the same side of the diaphragm, III—several sites on both sides of the diaphragm ($\pm$ local organ involvement), and IV—disseminated disease. Each stage is subclassified as "B" for presence of B symptoms as discussed earlier.

▶ **TREATMENT**

Which patients with NHL require treatment and how effective is it?

Some asymptomatic indolent lymphomas are not treated. For symptomatic or more aggressive tumors various combinations of radiation and chemotherapy are used. Overall, five-year survival is about 50%, but that does not tell the whole story. People with low-grade lymphomas live many years but are rarely cured, whereas patients with aggressive grades are cured about half the time.

K E Y   P O I N T S

▶ Suspect non-Hodgkin's lymphoma when diffuse or persistent lymphadenopathy is present.

▶ Non-Hodgkin's lymphoma is a common complication of HIV infection.

▶ Treatment decisions depend on grade, stage, and the age and condition of the patient.

PROSTATE CANCER

▶ ETIOLOGY

How many men have prostate cancer?

Prostate cancer is the most common newly diagnosed cancer in men (i.e., it has the highest incidence). About 30,000 men die of this disease each year in the U.S. It is unique in its high prevalence of "latent" disease: 70% of men in their eighties who die from something else have microscopic foci of prostate cancer. In contrast, only 3% of prostate cancers lead to death. The incidence is highest in blacks, less in whites, and least in Asians. Mortality per case is higher in African-Americans. Family history is a risk factor.

▶ EVALUATION

Should I screen my patient for prostate cancer?

There is insufficient evidence to recommend for or against screening. Digital rectal exams, prostate specific antigen, and transrectal ultrasound can detect tumors that would never cause symptoms or are already incurable. Treatments may also cause incontinence and impotence with unclear benefit. You must help your patient make a personal decision considering such uncertainty.

What symptoms suggest prostate cancer?

Early cancers often produce no symptoms. Some men report benign prostatic hyperplasia (BPH)-like symptoms of dysuria, hematuria, or trouble voiding, but this is relatively uncommon. The first sign may be metastatic bone pain. Sorting out the few men with treatable prostate cancer from the millions with symptomatic BPH is a clinical dilemma.

How is prostate cancer classified?

Prostate cancer is staged clinically by how far the cancer has extended (Table 29–7). Pelvic CT scan is not sensitive enough to detect extracapsular extension and pelvic node or seminal vesicle involvement; hence, some cancers are only fully staged at the time of surgery. Each cancer is assigned a Gleason grade based on histologic features. Tumors are graded 1–5 on two accounts: primarily on the level of differentiation, and secondarily on structural architecture. These two scores are then added, with the most well-differentiated tumors having the best prognosis and a score

TABLE 29-7	

Staging of Prostate Cancer

Stage	Criteria
T1	microscopic, not palpable on rectal examination
T2	palpable, confined to prostate gland
T3	protrudes beyond prostate capsule or into seminal vesicles
T4	tumor fixed, extends locally well beyond gland
Metastatic	tumor spread to pelvic nodes or bone

of 2–4, moderately differentiated tumors scoring 5–7, and poorly differentiated tumors with the worst prognosis scoring 8–10. Both stage and grade assist with treatment decisions and prognosis.

When and where should I look for metastatic prostate cancer?

Bone is the most common distant site, usually involving the pelvic girdle and vertebrae. Some physicians obtain radionuclide bone scan in all patients with a prostate cancer diagnosis, although others are more selective, ordering the test only when PSA is greater than 10, Gleason score is greater than 5, or there is palpable extension of tumor on rectal exam. Lung and liver are rarely sites of distant metastasis.

▶ TREATMENT

What treatment options are there for men with prostate cancer?

Treatment options include observation, radiation, surgery, and hormonal therapy. For disease limited to the gland, the decision to treat is usually based on Gleason score. Nonaggressive tumors are candidates for watchful waiting. More aggressive cancer limited to the gland may be cured with either radical prostatectomy or radiation therapy, although there is controversy among experts whether benefits outweigh risks of side effects. The treatment for tumor extending through the capsule is another area of controversy. Once lymph nodes, bone, lung, or liver is involved, the cancer cannot be cured. In contrast to breast and colon cancer, even a single positive lymph node makes recurrence nearly certain. Consequences of surgical or radiation therapy include urinary incontinence and impotence for a large number of patients. Radiation can also cause chronic proctitis. Long-term survivors of radiation therapy may have an increased risk of bladder and rectal cancers.

Is there a role for palliative therapy in patients with metastatic prostate cancer?

Palliative treatment is the rule for symptomatic metastatic disease. Since this tumor is responsive to androgens, antiandrogens, orchiectomy, estrogens, or luteinizing hormone releasing hormone (LHRH) analogues all reduce androgen synthesis and are effective in decreasing symptoms. Bone pain from metastases also responds well to anti-inflammatory agents but may require use of opioid analgesics. Chemotherapy has been shown to decrease pain and prolong palliation, but has not been shown to have an impact on survival.

How long will my patient live?

Five-year survival for local disease is over 90%. It drops to 80% for locally invasive disease, and 30% for metastases, which is better than for most other metastatic cancers. All of these rates are lower for African-Americans, who may have more aggressive tumors or may get less timely or aggressive treatment.

K E Y   P O I N T S

▶ **It is not known whether screening for prostate cancer is beneficial or harmful.**

▶ **The treatment tools are surgery and radiation, but some patients may be better off untreated.**

▶ **Metastatic disease cannot be cured, but antiandrogen therapies and anti-inflammatory medications may reduce bone pain symptoms.**

TUMORS IN YOUNGER ADULTS

What cancers of younger adults should I look for?

Hodgkin's disease is a tumor of lymphoid tissue, commonly occurring with painless, rubbery nodes. It is highly curable with radiation and/or chemotherapy, but staging must be done carefully. *Testicular cancer* is the most common cancer in men ages 15–35. It is highly curable and, because of the ignorance and embarrassment of patients and doctors, the diagnosis is often made later than need be. It is more common in whites and in those with undescended testes. Your patient may present with a painless testicular mass, or even supraclavicular nodes. Early stages are usually cured with excision. The cure rate in advanced stages is greater than 60% with chemotherapy and irradiation. Early stages of *ovarian cancer* are asymptomatic. Patients present late, often with ascites or pain from peritoneal spread. Most patients die, 14,000/year in the U.S., and there is no effective screening. Deaths from *cervical cancer* have dropped to less than 5000/year in the U.S., and most of these could be prevented with regular Pap smears. The major risk factor is infection with human papillomavirus, and the disease is particularly aggressive in patients with HIV.

CASE 29–3. A 61-year-old, 80-pack-year smoker presents with neck and upper back pain. CXR shows hyperinflation, flattened diaphragms, bullae, and a 2 cm right upper lobe nodule. Calcium is 10.5.

    A. What is your diagnostic plan?
    B. What are the characteristics of a lung nodule that suggest malignancy?
    C. What are possible explanations for his abnormal calcium level?

CASE 29–4. A 50-year-old woman reports feeling very tired. She used to play soccer with her daughters, but now she gets out of breath just unloading the car. She had a prolonged nosebleed yesterday for the first time in years.

    A. What diagnoses are you considering and what questions will you ask?
    B. What will you look for on exam? Will this pin down the diagnosis?
    C. What complications might occur?

CASE 29–5. A 40-year-old man reports chills for the last few days. He has smoked 2 packs per day since age 15, and "coughs all the time, but I think it has been worse." His 43-year-old brother had a bleeding adenoma removed from his colon last year. You see that he is tired and thin, and you find a clump of nodes in the left supraclavicular fossa. A CXR shows left hilar enlargement.

    A. What is a Virchow's node?
    B. What tests do you order?
    C. If he is cured by chemotherapy, will there be long-lasting effects?

CASE 29–6.
A 58-year-old woman elects to have a screening colonoscopy because her neighbor just died of colon cancer. You find a 2 cm ulcerating adenocarcinoma in her ascending colon. Liver tests, a CT scan of the abdomen, and CXR are normal. She undergoes hemicolectomy and tumor is found in two regional lymph nodes.

A. Should she have been screened earlier? If so, why and how?
B. What stage of colon cancer does she have?
C. Do you recommend any further treatment?

CASE 29–7.
A 70-year-old man comes to you for a routine physical exam. On rectal exam, you find that his prostate is mildly irregular and firm in one area. He tells you that his father had prostate cancer at age 57.

A. What evaluation do you suggest?
B. How can you help him decide on treatment?
C. He is concerned about his 35-year-old son and 92-year-old uncle and he hopes that you will see them for screening too. What do you say?

USEFUL WEBSITES

National Cancer Institute
http://www.cancer.gov/cancer_information/
This evidence-based NIH site has detailed and current information on the staging and treatment of all cancers, and much more.
The American Cancer Society
http://www.cancer.org
This site has information on many aspects of cancer, including statistics, decision tools, and patient support.

30

Infectious Diseases

BIOTERRORISM

▶ ETIOLOGY

What is bioterror?

Bioterror is the dissemination of potentially lethal biological agents—bacteria, viruses and toxins—with the intent of generating illness, death, and panic in a population. The degree of fear and anxiety generated may well be disproportionate to the number of individuals afflicted.

Why is it appropriate to include a review of bioterror agents in the medical curriculum?

Dissemination of anthrax spores by U.S. mail in the fall of 2001 infected 20–30 individuals, killed 5, and produced a high level of anxiety among the more than 200 million citizens of this country. Despite the fact that very few practitioners encountered a case of anthrax, many or most had to deal with personal, patient, and community anxieties about the threat. They also needed to be able to recognize an instance of cutaneous or inhalational anthrax had it appeared before them. Whereas it seems impractical to know the details of each otherwise rare agent, it seems appropriate to be aware of general principles relevant to the recognition and management of the most likely agents of bioterror.

What are the likely agents of bioterror?

Potential agents of bioterror are limited only by the imagination of the bioterrorist. Some of the features that might be sought in a bioterror agent include the following:

- Easy dissemination
- Infectious by aerosol route
- Civilian populations are susceptible
- High rates of morbidity and mortality

- Person to person transmission
- Unfamiliar to physicians—difficult to diagnose/treat
- High capacity to cause panic and social disruption
- Prior development for biological warfare by governmental entities

Those agents that are deemed to best fit the criteria above have been designated "Category A" agents and are listed in Box 30–1. A second and third tier of potential bioterror agents, designated "Category B" and "Category C," are listed in the CDC (Centers for Disease Control) website given later. We discuss here only anthrax, other agents of "ulceroglandular fevers," and smallpox.

What makes anthrax a Category A bioterror agent?

Anthrax is favored as a bioterror agent because of its special features. The initial presentation of inhalational anthrax is difficult for physicians to diagnose because it is a vague illness that is similar to a mild upper respiratory illness. By the time fulminant symptoms have developed, antibiotics are not effective, so morbidity and mortality of undiagnosed exposure is high. Anthrax exists in a spore (hibernating) form that is long-lived in the environment and withstands conditions that would kill growing bacteria. As to dissemination, mechanisms have been developed to disperse the spores finely, substantially reducing the inhaled dose required to cause infection. This has been termed "weaponizing." In the natural form, anthrax can also be aerosolized, but this is less effective as a bioterror agent because the spores tend to cluster and stick to environmental surfaces.

How deadly is smallpox and is vaccine effective at preventing disease?

Smallpox is a viral disease that affects only humans and that can be prevented by vaccination. As a consequence of a vig-

---

BOX 30-1

Likely "Class A" Agents for Bioterrorism*
Anthrax
Other ulceroglandular fevers
Plague
Tularemia
Smallpox
Hemorrhagic fever viruses
Ebola
Marburg
Botulinum toxin

*For class B and class C agents refer to http://www.bt.cdc.gov/

orous worldwide vaccination and isolation campaign, natural smallpox was eradicated in 1977. In the U.S., vaccinations were no longer administered after 1972. The CDC continues to hold a small supply of the virus, and concern remains that bioterrorists may choose to use this pox virus as a weapon. Smallpox is a devastating disfiguring disease that is associated with a mortality rate of approximately 30% in nonimmune populations. There is probably significant, but incomplete, immunity among individuals who have been vaccinated decades (up to 50 years) prior to exposure. Although smallpox is contagious by the aerosol route, infectivity does not emerge until the diagnostic features of the disease are evident, making quarantine of individuals with symptoms an effective strategy to prevent person-to-person spread of disease.

▶ EVALUATION

What are the clinical features of ulceroglandular fevers?

Ulceroglandular fevers have in common the following features. They are acquired by inoculation of bacteria into the skin usually either by microtrauma or by the bite of an arthropod vector. Local replication of the bacteria produces local inflammation and, later, tissue necrosis resulting in an ulcer—often with a black scar at the center. Lymph nodes that drain the affected area become swollen, hence the glandular component of the disease. The principal agents of ulceroglandular fevers are plague (*Pasteurella pestis*), tularemia (*Francisella tularensis*), and anthrax (*Bacillus anthracis*). Each of the agents of the ulceroglandular fevers has a natural life cycle in animals and is endemic, albeit at low levels, in the U.S. All of these agents are treatable with common antimicrobials when given early in the course of the disease. Each of the agents rarely can be acquired by an aerosol route producing an infection that is much more difficult to diagnose and more deadly.

How does anthrax present?

The clinical presentation of *cutaneous anthrax* produces an ulceroglandular fever syndrome that, in approximately 80% of cases, resolves without specific treatment. Antimicrobials are effective for the remaining 20% of individuals. A special feature of anthrax skin lesions is the remarkable degree of brawny edema at the margins of ulcers. The edema reaction is thought to be mediated by a particular toxin, edema toxin. *Inhalation anthrax* is characterized early by an upper respiratory illness with sore throat, mild fever, and myalgias, followed by mediastinal lymphadenopathy with lymph nodes growing so large as to produce pain, respiratory distress, and stridor. Large pleural effusions are also a prominent characteristic. Whereas naturally acquired inhalation disease rarely leads to pneumonia, inhalation anthrax associated with bioterror agents has resulted in pneumonias in about half of the cases. When inhalation disease is evident, blood cultures for gram-positive rod bacteria are usually positive. Death is usually associated with overwhelming sepsis and, often, with bacillary meningitis.

How does smallpox present?

Usually patients become severely ill with fever, headache, backache, and vomiting two to three days before onset of a rash. When the rash begins, the patient becomes infectious. The rash begins on the face, hands, and forearms (different from the truncal predominance in chicken pox) and involves the palms and soles, unlike most other viral exanthemas. Oropharyngeal virus is aerosolized through coughing. Symptoms suggestive of smallpox should prompt early communication with local health authorities and rapid quarantine to prevent spread of disease.

▶ TREATMENT

How do I treat anthrax?

Doxycycline and quinolones are effective if given early in the course of the disease. Ciprofloxacin is the only drug with a specific FDA treatment indication for anthrax.

How do I treat smallpox?

For close contacts of a smallpox patient, treat by vaccination, which is effective if given within a few days of exposure. There are no specific antimicrobials available.

What is the role of the practitioner in coping with bioterror agents?

It is impossible to know all about these ordinarily rare disorders. Rapid self-education through local CME resources and reliable websites such as the one maintained by the CDC, listed later, is appropriate (Box 30–2). The goals of self-education are to be able to recognize the more classical manifestations of an agent once it is identified. A key role is to communicate medical events of concern to local health authorities. Such events would include an increase in persons ill with a similar or unusual syndrome, an increase in unexplained diseases or deaths, a single case of a disease caused by an uncommon agent, an unexpected seasonal or geographic distribution of a disease, an unusual

BOX 30-2

Role of the Practitioner in Coping with Bioterror—The 5 R's
Rapid self-education
Recognition of syndromes
Reporting to public health agencies
Rx of patients
Realistic reassurance of worried well

age distribution (such as varicella or measles in adults), and an acquisition of a disease by an unusual route of transmission.

How do I provide psychological care to the worried well?

The first issue is to become knowledgeable about the bioterror agent of immediate concern and to gain a reasonable view of the epidemiological risks associated with that agent. If you personally can honestly be reassured and can speak with your patients in an informed manner, this may help significantly in providing truthful reassurance. Real risks should not be negated. For individuals who manifest extreme anxiety, anxiolytic drugs may be of benefit.

Prophylaxis or empiric treatment in the form of vaccines, antiserum, or prophylactic antibiotics should be restricted to circumstances set out in guidelines developed by public health authorities. Risks of vaccination or widespread prophylactic antibiotic therapy need to be balanced against the potential benefits. Public health guidance is critical in making these decisions.

USEFUL WEBSITE

The most important information about a specific agent of bioterror at any given time will be context dependent. A reliable resource is the CDC website at *http://www.bt.cdc.gov/*

ENCEPHALITIS

▶ **ETIOLOGY**

What is encephalitis and what causes it?

Encephalitis is inflammation of the brain tissue. Viral causes predominate, but fungus, rickettsial infection, toxoplasmosis and tuberculosis are also important etiologies. Without question, the most important cause of acute encephalitis in the U.S. is the herpes virus, especially HSV I. Note that HSV is an important cause of viral meningitis as well. Rare eastern equine encephalitis, St. Louis encephalitis, and rabies cases are reported each year. Recently West Nile virus cases have been reported in the United States. *Toxoplasma* encephalitis is common in HIV-infected patients with low CD_4 counts (see HIV Disease chapter). The mortality rate of untreated HSV encephalitis is 70%.

▶ EVALUATION

What are the typical clinical features of herpes encephalitis?

The clinical features of herpes encephalitis include fever, nausea, vomiting, headache, and alterations in level of consciousness with lethargy and confusion. HSV can involve the temporal lobe, causing personality change, temporal lobe seizures, and odd behavior. Other symptoms include speech disturbances, ataxia, cranial nerve defects, and visual field loss. Patients who present with coma, or in whom the diagnosis is missed, have a high likelihood of death. Neurologic sequelae are common in survivors.

What testing should be done to evaluate suspected encephalitis?

CSF in patients with HSV encephalitis usually shows a pleocytosis with both lymphocytes and polymorphonuclear cells (PMNs). PMNs may predominate early in infection. Red blood cells are frequently present in the CSF. In the past, definitive diagnosis has been made by brain biopsy, because culture of HSV from CSF is difficult. CT scan, MRI, or EEG can localize the area of brain involvement. HSV DNA polymerase chain reaction performed on CSF is replacing brain biopsy for diagnosis because it is rapidly performed and highly sensitive and specific.

▶ TREATMENT

How do you treat HSV encephalitis?

Treat with high dose intravenous acyclovir. Because of high mortality rates, begin therapy as soon as you consider the diagnosis. No treatment is effective for other viral encephalitides.

K E Y   P O I N T S

▶ HSV encephalitis may present with personality change, odd behavior, and confusion along with fever, headache, and vomiting.

▶ Early therapy with intravenous acyclovir is critical for decreasing mortality and diminishing the likelihood and severity of permanent neurologic sequelae.

▶ DNA PCR for HSV on cerebrospinal fluid is the preferred diagnostic test for HSV encephalitis.

ENDOCARDITIS

▶ ETIOLOGY

What causes endocarditis?

Endocarditis is an infection of heart valves. Endocarditis usually begins with seeding of a pre-existing valve abnormality during a period of transient bacteremia. Native valve disease is usually caused by *Staphylococcus aureus* in injection drug users and to streptococcal species in other patients. Prosthetic valve disease within two months of valve placement is likely due to *Staphylococcus epidermidis, S. aureus,* or a gram-negative organism, or if more than two months have passed, streptococcal species or *S. aureus. Streptococcus bovis* endocarditis is associated with colon cancer and so should prompt colonoscopy.

How serious is endocarditis infection?

Mortality from endocarditis ranges from 10%–50%. The highest mortality rates occur in patients infected in the two months after receiving their prosthetic valve.

▶ EVALUATION

How do I recognize the clinical presentation of endocarditis?

Most patients have a fever, although older patients may have a normal temperature. Endocarditis can present with acute symptoms such as high fever and systemic toxicity. Endocarditis can also be subtle, causing nonspecific symptoms such as cough, dyspnea, fatigue, arthralgias, and abdominal or back pain. Some patients present with complications such as congestive heart failure, stroke, arrhythmia, and lung abscesses. Ask about risk factors including injection drug use, prior valve abnormality, or recent invasive procedures (dental, upper respiratory, lower GI, GU) likely to cause transient bacteremic episodes. On exam, look for septic emboli in the fundi (Roth spots), the palms, and finger pads (tender Osler's nodes, red nontender Janeway lesions) and nail beds (splinter hemorrhages). Listen for a new murmur or abnormal lung sounds. Document a thorough neurologic exam as a baseline for potential future embolic events.

How do I diagnose endocarditis?

Diagnose with at least three sets of blood cultures drawn at least one hour apart within the first twenty-four hours, before starting antibiotics. Do not withhold antibiotics in the acutely ill. CXR may show multiple patchy peripheral and lower lobe infiltrates with tricuspid valve endocarditis. Echo can confirm the diagnosis by showing a valvular vegetation, but can't rule it out as the sensitivity of TTE is only 55%–65%. Transesophageal echo is more sensitive and is recommended for suspected prosthetic valve endocarditis, suspected myocardial abscess, or valve perforation. A TEE should be obtained despite a normal TTE if the suspicion of endocarditis remains high. Clinical criteria for the diagnosis have been proposed (Box 30–3).

▶ TREATMENT

What antibiotics are appropriate for endocarditis?

Treat with empiric bactericidal antibiotics based on the presentation. For patients using intravenous drugs, start gentamicin and nafcillin to cover presumptive *S. aureus*. Substitute vancomycin for nafcillin if the patient is penicillin allergic or if the patient resides in an area with a high rate of methicillin resistant *S. aureus*. Most native-valve streptococcal infections can be covered with penicillin or ceftriaxone. Prosthetic valve infections should be covered empirically with vancomycin, gentamicin, and rifampin. Narrow therapy when culture results are available and treat for four to six weeks with intravenous and oral antibiotics, depending on the clinical situation. Uncomplicated tricuspid valve *S. aureus* endocarditis can be treated with two weeks of nafcillin and an aminoglycoside.

BOX 30-3

Duke Criteria for the Diagnosis of Endocarditis
Major Criteria

(1) Two separate positive blood cultures with a typical microorganism
(2) New regurgitant murmur or characteristic echo findings: vegetation, myocardial abscess, partial dehiscence of a prosthetic valve

Minor Criteria

(1) Presence of a predisposing condition
(2) Fever greater than 38°C
(3) Embolic disease
(4) Immunologic phenomena: glomerulonephritis, Osler nodes, Roth spots, rheumatoid factor
(5) Positive blood cultures not meeting major criteria
(6) Positive echo not meeting major criteria

Definite diagnosis with 80% accuracy when there are:

2 major criteria OR
1 major criterion + 3 minor criteria OR
5 minor criteria

Endocarditis unlikely when there are:

none of the criteria AND
alternative explanation for illness found OR
fever defervesces within 4 days

K E Y   P O I N T S

▶ Endocarditis in IDUs is most frequently the tricuspid valve infected with *S. aureus.*

▶ Blood culture is the most important diagnostic procedure.

▶ Echocardiography provides useful confirmatory information, but TTE only has a sensitivity of 55%–65%.

REFERENCES

Giessel BE, Koenig CJ, Blake RL, Jr: Management of bacterial endocarditis. Am Fam Physician 61(6):1725–1732,1739, 2000.

Mylonakis E, Calderwood SB: Infective endocarditis in adults. N Engl J
    Med 345(18):1318–1330, 2001.

GENITAL INFECTIONS

 ETIOLOGY

What are the common causes of genital discharge?

In women, vaginal discharge is often normal and varies in amount
and quality through the hormonal cycle. In men, penile discharge
aside from ejaculation warrants further evaluation. In women,
pathologic causes of discharge are *cervicitis* and *vaginitis*, and in
men, *urethritis* (Table 30–1). In men and women, discharge may
be absent despite infection. In particular, chlamydia is often clinically silent; untreated chlamydia may cause infertility in women.

What is bacterial vaginosis (BV)?

BV is an overgrowth of normal vaginal flora. There is no infection
or inflammation, hence the term *vaginosis* rather than *vaginitis*.
This is not a dangerous or sexually transmitted condition, but the
increased discharge and postcoital fishy odor may be bothersome
to patients and, if so, merits treatment. In pregnancy, BV may be
associated with preterm labor and so should be treated.

What causes genital ulcers?

The most common cause of painful genital ulcers is herpes simplex virus infection (HSV). Particularly with primary infection,
patients may have accompanying fevers and myalgias. Painful

TABLE 30–1

Pathologic Causes of Genital Discharge		
Women	**Cervicitis**	**Vaginitis**
	Gonorrhea	Candida
	Chlamydia	Trichomonas
	Polymicrobial GNR, Streptococcus species	Bacterial vaginosis
		Atrophic vaginitis of low estrogen
Men	**Urethritis**	
	Gonorrhea	
	Chlamydia	
	Reiter's syndrome (rare)	

ulcers also occur with chancroid from infection with *Haemophilus ducreyi*, although these are usually deep, friable, and undermined at the edges, unlike the superficial ulcers of HSV. Painless, deep, and indurated ulcers are seen with primary syphilis. Toxic epidermal necrolysis is a rare, potentially fatal, drug reaction that can cause painful genital and oral ulcers.

What causes genital growths?

Human papilloma virus (HPV) causes genital warts or condyloma acuminata, which are broad-based and verrucous. These can appear at any location in the perineum, including perirectally. Condom use does not prevent transmission of this virus, which is easily spread from skin-to-skin contact. More than half of the general population has serologic evidence of exposure. Certain subtypes of HPV (16, 18, and others) play a causative role in cervical and other genital cancers. Genital growths may also be skin tags, molluscum contagiosum, or skin cancer.

My patient reports pelvic pain. What are common genitourinary causes?

In women, urinary tract infections, menstrual pain, ovarian cyst rupture, ectopic pregnancy, endometriosis, and PID can all cause pain. PID is a polymicrobial infection of the upper genital tract in women, usually caused by some combination of chlamydia, gonorrhea, enteric gram-negative rods, and/or streptococci. Chronic pelvic pain is closely associated with a history of sexual abuse. In men, deep pelvic or perineal pain can be caused by prostatitis or urinary tract infection.

▶ EVALUATION

What historical points are important in evaluating genital infections?

Ask about new sexual partners, previous infections, and unprotected or high-risk sex. Inquire into last menstrual period, irregular vaginal bleeding, new discharge, pain with intercourse, fevers, or new skin or genital lesions. History regarding specific symptoms is generally not reliable for diagnosis. The classic example is vaginal itching, which does not correlate with vaginal yeast infections.

What examination is necessary for patients reporting genital symptoms?

Examine the external genitalia for dermal or mucosal ulceration, redness, discharge, or new lesions. Include testicular and prostate examinations in men, pelvic speculum and bimanual exam in women, and inguinal lymph node exam in both sexes. For women with discharge or pain on exam, obtain CBC, urine pregnancy test, and perform a wet prep and KOH microscopic exam on secretions from the vaginal wall, as well as a Gram stain on any cervical discharge. For both sexes, order urinalysis and gonorrhea and chlamydial testing. This can be performed by urethral or cervical swab for culture. A DNA-based test called LCR, ligase chain reaction, is extremely sensitive and specific when used to detect chlamydia or gonorrhea on swab or urine samples. The urine test requires "dirty urine," or the first 10–20 mL of void urine, to accurately sample urethral pathology. This collection technique is very different from the clean catch midstream sample most patients are accustomed to obtaining, so be sure to instruct them carefully, as samples will not be processed if sent to the lab with more than 20 mL in the cup. Consider RPR and HIV testing in patients with genital symptoms, or any other STD diagnosis, including *Trichomonas*, HSV, genital warts, gonorrhea, and chlamydia infections.

How do I perform a microscopic exam of vaginal discharge?

In a woman with new or symptomatic discharge, studies show that routine office pelvic examination is not adequate to determine the cause. Further sampling is required. Using a cotton swab, obtain fluid from the vaginal wall and place in a small amount of saline. The swab must stay moist because even a few seconds of drying can decrease sensitivity for *Trichomonas*. Use this swab to prepare saline KOH slides. The saline slide may reveal WBCs suggesting inflammation of any cause, clue cells suggesting bacterial BV (grainy-appearing squamous cells coated with bacteria), or trichomonads that are motile and slightly larger than WBCs. The KOH slide may show candidal hyphae after the normal cells have lysed. Because yeast colonization is common, WBCs should also be seen on the saline slide to help confirm the diagnosis. Vaginal pH is normally 4.5 and can be tested directly using pH paper along the vaginal wall; pH is above normal with BV, *Trichomonas*, and estrogen deficient states.

How do I diagnose PID?

Diagnosis of PID can be tricky owing to a range of presenting symptoms from subtle to severe. Minimum criteria for diagnosis include pelvic pain or cervical motion tenderness, although presence of fever greater than 38.3°C, cervical discharge, elevated ESR or C-reactive protein, or positive cervical or endometrial cultures enhance diagnostic specificity. Endometrial biopsy, imaging, or laparoscopy can also help make the diagnosis of PID more definitively.

Should I perform routine screening for any of these infections?

Chlamydial screening is indicated in high-risk populations of women younger than age 25 and women with two or more new sexual partners per year. HPV, BV, and gonorrhea are not routinely screened. Annual pap smear is indicated for women with new partners in the prior several years to screen for cervical atypia that may arise in the setting of HPV infection, whereas women in a single, long-term, monogamous relationship with three prior normal annual paps can safely undergo screening every three years.

▶ TREATMENT

What are current therapies for genital infections?

See Table 30–2 for pathogens, diagnosis, and treatment of common genital infections.

Gonorrhea, chlamydial infection, and trichomoniasis are reportable conditions in most states and partners require evaluation and treatment. BV only requires treatment if the patient is pregnant or is bothered by the symptoms. HSV can be treated acutely to shorten duration of outbreaks, or with daily suppressive therapy for severe or frequent outbreaks. Genital warts are easily removed with cryotherapy or topical podophyllin, although the underlying HPV infection cannot be eradicated.

What are the potential complications of PID infection?

Even with treatment, up to 25% of women with PID experience repeat infections, chronic pelvic pain, dyspareunia, ectopic pregnancy, and infertility.

Can I treat a vaginal yeast infection empirically?

Yes, if the patient has been on antibiotics recently. Otherwise, it is best to perform a full examination as several studies have shown inaccurate diagnoses by physicians and patients alike based on history and inspection alone. Microscopic examination is especially important in patients with recurrent symptoms because the diagnosis may be incorrect, or the yeast may be resistant to routine therapy. Send vaginal swab for culture and sensitivity in these cases. Screen for elevated blood sugar and consider HIV testing in patients with recurrent yeast infections, as diabetes and HIV infection are risk factors. Topical treatment may provide relief more rapidly than oral fluconazole therapy.

TABLE 30–2

Pathogens, Diagnosis, and Treatment in Genital Infections

Pathogen	Diagnosis	Treatment (oral unless otherwise noted)
Cervix/endometrium/urethra		
Chlamydia	LCR or culture	azithromycin 1000 mg × 1
Gonorrhea	LCR or culture	ceftriaxone 125 mg IM, OR
		cefixime 400 mg × 1
PID	Pelvic pain, fever	*Inpatient*:
	CMT	cefoxitin 2g IV q6h, OR cefotetan IV 2g q12h
	Elevated WBC, ESR, CRP	AND
	Cervical cultures	doxycycline 100 mg IV or PO bid × 14d
	Imaging, laparoscopy	*Outpatient*:
	Endometrial biopsy	ofloxacin 400 mg bid × 14 d AND
		metronidazole 500 mg bid × 14 d, OR
		ceftriaxone 250 mg IM 1X AND
		doxycycline 100 mg bid × 14 days
Vagina		
Candida	Hyphae, WBC on KOH	Fluconazole 150 mg × 1, may repeat × 1
	pH < 4.5	Topical antifungal
Trichomonas	Flagellates on wet mount	Metronidazole 2g × 1
	pH > 4.5	
Bacterial vaginosis	Clue cells, WBC on wet prep	Metronidazole 500 mg bid × 7d OR
	pH > 4.5	Metronidazole vaginal gel 0.75% bid × 5d
	Positive whiff test	
Genital mucosa		
Herpes simplex virus	Tzanck prep or culture serology*	Suppressive: acyclovir 400 mg bid†
		Acute: acyclovir 400 mg tid × 5-10d
Human papillomavirus	Exam, biopsy if needed	Cryotherapy
		Topical imiquimod or podophyllin

*Does differentiate type 1 from type 2, but does not distinguish past from new infection, and so is not diagnostic for a current lesion.
†Valacyclovir and famcyclovir are also effective but more expensive.

K E Y   P O I N T S

▶ In any patient with new discharge, perform a genital exam, a microscopic exam in women, chlamydial and gonorrhea tests, and consider rapid plasma reagin (RPR) and HIV tests.

▶ In asymptomatic high risk women, perform pap and screen for chlamydia annually.

▶ Urine LCR is a highly sensitive and specific test for both gonorrhea and chlamydia.

▶ Suspect PID in women with pelvic pain, especially if other suggestive features are present.

▶ Genital warts may be easily removed although the underlying infection persists.

▶ HPV is easily transmitted and is associated with cervical and rectal cancer.

▶ HSV outbreaks can be treated episodically or prevented with daily suppressive therapy, depending on frequency and severity of episodes.

CASE 30–1. A 47-year-old woman presents

with vaginal itching and states that she has a yeast infection that has not responded to over-the-counter creams. She has heard of a pill and wonders if you will prescribe it.

A. What is your differential diagnosis?
B. What tests will you obtain?

REFERENCE

1998 guidelines for treatment of sexually transmitted diseases. MMWR Morb Mortal Wkly Rep 47(RR-1):79, 1998.

USEFUL WEBSITE

CDC STD prevention website that includes treatment guidelines for STDs: *http://www.cdc.gov/nchstp/dstd/dstdp.html*

HIV INFECTION PRIMARY CARE

▶ ETIOLOGY

What terminology is useful in categorizing HIV infection?

HIV infection is classified by numbers 1, 2, or 3 depending on the CD4 count, and by letters A, B, or C depending on the occurrence of specific conditions (Table 30–3). AIDS is defined as category C disease or a CD4 count less than 200 (A3, B3). Begin your oral presentation of any HIV-infected pàtient by giving the classification, last CD4 count, and viral load.

Why are CD4 cell counts and HIV viral load important?

CD4 count indicates the severity of immune suppression and is used to determine 1) disease classification; 2) when to start or change antiretroviral therapy; 3) when certain opportunistic infections are likely (Figure 30–1); and 4) when to start opportunistic infection prophylaxis. Quantitative HIV viral load gives prognostic information beyond that provided by the CD4 count. The higher the viral load, the more rapidly the patient is becoming immune-suppressed. Viral load is used to assess efficacy of antiretroviral therapy within weeks of any change.

TABLE 30–3

Classification of HIV Infection

CD4 count per mm^3	A Asymptomatic, or persistent generalized lymphadenopathy	B* Symptomatic, not category C	C** AIDS-indicator conditions
> 500	A_1	B_1	C_1
200-499	A_2	B_2	C_2
< 200	A_3	B_3	C_3

*Examples of category B conditions include bacillary angiomatosis, oral thrush, cervical dysplasia/carcinoma, oral hairy leukoplakia, herpes zoster (recurrent or multi-dermatomal), and ITP.

**Examples of category C conditions include PCP, cryptococcal meningitis, toxoplasmosis, CMV retinitis, AIDS dementia complex, TB recurrent bacterial pneumonias, Kaposi's sarcoma, CNS lymphoma, and other non-Hodgkin's lymphomas.

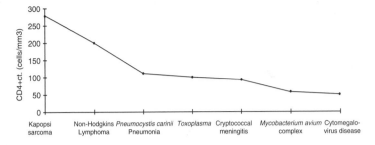

From the New England Journal of Medicine (324: 1332-B, 1992)

Figure 30–1. Occurrence of AIDS-indicating conditions in the natural history of HIV infection, according to mean CD4+ cell count.

What is the risk of acquiring HIV infection from a needle stick injury?

Fear of contracting HIV in the health care setting through needle stick or mucosal splash accidents is a significant stress factor for all health professionals. The risk of infection is low, estimated in a CDC study to be 0.5% for percutaneous exposure (3/860). Based on other data, the risk is probably somewhat less (~0.2%) than that reported by the CDC. The risk for HIV transmission is greater if blood is seen on the needle, if the needle stick is a deep wound from a hollow bore needle, if gloves were not worn, or if the source patient has advanced HIV disease.

▶ EVALUATION

How do I diagnose HIV infection?

Screen for HIV infection with an ELISA test. This detects HIV antibodies with sensitivity and specificity of greater than 99%. The positive predictive value of the ELISA (i.e., the likelihood that a patient with a positive test actually has HIV infection) ranges from 20% in very low risk populations to greater than 95% in patients with strong risk factors. Because the ELISA is not 100% specific, use a Western blot to confirm any positive ELISA. This test detects serum antibodies directed against specific HIV-1 proteins of various molecular weights and is defined as positive when two or more of the following antibody bands are present: p24, gp41, or gp120/160. Indeterminate Western blots are not uncommon;

without p24, gp41, or gp 120/160 bands, the patient does not need further evaluation and does not have HIV infection.

What is the window period?

This is the period of time between acquiring infection and development of antibodies. Antibody-based test results remain negative in this window period. Over 90% of patients undergo seroconversion within four weeks of infection. Three tests can detect HIV infection before the appearance of antibody: viral p24 antigen and viral load testing with nucleic acid polymerase chain reaction or branch chain DNA assays. The p24 antigen is transiently positive and less sensitive for acute HIV infection than are the viral load tests (PCR or branch chain DNA assay). Occasionally when risk of acute infection is high and a patient is still within the "window" period, viral load testing may be used for diagnosis instead of the usual antibody-based tests.

What key questions should I ask of patients with HIV infection at clinic visits?

Your main goal is to assess the immune status of your patient. In patients with high CD4 counts, focus on skin or mouth symptoms, side effects from any medications, general health (weight loss, fatigue, itching, loss of appetite), and any patient concerns.

In patients with low CD4 counts below 300 the risk of opportunistic infection is much greater. Mean CD4 count is less than 100 for most common opportunistic infections. Ask these patients about diarrhea, dysphagia, thrush, headache, fever, or changes in vision (Table 30–4).

What are the important parts of the physical exam to include in all visits?

Perform skin and oral exams at each visit in all patients. Look for any of the three forms of candidiasis: pseudomembranous candidiasis causes well-recognized thick white plaques on the tongue and palate; atrophic candidiasis causes a painful red shiny tongue or hard palate; angular cheilitis causes cracking and fissuring at the corners of the mouth. Look for hairy leukoplakia, aphthous ulcers, Kaposi's sarcoma, and gingivitis as well. Perform careful skin exam. Test for peripheral neuropathy in patients on ddI/ddC/D4T. This can be done easily by breaking a cotton-tipped applicator and using the sharp broken end and the soft cotton end to distinguish sharp from light touch sensation. Examination of the anal and perineal area should be done annually in patients with a history of receptive anal intercourse. These patients are at an increased risk for anal cancer due to HPV infection.

TABLE 30–4

History Questions to Ask HIV-Infected Patients at Routine Clinic Visits

Patient with High CD4 Count (>300)	Diseases Concerned About
Medication side effects	Pancreatitis: ddl, d4T, ddC
	Neuropathy: ddl, ddC, d4T
	Myositis: AZT
	Kidney stones: indinavir
	Diarrhea: Nelfinavir, ritonavir
	Hepatitis: all protease inhibitors, nevirapine
Skin changes	Seborrheic dermatitis
	Generalized pruritus
General health (fatigue, weight change, anorexia)	Medication side effects, depression, TB
Patient with Low CD4 Count (< 300)	
Headache, seizure, weakness, general fever, weight loss, night sweats	MAC, AIDS wasting syndrome, toxoplasmosis, *Cryptococcus*
Dysphagia	Candidal esophagitis (CMV/HSV esophagitis less commonly)
Diarrhea	*C. difficile, Cryptosporidium*, MAC
Abdominal pain	MAC, lymphoma, acalculous cholecystitis
Cough, dyspnea	Pneumonia, especially PCP
Visual changes	CMV

When should I obtain HIV RNA viral load and CD4 counts?

Current recommendations for obtaining quantitative measurement of HIV RNA are 1) before starting antiretroviral therapy; 2) four weeks after starting a new antiretroviral regimen; and 3) every three to four months during antiretroviral therapy to assess whether modifications are needed. Check CD4 counts every six months when CD4 is greater than 500 and every three months when CD4 is less than 500.

▶ TREATMENT

When should I start antiretroviral therapy?

Patients who present with acute HIV infection should be enrolled in trials looking at the efficacy of aggressive antiretroviral therapy shortly after infection occurs. Some providers treat acute infection regardless of CD4 count and viral load with triple drug combinations including protease inhibitors, although we do not know long-term outcomes with this approach. In patients with CD4 counts greater than 500 and an undetectable viral load, monitoring without antiretroviral therapy is appropriate. A high viral load greater than 55,000 is reason to start antiretroviral therapy regardless of CD4 count. When the CD4 count is less than 500 antiretroviral therapy can be considered and should be encouraged if the viral load is high (greater than 55,000). Watching closely without antiretroviral therapy is a very reasonable approach in patients with CD4 counts above 350 but with low or nondetectable viral loads. Antiretroviral therapy should be started only when patients can commit to making all follow up visits and taking medications without missing doses so as to decrease the risk of developing viral resistance.

What antiretroviral drug should I use?

Combination therapy is the rule. The most potent combination is two nucleoside reverse transcriptase inhibitors (AZT, ddI, ddC, d4T, 3TC, tenofovir, or abacavir) with a protease inhibitor. Another option is two reverse transcriptase inhibitors with a non-nucleoside drug, efavirenz or nevirapine (Table 30–5).

TABLE 30–5

Antiretroviral Medications, Dose, and Side Effects

Drugs	Typical Dose	Side Effects
Nucleoside reverse transcriptase inhibitors (NRTI)		
• Zidovudine (AZT)	300 mg bid	Nausea, headache, myopathy, anemia, Neutropenia
• Didanosine (ddI)	400 mg qd	Neuropathy, pancreatitis
• Zalcitabine (ddC)	0.75 mg tid	Neuropathy, pancreatitis, mucosal ulcer
• Stavudine (d4T)	40 mg bid	Neuropathy, pancreatitis
• Lamivudine (3TC)	150 mg bid	Minimal
• Abacavir	300 mg bid	Life threatening hypersensitivity
• Tenofovir	300 mg qd	Nausea, asymptomatic CPK↑
Non-nucleoside reverse transcriptase inhibitors (NNRTI)		
• Nevirapine	200 mg bid	Rash, liver failure
• Efavirenz	600 mg qd	Rash, agitation, confusion
Protease inhibitors (PI)		*All PI's can raise cholesterol, triglycerides, transaminases*
• Indinavir	800 mg q8 hrs	kidney stones, elevated bilirubin
• Nelfinavir	750 mg tid	Diarrhea
• Ritonavir	400 mg bid with saquinavir	Nausea, vomiting, perioral paresthesias
• Saquinavir	400 mg bid with ritonavir	Nausea, diarrhea
• Amprenavir	1200 mg bid	Nausea, diarrhea
• Kaletra (lopinavir/ritonavir)	3 capsules bid	Nausea, diarrhea

What are the side effects of antiretroviral agents?

Zidovudine (AZT) can cause headaches, nausea, and vomiting when first started. Anemia and neutropenia occur with longer-term use and are more common in patients who have lower CD4 counts. Patients on the drug for more than six months can develop myopathy. All the drugs that begin with "D" (ddI, ddC, D4T) can cause peripheral neuropathy and pancreatitis. In addition, ddC can also produce mucosal ulceration. Abacavir can cause a life-threatening allergic reaction. The non-nucleoside drug nevirapine is responsible for rash in 15% of patients and can rarely cause liver failure. The non-nucleoside drug efavirenz can cause insomnia, nightmares, and problems concentrating. All the protease inhibitors (indinavir, ritonavir, nelfinavir, amprenavir, lopinavir, and saquinavir) can result in transaminase elevations. Indinavir is known for its propensity to produce kidney stones. Patients on this drug should be counseled to stay well hydrated. All protease inhibitors can raise triglycerides and lower HDL cholesterol levels as well as cause glucose intolerance, so lipids and glucose should be monitored regularly (see Table 30–5).

What is lipodystrophy?

Patients on protease inhibitors or D4T can develop changes in body fat distribution referred to as lipodystrophy. Typical features are temporal wasting and sunken cheeks, thin arms and thin legs with a protuberant abdomen ("protease paunch"). Veins on the arms and legs become prominent and there is an increased incidence of paronychia. Metabolic abnormalities include increased glucose and triglycerides and low HDL cholesterol level.

When should I start prophylaxis against *Pneumocystis carinii* pneumonia (PCP)?

Patients who have any of the following conditions should receive PCP prophylaxis: CD4 count under 200, previous PCP, oral candidiasis. Trimethoprim-sulfamethoxazole (TMP/SMX) is by far the most effective agent. It is also prophylactic against toxoplasmosis and may prevent bacterial sinusitis and bacterial pneumonias. For patients who cannot tolerate TMP/SMX, dapsone is a reasonable option. Atovaquone and aerosolized pentamidine are third-line options, but are less effective than TMP/SMX or dapsone. Because aerosolized pentamidine is not a systemic therapy, patients may develop *Pneumocystis* at sites other than their lungs. *Pneumocystis* prophylaxis can be stopped in patients on highly active antiretroviral therapy (HAART) with CD4 counts that have risen above 200 and nondetectable viral loads for at least six months.

When should patients receive *Mycobacterium avium* complex (MAC) prophylaxis?

Current recommendations start MAC prophylaxis when CD4 count is under 50. Favored regimens are azithromycin 1200 mg weekly or clarithromycin 500 mg bid. MAC prophylaxis can be stopped in patients on HAART who have CD4 counts above 100 and non-detectable viral loads for at least six months.

What do I do if I get a needle-stick from an HIV-infected patient?

First of all, try to prevent this by wearing gloves whenever you draw blood, manipulate intravenous lines, or examine a mucosal surface. Wear eye protection for any procedure (endoscopy, bronchoscopy, surgery). *NEVER* recap needles: this is the most common cause of needle stick injury. Use of AZT after needle-stick injury appears to decrease the risk of transmission. Current practice is to give AZT plus 3TC for lower risk exposures, and to add a third drug, usually a protease inhibitor, for high-risk exposures. If the source patient has known AZT resistance, substitute D4T, abacavir, or ddI for the AZT in the prophylactic regimen.

K E Y   P O I N T S

▶ Perform skin and oral cavity exam at all visits.

▶ Use HIV viral load to decide when to start antiretrovirals and assess response to treatment.

▶ Use combination therapy, beginning with two nucleoside reverse transcriptase inhibitors and a protease inhibitor; alternately, a non-nucleoside reverse transcriptase inhibitor can be substituted for a protease inhibitor.

▶ Prevent needle-sticks: never recap needles, always wear gloves, and discard all sharps appropriately.

▶ Typical features of lipodystrophy syndrome are temporal wasting, thin arms and legs, increased central fat deposition, low HDL, high triglycerides, and glucose intolerance.

CASE 30–2. A 27-year-old HIV infected man with A2 HIV disease comes to establish primary care. He was diagnosed with HIV three years ago, and believes he was infected about six years ago. His CD4 count done two months ago was 405 and viral load was 75,000. He reports no symptoms. He has had only sporadic, routine care in the past and was previously on AZT + ddI for about six months.

A. Would you start antiretroviral therapy? If so, what combination would you use?

B. What tests would you want to obtain?

REFERENCE

Antiretroviral therapy in adults: Updated recommendations of the international AIDS society-USA panel. JAMA 283(3):381–390, 2000.

USEFUL WEBSITES

2001 USPHS/IDSA Guidelines for the Prevention of Opportunistic Infection in Persons with Human Immunodeficiency Virus:
http://www.hivatis.org/trtgdlns.html#opportunistic
Postexposure prophylaxis information:
http://www.cdc.gov/mmwr/preview/mmwrhtml/rr5011a1.htm
Online AIDS text (Medical management of HIV infection):
http://www.hopkins-aids.edu/

HIV INFECTION COMPLICATIONS

▶ ETIOLOGY

What types of skin problems affect patients with HIV infection?

Skin findings that occur at higher CD4 counts include seborrheic dermatitis, allergic reactions (to medications, insect bites) and exacerbations of psoriasis. Later in the course of HIV infection, patients can develop Kaposi's sarcoma (KS) and *Molluscum contagiosum.* In patients with HIV infection, molluscum can cluster to form giant molluscum up to 1–2 cm across. This form is an indication of a markedly depleted immune system. Patients with very low CD4 counts, less than 50, can develop large cutaneous ulcers, often in the perirectal region, which should be considered herpes simplex virus until proved otherwise.

My patient with HIV infection has a mouth lesion. What could this be?

Possibilities include hairy leukoplakia, candida infection, aphthous ulcers, gingivitis, and KS. Hairy leukoplakia (HL) appears as white plaques on the side of the tongue and is due to Epstein-Barr virus. HL is specific for HIV infection and indicates a higher risk for disease progression to AIDS. In one study of CD4-count-matched patients, 22% of patients with HL progressed to AIDS within two years compared with 9% of patients without HL. Candidiasis, "thrush," occurs generally when the CD4 count is less than 300 and is a marker of immune deficiency. Patients with oral candidiasis are at higher risk for developing other opportunistic infections and should therefore receive *Pneumocystis* prophylaxis. About 30% of patients with KS have mouth involvement.

My patient is short of breath. What diseases do I need to consider?

Approximately 95% of cases of *Pneumocystis carinii* occur with CD4 counts less than 200 and a mean CD4 count less than 100. TB is more common in patients with HIV, especially in the presence of intravenous drug use, homelessness, or origin from an endemic area such as Africa, Latin America, and Southeast Asia. With HIV infection and positive PPD, the yearly risk of developing TB is 7%. This compares with a lifetime TB risk with positive PPD but no HIV infection of 10%. Bacterial pneumonia is more common also. It occurs at high CD4 counts and may be the first hint to the presence of HIV disease. *Pneumococcus* and *Haemophilus influenzae* are the most common organisms involved. Estimated annual rates of pneumococcal pneumonia in HIV infected individuals are as high as 10%. *Pseudomonas aeruginosa* is another important cause of community-acquired pneumonia when CD4 count is below 50. Bacteremia and recurrent pneumonias are more likely in the setting of HIV infection. HIV infection also causes cardiomyopathy, which may appear as dyspnea.

What causes headaches in HIV-infected patients?

Headache is common. If the CD4 count is over 500, nonopportunistic infections are more likely (sinusitis, HIV meningitis). When the CD4 is below 200, consider the big three opportunistic diseases: cryptococcosis, toxoplasmosis, and lymphoma. Sinusitis, HIV meningitis, or tuberculous meningitis can also occur at these lower CD4 counts.

My patient has diarrhea. What causes do I need to consider?

Approximately 50% of AIDS patients have GI problems, with diarrhea from enteric pathogens being the most common. Common pathogens include CMV, *Cryptosporidium*, *Giardia*, MAC, and *Clostridium difficile*. *Cryptosporidium* is a small noninvasive parasite of animals and was a rare cause of self-limited diarrhea in immunocompetent patients prior to the AIDS epidemic. Cryptosporidiosis is characterized by a persistent watery diarrhea, cramping abdominal pain, anorexia, and weight loss. *Giardia* is the most common nonopportunistic protozoan parasite in AIDS patients. It is seen in up to 15% of AIDS patients with symptomatic diarrhea. *C. difficile* is extremely common in patients with HIV disease because frequent hospitalizations result in colonization, and antibiotic use leads to overgrowth. HIV infection itself can also cause diarrhea but is a diagnosis of exclusion.

What are the causes of esophagitis?

Dysphagia, difficulty swallowing, and odynophagia, painful swallowing, are symptoms suggesting esophagitis in AIDS patients. These symptoms can significantly decrease food intake and worsen nutritional status. *Candida* esophagitis is the most frequent cause especially when oral candidiasis is present. CMV, herpes simplex, and the drug ddC can also cause symptomatic esophageal ulcerations.

What causes fever in HIV-infected patients?

When CD4 count is above 500, nonopportunistic causes are more common: bacterial pneumonia, pulmonary TB, and sinusitis, which is an almost universal problem in patients with HIV. In patients with lower CD4 counts, especially under 200, opportunistic infections are more likely. With diarrhea, consider the enteric pathogens *C. difficile*, *Salmonella*, and MAC. For fever with pulmonary symptoms, consider bacterial pneumonia, TB, or *Pneumocystis*. If no focal signs accompany fever, think of cryptococcal meningitis because 10%–20% of patients do not have headache. Other poorly localized conditions causing fever in HIV-infected patients include lymphoma; extrapulmonary TB, common with low CD4 counts; MAC, which can cause night sweats and anemia; hepatitis, either caused by hepatitis B or C or toxin effect (e.g., from TMP/SMX); CMV infection; or sinusitis. Don't forget the possibility of drug fever, especially if associated with TMP/SMX. The drug abacavir can cause a life threatening allergic reaction with fever.

▶ **EVALUATION**

When should I suspect pneumonia in an HIV-infected patient?

The symptoms of bacterial pneumonia in HIV-infected patients are similar to those in non–HIV-infected individuals: dyspnea, productive cough, high fever, fatigue. Tachycardia, tachypnea, and hypoxia may be present on exam, although lung exam may be unrevealing. In patients with *Pseudomonas* and CD4 counts under 100, CXR may show cavitary lesions.

Does TB present differently in HIV-infected patients?

Clinical manifestations of TB vary by the CD4 count. At CD4 counts above 300, symptoms and x-ray findings are more typical: weight loss, night sweats, fevers, productive cough, with upper lobe infiltrates, pleural effusions or cavitary lesions on x-ray. At CD4 counts under 200 clinical manifestations are less typical, extrapulmonary TB becomes common (two thirds of cases), and CXR findings are atypical with bilateral hilar adenopathy and lower lobe disease. Upper lobe infiltrates and pulmonary cavities are rare in patients with frank AIDS.

How do patients with PCP pneumonia present?

Patients with PCP usually present with dry, nonproductive cough, low-grade fever, and progressive dyspnea and fatigue over two to three weeks. Exam is often unrevealing except for an increased respiratory rate. ABG often shows a decreased PO_2 and a widened A-a gradient. LDH is commonly elevated and is a prognostic factor for severity of illness. Bilateral interstitial infiltrates are typical on x-ray, but in severe cases alveolar/lobar infiltrates occur as well. In up to 20% of cases, the CXR is normal. Spontaneous pneumothorax in a patient with HIV disease is usually a sign of underlying PCP.

What tests are warranted in patients with headache in the setting of HIV infection?

Work-up of patients with headache and low CD4 count, less than 200, consists of an imaging procedure, MRI or contrast CT scan, followed by a lumbar puncture. Characteristic CT findings are listed in Table 30–6. Send CSF for cell count, protein, glucose, Gram stain, cryptococcal antigen, and bacterial culture, and strongly consider mycobacterial culture. Serum cryptococcal antigen is 99% sensitive for cryptococcal meningitis. Review if the patient has had toxoplasmic titers checked—if negative, toxo is

TABLE 30-6

Patterns Seen on Head CT Scan in HIV-Related CNS Disease

Disease	Pattern	Enhancement	Location
Toxoplasmosis	Ring mass	++	Basal ganglia
Lymphoma	Solid mass	+++	Periventricular
Progressive multifocal leukoencephalopathy	No mass	None	Subcortical white matter

unlikely because greater than 90% of patients with CNS toxo have had a prior positive IgG with a reactivation of previous infection. CNS lymphoma requires brain biopsy for diagnosis, although it is usually diagnosed by exclusion after an unsuccessful trial of therapy for toxoplasmosis.

How should I evaluate my HIV-infected patient who has a fever?

Look for a focal process and let history and exam guide your work-up. The CD4 count is the single most important factor in determining risk of opportunistic infection. Obtain CBC with differential, CXR, blood cultures, urinalysis, and SGOT/SGPT. Hepatitis C is common with intravenous drug use; hepatitis B is common in patients with intravenous drug use or male-male sex. If no focal signs exist, consider additional tests including blood cultures for mycobacteria and serum cryptococcal antigen. Other tests such as head CT with contrast, lumbar puncture, stool cultures, and sinus CT should all be based on symptoms suggesting focal abnormalities. If the patient has diarrhea, obtain stool *C. difficile* toxin, and stool culture for enteric pathogens and atypical mycobacteria. Consider colonoscopy if etiology remains unclear. With pulmonary symptoms, obtain chest film, sputum Gram stain, and sputum cultures for TB. Pulmonary disease is usually one of three—bacterial pneumonia, TB, or PCP. PCP prophylaxis makes PCP unlikely, and fluconazole use makes cryptococcosis unlikely.

My patient has persistent dysphagia after two weeks of fluconazole. What should I do next?

Obtain endoscopic biopsy with viral cultures to identify infection other than *Candida*. CMV appears on endoscopy as large shallow superficial ulcerations often involving most of the esophagus. Stop ddC, as this medication can cause esophageal ulceration.

▶ TREATMENT

How do I treat PCP infection?

Treatment is with high-dose TMP/SMX (first choice), pentamidine, trimethoprim-dapsone (for mild disease), Atovaquone, or clindamycin-primaquine. All these regimens appear to have equivalent efficacy. Side effects are common, occurring in 50% of cases treated with TMP-SMX or pentamidine. The major side effects with pentamidine are renal insufficiency, pancreatic islet cell destruction, which can cause transient hypoglycemia or permanent hyperglycemia, and hypotension. Early use of corticosteroids in patients with moderate to severe PCP can improve survival and decrease the occurrence of respiratory failure. Give steroids to patient with PO_2 less than 75 or an alveolar-arterial oxygen gradient greater than 35.

What treatments are used for the various causes of diarrhea?

Ganciclovir decreases CMV-induced nausea and diarrhea. *Giardia* and *C. difficile* infections are treated with oral metronidazole. Common enteric bacteria respond to appropriate antibiotics with gram-negative coverage. *Cryptosporidium* is harder to eradicate. (Azithromycin, paromomycin are used.) These patients may benefit from a hypomotility agent such as loperamide or diphenoxylate/atropine

How do I treat esophagitis?

Patients with oral candidiasis and dysphagia can be given empiric ketoconazole 200 mg qd, or fluconazole 100–200 mg qd. Treat endoscopically diagnosed CMV with ganciclovir, herpes with high dose acyclovir, and documented *Candida* with fluconazole or ketoconazole.

How do I treat cryptococcal meningitis?

Treat initially with intravenous amphotericin B, usually for two weeks. Follow with suppressive therapy using oral fluconazole.

■

KEY POINTS

▶ Pneumothorax in an AIDS patient should make you think of *Pneumocystis* pneumonia.

▶ When the CD4 count is greater than 300, patients with TB present typically with cough, fever, sputum, upper lobe infiltrates. When CD4 count drops, the presentation is more atypical with hilar adenopathy, lower lobe disease, or miliary TB.

▶ Bacterial pneumonias are common, usually caused by *Pneumococcus* and *H. influenzae*. When the CD4 count is less than 100, *P. aeruginosa* becomes a possible pathogen.

▶ Patients with oral candidiasis and dysphagia have a greater than 90% likelihood of candidal esophagitis and should receive empiric fluconazole or ketoconazole.

▶ Consider *C. difficile* as an important cause of diarrhea with HIV infection.

▶ Remember to consider drugs as causes of fever, especially TMP/SMX.

CASE 30–3. A 30-year-old man with C3 HIV disease, CD4 count 60, presents with severe headaches and confusion that have progressed over the past two weeks. He has had intermittent fevers for the past three weeks. His friends state he has been more forgetful, and on the day of admission he became belligerent and did not recognize his partner. He takes AZT 200 tid, 3TC 150 bid, indinavir 800 q 8°, and dapsone 100 mg qd. Exam shows severe seborrheic dermatitis, molluscum contagiosum, oral hairy leukoplakia, and left lower extremity weakness with a left up-going toe. HCT 31, WBC 2.0, Na 134, K 3.9, Cl 98, HCO_3 26, Cr 1.0, BUN 18.

A. What does the seborrheic dermatitis tell you?
B. What is the importance of molluscum contagiosum and oral hairy leukoplakia in patients with HIV disease?
C. What is the differential diagnosis for this patient?
D. What work-up would you pursue?

MENINGITIS

▶ **ETIOLOGY**

What is the definition of meningitis?

Meningitis is inflammation of the meninges from *infectious* (bacterial, viral, or fungal) or *noninfectious* causes (sarcoid, malignancy, or hemorrhage from vasculitis).

What are the most common causes of infectious meningitis?

Viral meningitis is much more common than bacterial meningitis, with enteroviruses in 70% of all patients with viral meningitis. Herpes simplex meningitis is usually associated with episodes of primary HSV II infection. Acute HIV infection can cause meningitis and is under-diagnosed. In adults with *bacterial meningitis*, the most common etiologic agent is *Streptococcus pneumoniae*, occurring in 30% to 50% of patients. *Neisseria meningitidis,* meningococcus, is the second most common cause occurring in 10%–35% of adult patients with bacterial meningitis. *H. influenzae*, a very common cause of bacterial meningitis in children, is rare in adults, causing only 1%–2% of adult meningitis cases (Table 30–7).

What are the risk factors for the different organisms causing bacterial meningitis?

Pneumococcal meningitis may occur in the presence of pneumococcal pneumonia (15%–25% of cases), otitis media, or CSF leaks following trauma. Risk factors for pneumococcal meningitis, as for pneumococcal pneumonia, include alcoholism, cirrhosis, sickle cell anemia, asplenism, multiple myeloma, and chronic lymphocytic leukemia. Neisserial meningitis usually occurs in young

TABLE 30–7		
Causes of Bacterial Meningitis in Adults		
Common	**Uncommon**	**Special Circumstances**
Streptococcus pneumoniae *Neisseria meningitidis*	*Haemophilus influenzae*	Neurosurgical patients *Staphylococcus aureus* gram- negative rods Alcoholics or immunosuppressed *Listeria*

adults, is rare after age 45, and is the most common cause for epidemic bacterial meningitis. Complement deficiency increases the risk, particularly with deficient terminal components (C-5 through C-8). *Listeria monocytogenes* is a gram-positive rod that is more prevalent in the setting of alcoholism, pregnancy, or hematologic malignancy. Twenty to thirty percent of adults with *Listeria* infections have no risk factors.

▶ EVALUATION

What are the typical symptoms of bacterial meningitis?

Classic symptoms seen in greater than 85% of adults include fever, headache, cerebral dysfunction, and meningismus. More nonspecific symptoms include nausea, vomiting, rigors, profuse sweats, weakness, myalgias, and photophobia. The presenting signs can be variable depending on the infecting organism and the underlying immune status of the patient. Presence of mental status change, occurring in 95% of patients, is the single strongest indicator of bacterial meningitis.

What signs should I look for if I suspect meningitis?

Kernig's and Brudzinski's signs are present in 50% of bacterial meningitis cases. Perform these tests as follows. For Kernig's sign, attempt to extend the knee with the hip flexed. This is positive when radicular pain in the back or leg causes resistance to further extension. For Brudzinski's sign, flex the patient's neck. In a positive test, this maneuver produces flexion in the hip. Perform a careful skin exam, as 66% of patients with meningococcus have a violaceous rash.

Does meningitis present differently in elderly and immunosuppressed patients?

The usual signs of meningeal inflammation, nuchal rigidity, headache, Kernig's and Brudzinski's signs, and fever may not be present in the elderly or patients with immune dysfunction, such as neutropenia or HIV disease. In the elderly, confusion and mental status changes are the most reliable findings, 80%–90%, although these are very nonspecific as they occur with many other conditions.

What are the typical clinical features of viral meningitis?

The clinical features of viral meningitis include a prodrome of headache, malaise, and fever with normal mental status. Viral meningitis is particularly common in individuals younger than age 40. Exam is usually unrevealing. Look for genital ulcers or blisters suggesting HSV II, generalized adenopathy suggesting HIV, or parotitis suggesting mumps.

Should I obtain a CNS imaging test before lumbar puncture?

The question frequently arises whether CNS imaging is required preceding lumbar puncture (LP). Obtain a CT scan or MRI prior to LP in any patient with a focal neurologic exam, papilledema or loss of venous pulsations on funduscopic exam, seizures or HIV infection, with a CD4 count below 200. HIV infected patients more commonly have mass lesions caused by toxoplasmosis, TB, or lymphoma. Look for evidence of midline shift, indicating CNS mass lesion and increased intracranial pressure. If present, risk for herniation and subsequent death with LP is approximately 6%.

What tests do I order on CSF?

Send CSF for glucose, protein, cell count with differential, bacterial culture, and Gram stain. In patients at high risk for TB or fungal meningitis, test for TB with an AFB smear and culture and for cryptococcal disease with cryptococcal antigen and India ink prep. An important point here is that not all patients need AFB and fungal testing of the CSF.

What does the CSF look like in patients with bacterial meningitis?

CSF in bacterial meningitis shows greater than 500/mm^3 polymorphonuclear cells (PMNs), protein greater than 100 mm/dL, and glucose less than 40% of serum glucose (Table 30–8). About 80% of patients have a positive Gram stain (*S. pneumoniae* 83%, *H. influenzae* 76%, *N. meningitidis* 66%).

What tests are useful if you suspect bacterial meningitis and the gram stain and culture are negative?

Counter immunoelectrophoresis (CIE) can detect the presence of capsular polysaccharide from *H. influenzae, S. pneumoniae*, and *N. meningitidis*. This is particularly useful for evaluating patients who have received antibiotics because the polysaccharide persists after bacterial lysis.

What does the CSF test look like in a patient with viral meningitis?

In contrast to the high PMN count of bacterial meningitis, the typical pattern of viral meningitis is a total cell count less than

TABLE 30-8

CSF Findings with Meningitis of Various Causes

Etiology	WBC	WBC Differential	Protein mg/dL	Glucose* mg/dL	Gram Stain
Viral	5-500	>50% monos	30-150	Normal	No organisms
Bacterial	100-2000	>90% PMNs	80-500	<35	80% Gram stain positive
Cryptococcal	40-400†	>80% monos	40-150	Normal	>90% cryptococcal Ag 50% india ink positive
TB	100-1000	>80% monos	40-150	Normal or lower	AFB smear positive
Subdural or epidural abscess	50-300	Variable	75-300	Normal	No organisms

*Normal glucose is >40 mg% or >50% of simultaneous blood glucose; glucose may be decreased in viral, fungal, or parameningeal infections.
†Lower in immunocompromised patients with HIV.

$500/mm^3$ with a mononuclear predominance, protein less than 80–100 mm/dL, and normal glucose level. Early in the course of viral meningitis, PMNs may predominate. A repeat lumbar puncture within six to eight hours often shows a shift to mononuclear predominance.

▶ TREATMENT

What therapy should be used for suspected bacterial meningitis?

With the increase in pneumococcal resistance to penicillin, empiric therapy for meningitis must cover penicillin-resistant organisms. Vancomycin, in addition to a third generation cephalosporin, ceftriaxone or cefotaxime, is recommended. If the patient has risk factors for *Listeria* or if this organism is seen on Gram stain, add ampicillin as well. A third generation cephalosporin alone is adequate when meningococcus is seen on Gram stain, in elderly patients with probable gram-negative meningitis, or postneurosurgical patients in whom gram-negative meningitis or *S. aureus* meningitis is possible. Do not use cefoperazone or ceftazidime as they have very poor CNS penetration. Narrow the spectrum of coverage once an organism is identified. If you need to obtain a CT scan before a lumbar puncture in a patient with a high suspicion index for bacterial meningitis, give antibiotics *before* sending the patient for the CT scan.

K E Y   P O I N T S

- ▶ Obtain CSF to look for meningitis in patients with mental status changes, headache, and fever.

- ▶ Mental status changes or seizure may be the only symptoms of meningitis in the elderly.

- ▶ Obtain contrast CT before LP if the patient has a seizure, papilledema, or focal neurologic exam, or in HIV patients with CD4 less than 200.

- ▶ Viral meningitis may elevate PMNs in the CSF early in the course of the disease. Treat patients with antibiotics until CSF cultures are negative (twenty-four hours is sufficient).

- ▶ Treat suspected pneumococcal meningitis with vancomycin plus third generation cephalosporin until cultures/sensitivity return.

CASE 30-4. A 73-year-old man is brought by his daughter to the ED with mental status changes over the past twenty-four hours. He reports no concerns or symptoms. PMH is significant for CAD, CHF, and BPH. Exam reveals BP 100/60, P 110, T 39°C, no rash, chest is clear, heart is without murmur, abdomen is nontender. Labs: HCT 38, WBC 23,000 with 90% polys, Na 136, K 4.9, Cl 100, HCO$_3$ 18, BUN 30, Cr 2.0.

A. What tests would you order?
B. What is the most likely diagnosis for this patient?

CASE 30-5. A 37-year-old alcoholic man presents with obtundation and fever. He was found seizing on a downtown sidewalk. His old chart shows multiple ED visits for alcohol intoxication, lacerations, and one episode of pancreatitis. On exam BP 90/60, P 120, T 40.8°C. Skin is without rash, neck is stiff with a positive Brudzinski's sign. Breath sounds are decreased at the right base, and heart is without murmur. He is sleepy with symmetric neurologic exam and toes up-going bilaterally. Labs: Na 128, K 3.8, Cl 96, HCO$_3$ 12, HCT 39, WBC 2.9, CXR shows RLL infiltrate.

A. What tests would you order?
B. What is your differential diagnosis?
C. What treatment would you start?

REFERENCES

Durand ML, Calderwood SB, Weber DJ, et al: Acute bacterial meningitis in adults. N Engl J Med 328:21, 1993.
Sigurdardottir B, Bjornsson OM, Jonsdottir KE, et al: Acute bacterial meningitis in adults. A 20-year overview. Arch Intern Med 157:425, 1997.

PNEUMONIA

▶ ETIOLOGY

How common and how dangerous is pneumonia?

Community acquired pneumonia is common, with over four million cases annually in the U.S. Most patients are treated as outpatients with a mortality rate of about 1%, although 20% of patients require hospitalization, where death rates are as high as 25%. Pneumonia is the 6th leading cause of death overall.

How do people get pneumonia?

Pneumonia is inflammation of lung parenchyma from infection. Organisms reach the lung by oropharyngeal aspiration, inhalation, or hematogenous spread. Defects in host defenses often contribute, e.g., impaired glottic reflex, insufficient cough, impaired ciliary function usually from smoking, and deficient immunity. Important risk factors for pneumonia are listed (Table 30–9).

What organisms cause community-acquired pneumonia?

Microbiologic confirmation of cause is only obtained in about 50%–70% of cases at best, even using invasive studies. *Streptococcus pneumoniae*, then *H. influenzae* are most common: both occur in patients with predisposing conditions (see Table 30–9), although these are not always present. *Mycoplasma pneumoniae* is probably the most common cause in young, otherwise healthy adults. Anaerobic pneumonias occur with periodontal disease because anaerobes flourish amid rotting teeth and gums. Edentulous patients rarely get anaerobic infections. Anaerobic infections are also more common with aspiration of mouth flora during periods of unconsciousness or with swallowing disorders. Aspiration is a common cause for pneumonias in injection drug users (heroin decreases the gag reflex, cocaine can cause seizures) and alcoholics. Bacterial pneumonia can occur after viral upper respiratory infections, usually soon after symptoms of the viral infection begin to improve. *Pneumococcus* and *S. aureus* are the most common causes of pneumonia after a preceding viral upper respiratory infection.

How is hospital-acquired different from community-acquired pneumonia?

Hospital-acquired pneumonia occurs in up to 10% of hospitalized patients. Common culprits are gram-negative rods, often resistant

TABLE 30-9

Organisms and Mechanisms Causing Pneumonia in Patients with Specific Risk Factors for Pneumonia

Risk Group	Specific Likely Organisms	Mechanisms of Acquiring Pneumonia
Alcoholism	*Streptococcus pneumoniae* Anaerobes *Haemophilus influenzae* *Klebsiella pneumoniae* *Mycobacterium tuberculosis*	Decreased glottic reflex Seizures Stupor Aspiration of oral and gastric flora Poor WBC function and humoral immunity
Injection drug use	*Streptococcus pneumoniae* Anaerobes *Staphylococcus aureus* *Mycobacterium tuberculosis*	Aspiration during times of altered consciousness (heroin) or seizures (cocaine) Septic pulmonary emboli (tricuspid endocarditis)
Smoking-induced lung disease	*Streptococcus pneumoniae* *Haemophilus influenzae* *Moraxella catarrhalis* *Legionella*	HIV infection Impaired mucocilliary transport Colonized lower respiratory tract Resistance due to prior frequent antibiotics
HIV infection	*Streptococcus pneumoniae* *Haemophilus influenzae* *Pneumocystis carinii* *Pseudomonas aeruginosa*	Impaired cellular immunity Prophylactic antibiotics and CD4 < 100 make pseudomonal infection more likely
Nursing home residence	*Klebsiella pneumoniae* *Staphylococcus aureus* *Mycobacterium tuberculosis* (reactivation or primary)	Lowered immunity Predisposing illness Institutional exposures Neurologic disease or medication cause Altered cognition and aspiration Colonization with gram-negative rods
Postviral super-infection	*Streptococcus pneumoniae* *Staphylococcus aureus* *Haemophilus influenzae*	Viral infections disrupt mucociliary function Viruses interfere with cell-mediated host defense mechanisms (influenza, cytomegalovirus) Develops 7-19 days after viral infection

to multiple antibiotics, and *S. aureus,* followed by anaerobes and *S. pneumoniae.* Gram-negative pneumonias carry a high mortality (40%) because the organisms are aggressive and concurrent underlying medical conditions complicate recovery. Mortality in patients with nosocomial pneumonias can be as high as 50%, partially related to the presence and severity of comorbid conditions.

What are some uncommon causes of pneumonia?

Legionella occurs sporadically or epidemically. Those with underlying lung disease are at greatest risk. Consider psittacosis,

Chlamydia psittaci, with exposure to birds, especially in pet shop workers or bird keepers. Chlamydia pneumonia, occurs in young adults. Q-fever from inhalation of aerosolized *Coxiella burnetii* is seen in livestock handlers.

What causes pleural effusions in patients with pneumonia?

Exudative pleural effusion accompanies about 40% of pneumonias and is due to pleural inflammation. Most of these parapneumonic effusions are small, sterile, and resolve with treatment of the pneumonia. Some become infected, creating a purulent empyema, which can cause persistent infection, sepsis, and permanent scarring if left untreated.

▶ EVALUATION

What questions should I ask when I suspect pneumonia?

Classic symptoms of bacterial pneumonia include cough producing bloody or purulent sputum, high fever many times accompanied by rigors or chills, dyspnea, and pleuritic chest pain. Patients with pneumococcal pneumonia classically present with a single shaking chill at onset followed by high fever, pleuritic chest pain, and cough productive of bloody or "rusty" sputum. *Legionella* may cause myalgias, headache, confusion, and diarrhea as well. "Atypical" presentations are more subdued and suggest less inflammatory organisms such as viruses, *Mycoplasma, Pneumocystis, Chlamydia,* and uncommonly Q-fever or psittacosis. For atypical presentations, cough (when present) is usually nonproductive, fevers are lower grade, and myalgias or severe headache may be present. Extra-pulmonary manifestations may be prominent with *Mycoplasma,* such as meningitis, cerebellar ataxia, and erythema multiforme. Hoarseness or sore throat suggests *Chlamydia pneumoniae.* Ask about occupational or animal exposure, especially when symptoms are atypical, an organism cannot be found, or the patient does not respond to empiric therapy for common organisms. Foul-smelling sputum suggests anaerobes. Weight loss, anorexia, and night sweats are clues to TB infection.

In what situations might typical pneumonias present atypically?

Elderly patients may have few symptoms referable to the chest, and the main finding is confusion, disorientation, or anorexia. Neutropenic patients rarely have productive cough because there are no WBCs to produce sputum. Their earliest and most pronounced symptom of pneumonia is isolated fever. Some lower lobe pneumonias may occur with minimal chest symptoms and abdominal pain caused by irritation of the diaphragm.

What exam findings support a diagnosis of typical lobar pneumonia?

Tachypnea, tachycardia, and fever are common. With early lobar pneumonia, breath sounds may be decreased over the affected parenchyma, although occasionally are louder due to better transmission of tracheal airway sounds through consolidated lung, called bronchial breath sounds. Always compare breath sounds from side to side to detect subtle asymmetry. Dullness to percussion can represent consolidation or pleural effusion. Rales may be heard over the affected lobe and are most prominent with resolving pneumonia as air passages begin to open up again. Other signs of lobar consolidation include whispered pectoriloquy and tactile fremitus. Whispered pectoriloquy is elicited by having the patient whisper something such as their phone number or Social Security number. Transmission of sound is very good through consolidated lung, and you can easily hear the whispered words when your stethoscope is placed over the area. Elicit tactile fremitus by having the patient say "toy boat" while you place your hands symmetrically on the chest. Vibrations are increased over areas of consolidation and are decreased when fluid or air is present in the pleural space. Use this technique when dullness to percussion is present to differentiate effusion from infiltrate.

What lab tests are warranted if I suspect pneumonia?

Check O_2 saturation, CBC, sputum Gram stain and culture, electrolytes, and kidney function. In typical bacterial presentations, the WBC count rises, often with a left shift (excess immature forms or bands). In contrast, WBC count is often normal in viruses, *Mycoplasma,* or *Chlamydia.* Low WBC in the presence of pneumonia is a poor prognostic sign. In particularly ill-appearing patients, consider blood cultures and ABG. Positive blood cultures occur in up to 25% of pneumococcal pneumonias and are associated with poorer prognosis (20%–40% mortality). ABG may reveal hypoxia and respiratory alkalosis. *Mycoplasma* is suggested by hemolytic anemia or cold agglutinins, seen in 50% of patients. Confirm diagnosis by a rise in convalescent antibody titers. *Mycoplasma* and *Chlamydia* are often treated empirically without confirming a diagnosis. *Legionella* causes hyponatremia and a sputum Gram stain with leukocytes but no organisms. Diagnose *Legionella* by urinary antigen (type 1 only), DNA probe, direct fluorescent antibody, culture, or increase in convalescent antibody titer.

How do I interpret sputum gram stain and cultures?

Unfortunately, sputum specimens are often contaminated with saliva and oral flora, as indicated by epithelial cells and multiple organisms on Gram stain: greater than 25 epithelial cells per low power field correlates with an inadequate specimen. An adequate specimen from deep in the chest, with fewer than 10 epithelial cells and more than 25 WBCs per low power field, and with one dominant organism (more the exception than the rule) can guide initial empiric therapy. Gram stain is most reliable for *S. pneumoniae* and least reliable for the difficult-to-see pleomorphic gram-negative rods of *H. influenzae*. If you see WBCs with no organisms consider *Legionella, Mycoplasma, Chlamydia*, TB, or psittacosis. Sputum culture is less useful than stains, as it is negative in up to 50% of those with blood culture positive pneumonia. Sputum culture is more useful in the diagnosis of TB, as stains may not identify this disease.

How can CXRs help with the diagnosis of pneumonia?

The causative organism cannot be accurately predicted by CXR, but certain appearances are more typical of some organisms than others (Table 30–10).

TABLE 30–10	
Likely Organisms as Suggested by Specific Chest Film Findings in Pneumonia	
Chest Film Findings	**Likely Organisms**
Alveolar/air space lobar infiltrate with air-bronchograms,* silhouette sign†	*Pneumococcus, Haemophilus*, other typical organisms
Upper lobe infiltrates	TB, *Klebsiella*
Apical scarring	prior TB
Bilateral lower lobe infiltrates	anaerobes (aspiration)
Upper lobe posterior segment or lower lobe superior segment R > L	anaerobes (aspiration) right lung > left (right mainstem bronchus more straight)
Patchy bilateral infiltrates	*Mycoplasma pneumoniae*
Patchy unilateral segmental infiltrates	*Chlamydia pneumoniae, Mycoplasma pneumoniae*
Diffuse interstitial infiltrates	*Pneumocystis* and viral pneumonias
Cavitation‡	*M. tuberculosis, S. aureus*, or gram-negative rods

*bronchus remains aerated and dark while surrounding alveoli are fluid filled and bright.
†silhouette sign is the loss of a heart border or diaphragm shadow due to focal adjacent lung consolidation.
‡appearance of a hollow round cavity due to necrosis and liquefaction of lung parenchyma.

▶ **TREATMENT**

How do I choose empiric treatment for a patient with pneumonia?

Identify and target the most likely organism (Table 30–11). Switch to narrow spectrum antibiotic when or if sensitivities become available. For nosocomial pneumonia with gram-negative rods on sputum Gram stain, cover dually with an aminoglycoside and an extended spectrum antipseudomonal penicillin (ticarcillin, mezlocillin, piperacillin), an antipseudomonal third generation cephalosporin (ceftazidime or cefoperazone), or a quinolone with activity against *S. pneumoniae* (levofloxacin, gatifloxacin, or moxifloxacin). With clusters of gram-positive cocci in a nosocomial pneumonia, cover empirically for *S. aureus* as well as gram-negative rods until culture results are back.

TABLE 30–11

Empiric Antibiotic Treatment Options for Pneumonia by Risk Factor and Suspected Pathogens

Risk Factor	Empiric Therapy Options
COPD	Cefuroxime (oral)
	Ceftriaxone (IV)
	Ampicillin/clavulanate
	Quinolone (levofloxacin, gatifloxacin, moxifloxacin)
Aspiration	Clindamycin
	Amoxicillin/clavulanate or ampicillin/sulbactam
Nosocomial infection	Aminoglycoside + antipseudomonal penicillin or 3rd generation cephalosporin or quinolone

Suspected Pathogen	
Pneumococcus or	2nd or 3rd generation cephalosporin
Haemophilus	Amoxicillin/clavulanate or ampicillin/sulbactam
Mycoplasma	Erythromycin (also clarithromycin or azithromycin)
Legionella	Erythromycin in high dose (1 gm IV q6 hours)
	Quinolones
Staphylococcus	Nafcillin + aminoglycoside substitute vancomycin if penicillin allergic or MRSA suspected
Anaerobes	Clindamycin
	Metronidazole
	Amoxicillin/clavulanate or ampicillin/sulbactam
Psittacosis	Tetracycline/Doxycycline
	Erythromycin
Chlamydia pneumonia	Tetracycline/Doxycycline
Q-fever	Tetracycline/Doxycycline
	Chloramphenicol

What should I know about resistance to antibiotics?

Most strains of pneumococcus are penicillin sensitive and low-dose penicillin (600,000–1,200,000 units/day) is effective once the diagnosis is made. Pneumococcal resistance to penicillin and cephalosporins is up to 30% in some areas. Pneumococcal resistance to penicillin is due to alterations in penicillin binding protein. β-Lactamase production is not a factor in Pneumococcal penicillin resistance but is important in *S. aureus* and anaerobe resistance. Third generation cephalosporins and advanced generation quinolones (gatifloxacin, levofloxacin, and moxifloxacin) have reasonable activity against pneumococcal strains with intermediate resistance to penicillins. Vancomycin is the most active antibiotic against penicillin-resistant pneumococcus.

How do I manage a parapneumonic effusion?

Pleural tap is indicated to differentiate a sterile parapneumonic effusion from an infected empyema. Empyema must be drained expeditiously by chest tube or surgery to cure the infection, prevent sepsis, and avoid loculation, fibrosis, and permanent impairment of lung function. Treat for empyema if pleural fluid WBC and LDH are high, pH is less than 7.1, glucose is less than 40 or if cultures of pleural fluid grow organisms. If parameters are borderline, retap fluid in twelve hours.

Is there any way of preventing pneumonia?

Pneumococcal vaccine prevents pneumococcal pneumonia in high-risk patients, those older than age 65, institutionalized elderly, and HIV-positive patients, and in those with other severe underlying illness.

How long does it take patients to respond to treatment?

Patients generally improve after seventy-two hours. X-ray findings can worsen despite clinical improvement, and resolution of these abnormalities lags behind clinical improvement, often taking six weeks or more. If a patient is not responding to appropriate therapy, look for a resistant or unexpected organism, an alternate cause of fever, or a complication such as empyema.

Who should be hospitalized for treatment?

Admit patients with multiple lobe involvement, low initial WBC count, multiple sites of infection, severe underlying disease, alcoholism, or advanced age. Additionally, admit for signs of early sepsis such as hypotension, orthostasis, tachycardia, tachypnea, or hypoxia.

K E Y	P O I N T S

▶ Assess patients with pneumonia for predisposing risk factors such as HIV, alcohol use, smoking.

▶ Risk factors for poor outcome include low WBC count, multiple lobe involvement, extrapulmonary infection, severe underlying disease (CHF/cancer) and advanced age.

▶ A good sputum Gram stain is more predictive of a true pathogen than sputum culture.

▶ Injection drug users are at high risk of *S. aureus* pulmonary infection.

▶ Two common causes of pneumonia in healthy young adults are *Mycoplasma* and *Chlamydia.*

▶ Pneumococcal strains resistant to penicillin are on the increase.

CASE 30–6. A 66-year-old woman with a long history of cigarette use and recent onset of diabetes reports two days of worsening cough that started as she was gardening and became productive of purulent, rusty sputum yesterday. She had a severe shaking chill last night. T=101.9°F, HR=80, BP=120/60, RR=32.

A. What are the most likely organisms causing her symptoms?
B. What other information would you like?
C. What empiric treatment is appropriate?
D. After thirty-six hours, fevers continue to 102°F and WBC remains high. What should you do?
E. Five days into her stay, her fever reaches 103°F. How do you interpret this and what will you do?

CASE 30–7. An 80-year-old woman is brought to your office from her nursing home because she is more confused than usual today. She had been complaining of abdominal pain. T=98.5°F, WBC=4.

A. What could this be (list at least 7 possibilities)?
B. Name at least 7 tests to help you figure out her diagnosis.
C. If this is pneumonia, what organisms do you need to consider?
D. If this is pneumonia, explain her abdominal pain and lack of fever or leukocytosis.

REFERENCES

Bartlett JG, Dowell SF, Mandell LA, et al: Practice guidelines for the management of community-acquired pneumonia in adults. Clin Infect Dis 31:347, 2000.

Marie TJ: Pneumococcal pneumonia: Epidemiology and clinical features. Semin Respir Infect 14:227, 1999.

Niederman MS, Mandell LA, Anzueto A, et al: Guidelines for the management of adults with community-acquired pneumonia. Diagnosis, assessment of severity, antimicrobial therapy, and prevention. Am J Respir Crit Care Med 163:1730, 2001.

TUBERCULOSIS

▶ ETIOLOGY

What causes TB?

TB is an infection caused by a slow growing aerobic bacillus, *Mycobacterium tuberculosis*, which is not decolorized by acid alcohol, and thus is an "acid fast bacillus."

What are the risk factors for tuberculosis?

The major risk factors for TB are listed in Box 30–4.

Who is at risk for multidrug-resistant TB?

Most multidrug-resistant TB in the U.S. has occurred in those in institutions such as prisons and nursing homes, and in HIV-infected individuals.

BOX 30–4

Risk Factors for TB Infection

Major risk factors for TB infection
Close contact with smear-positive patient
HIV infection
Homelessness

Injection drug use
Institutionalization (prison)
Prior residence in endemic area
Africa, SE Asia, Central America

Minor risk factors for TB infection
Diabetes mellitus
Gastrectomy
Silicosis

> ▶ **EVALUATION**

What is the purpose of PPD screening in healthy-appearing patients?

PPD screening identifies patients who have been exposed to TB. A small sample of purified protein derivative is placed under the skin and incites an inflammatory reaction if the patient already has immune response against TB, indicating exposure. As live organisms are effective at evading normal host responses, a positive PPD result also suggests dormant, live bacteria are present as latent infection, waiting for a time of immunosuppression to cause reactivation TB. PPD interpretation depends on the host characteristics and diameter of induration present (Table 30–12). Once a patient has a known positive PPD reaction, never retest, as subsequent reactions may cause painful inflammation and skin necrosis.

My patient's screening PPD is positive. What should I do next?

Rule out active infection, because treatment of active infection requires multidrug therapy, whereas exposure with latent infection can be treated with INH alone in most cases. Ask about symptoms of TB, including constitutional, pulmonary, GI, and GU symptoms, as well as about joint pains. Perform full exam and CXR. Any signs or symptoms that could represent active pulmonary or nonpulmonary TB infection require further work-up.

TABLE 30–12

Interpreting Induration Reaction to PPD Testing

Reaction	Reading	Patient to Whom Positive PPD Reading Applies
<5 mm	Negative	All patients
5 mm or greater	Positive	HIV infected patients Organ transplant patients Patients on chronic prednisone Recent contacts with TB-infected patients X-ray findings suggesting prior TB infection
10 mm or greater	Positive	Children < 4, children exposed to high risk adults Injection drug users without HIV infection Patients with gastrectomy, malignancy, diabetes, silicosis, renal insufficiency Recent immigrants from country with high prevalence of TB Staff from AFB lab Staff from prisons, nursing homes, hospitals, shelters
15 mm or greater	Positive	No known risk factors for TB

What are the typical symptoms of active TB infection?

Classic symptoms are fever, night sweats, weight loss, and cough productive of thick sputum. Hemoptysis and dyspnea are symptoms of advanced disease. In elderly and HIV-infected patients, symptoms may be more subtle (anorexia, fatigue, confusion, weakness).

When should I think of TB in the differential diagnosis?

Patients who present with typical symptoms and major risk factors should have a work-up for TB. Anyone with an upper lobe infiltrate on CXR should also be considered for work-up. Think of TB, especially reactivation TB, in elderly patients who have infiltrates on CXR that do not respond to standard antibiotic therapy. Alcoholics are at higher risk for TB due to a higher likelihood of homelessness or incarceration.

What is the work-up for TB?

Order a CXR first. If infiltrates are present, especially in the upper lobe, obtain three separate morning sputum samples for AFB smear and culture. Patients admitted to the hospital and undergoing TB work-up should be kept in respiratory isolation until three smears are negative. TB skin testing (PPD) is most helpful when the presentation is atypical. In patients with typical presentations and suggestive CXR, obtain sputum samples first to avoid a painful, large positive PPD. Work-up for nonpulmonary TB infection is rarely needed and more invasive, requiring the sampling of affected tissues only as indicated: urinalysis for sterile pyuria, urine AFB culture, joint aspiration, liver biopsy, gastric secretion collection, bone marrow biopsy, or bone sampling.

What are the typical x-ray findings of TB?

Most TB is reactivation TB with upper lobe infiltrates, cavitation, and pleural thickening (Figure 30–2). Patients with primary infection can develop hilar adenopathy, pleural effusion, or miliary pattern (diffuse small nodules in the lungs, named after millet seeds). HIV-infected patients can have varying x-ray presentation (see HIV chapter).

▶ TREATMENT

Who should receive INH prophylaxis for latent infection?

In general, patients with a newly positive PPD or close contacts with smear-positive patients should receive prophylaxis (Box 30–5).

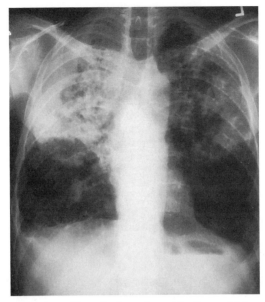

Figure 30–2. Chest film of tuberculosis. Findings of bilateral upper lobe pleural thickening, cavities, and infiltrates (more extensive in the right upper lobe).

BOX 30–5

Indications for INH Prophylaxis
PPD positive without prior treatment and old positive PPD and
  age younger than 35
Recent PPD conversion to positive, any age
Low risk criteria, any age
  Health care worker
  Homeless
  No risk factors
  Nursing home or prison resident
  Prior residence in endemic country
High-risk criteria, any age
  CXR consistent with old TB
  Close contact with a smear-positive patient
  HIV-infected
  Injection drug user
  Prolonged steroid use
  Immunocompromised conditions (diabetes, silicosis, ESRD)

Patients with HIV disease should receive prophylaxis if the PPD test shows 5 mm or more of induration.

What treatment is warranted for latent TB infection?

If evaluation for active TB is negative in a patient with positive PPD, proceed with nine months of INH prophylaxis, 300 mg/d. Liver function tests (AST, ALT, bilirubin) should be obtained at baseline, and if abnormal at baseline should be repeated monthly while on therapy. All patients on INH should be monitored monthly for adherence to the medication and asked about symptoms of hepatitis (nausea, vomiting, anorexia, and abdominal pain). INH can also interfere with pyridoxine metabolism, causing peripheral neuropathy. To prevent this complication, many prescribe 25–50 mg/d of vitamin B_6.

What therapy should a patient with active TB receive?

Multiple drug therapy is the rule due to the risk of drug resistance. Start with four drugs, usually isoniazid (INH), rifampin, pyrazinamide, and ethambutol. Directly observed therapy has a much greater success rate. If the organism turns out to be sensitive to INH and rifampin, then ethambutol can be discontinued after two months and the six-month course finished with INH and rifampin. Thrice weekly therapy with isoniazid, rifampin, pyrazinamide, and ethambutol under direct observation for six months is highly effective. Give B_6 as mentioned to avoid neuropathy from INH.

K E Y   P O I N T S

▶ Major risk factors for TB include recent exposure to a patient with active TB, injection drug use, HIV infection, homelessness, history of residence in a prison, or emigration from a country where TB is endemic.

▶ If TB is a possibility in a hospitalized patient, place the patient in an isolation room while you wait for results of three consecutive morning sputum AFB smears.

▶ Strongly consider TB when a patient has an upper lobe infiltrate on CXR.

▶ Directly observed therapy has a higher success rate and should be used if there are any concerns about adherence to the regimen or problems with follow-up.

CASE 30–8. A 48-year-old man presents with three months of 15 pounds of weight loss and cough, with occasional hemoptysis. He is a heavy alcohol drinker, has been homeless for the past two years, and has spent most of that time in homeless shelters. He was in jail briefly four years ago. He has a 40-pack-year smoking history.

  A. List possible causes of his symptoms.
  B. What features on a CXR would suggest TB?
  C. If his work-up reveals TB, what treatment would you choose?

REFERENCE

Small PM, Fujiwara PI: Management of tuberculosis in the United States. N Engl J Med 345:189, 2001.

URINARY TRACT INFECTIONS

▶ ETIOLOGY

My patient has dysuria. What is the likely cause?

Dysuria, urgency, frequency, and occasionally incontinence are symptoms of urethral irritation from urinary tract infection (UTI). Similar symptoms can occur with vaginitis or urethritis (*Candida* or herpes simplex infection, respectively). In men, prostatitis can occur with dysuria.

What causes urinary tract infections?

Up to 20% of women will have a UTI during their lifetime. In young women with *acute cystitis*, the most common bacterial pathogens are *E.coli* and *Staphylococcus saprophyticus.* Sexual intercourse and diaphragm use increase risk. *Complicated cystitis* is a broad category that affects young women at risk for resistant organisms, elderly or immunocompromised women with acute cystitis, pregnant women, and patients with indwelling catheters. *Uncomplicated pyelonephritis* is by definition community acquired and has no urologic abnormalities. As with cystitis, *E. coli* is the most common pathogen. *Complicated pyelonephritis* is a UTI occurring in the setting of urinary catheters, stones, obstructions such as BPH, or recent urinary procedures. Resistant gram-negative rods and *Enterococcus* are important organisms in this condition. Consider *Pseudomonas* with indwelling catheters and recent urologic procedures (TURP, cystoscopy) and enterococcus when recent broad-spectrum antibiotics such as cephalosporins have been used.

▶ EVALUATION

How is urinalysis interpreted?

In patients with dysuria, obtain clinic dipstick and lab microscopic analysis of a spun urine sediment. Many dipstick results include leukocyte esterase (LE), which correlates with the presence of pyuria with 95% sensitivity. This does not denote UTI. LE and WBCs are nonspecific, occurring also in cervicitis, vaginitis, and urethritis. Microscopic hematuria is present in 40%–60% of patients with acute cystitis and is uncommonly found in other causes of acute dysuria, making it a modestly specific indicator of cystitis.

When is urine culture useful?

There is no role for culture in acute cystitis. Send urine for culture and sensitivity in suspected pyelonephritis, recurrent urinary tract infection, or equivocal urinalysis. A positive culture is defined as greater than 100,000 colonies of a single organism. Lower counts, 10^2–10^4, can still be associated with infection. This is termed "acute dysuric syndrome."

How are symptoms of cystitis different from pyelonephritis?

Patients with cystitis usually present with dysuria, frequency, urgency, and suprapubic pain, sometimes accompanied by frank hematuria. Fever is not a symptom of isolated cystitis. Patients suspected of cystitis should also be asked about risks for sexually transmitted disease, as well as about vaginal discharge. If STD is possible by this history, perform pelvic exam. Pyelonephritis is important to distinguish from cystitis because a longer duration of therapy may be indicated, and treatment failures and complications are more likely. Although identified as having *upper tract infection*, patients with pyelonephritis commonly present with fever, back or abdominal pain, and costovertebral angle or flank tenderness. Concurrent cystitis symptoms may be present. Other symptoms seen with pyelonephritis are nausea, vomiting, headache, and malaise. Pyelonephritis can be subclinical, without classic symptoms, and should be suspected in patients with risk factors (Box 30–6).

BOX 30-6

Factors Suggesting Occult Pyelonephritis or Otherwise Complicated UTI
Diabetes
Pregnancy
Male patient
Childhood UTI
Elderly patient
Indwelling catheter
Immunosuppression
Urologic anatomic abnormality
Symptoms for more than seven days
Recent urinary tract instrumentation or antibiotics

▶ **TREATMENT**

What is the best antibiotic for cystitis?

For uncomplicated cystitis in young women, short course therapy with three days of TMP-SMX or a quinolone has an excellent cure rate and few side effects. Short course therapy is not recommended for patients with diabetes or for men. Treat these patients for seven days.

How does treatment for complicated pyelonephritis differ?

Treat complicated infections with drugs effective against resistant gram-negative rods, including *Pseudomonas*. If urine Gram stain shows gram positive cocci, cover for enterococcus as well. For empiric therapy, use an aminoglycoside and an antipseudomonal third generation cephalosporin. The best treatment option for enterococcus is ampicillin, but resistance is common. Remove urinary catheters if possible. Once cultures are available, narrow antibiotics. For *Pseudomonas*, use two drugs to limit emergence of resistance. Septic shock often accompanies complicated UTIs. Support blood pressure with IV fluids and treat refractory hypotension with vasoactive medications. Relieving any urinary obstruction is a critical part of therapy.

How do I treat cystitis in pregnant women?

Antibiotics to use in pregnancy include amoxicillin, amoxicillin-clavulanate, nitrofurantoin, cephalexin, cefixime, fosfomycin, and sulfisoxazole. Quinolones are contraindicated owing to adverse effect on cartilage development. Sulfonamides should be avoided in the

3rd trimester. Optimal length of treatment is not clear. Single dose, three-day therapy and seven-day regimens have all been used.

How are recurrent UTIs managed?

Recurrence is due either to relapse of the same organism or reinfection with a new organism. Relapse immediately following short course therapy warrants a two week treatment for presumed upper tract disease. For reinfection, self-treatment by patients is reasonable, as studies show excellent correlation between patients' symptoms and bacteriologic evidence of UTI. For patients with two to three recurrences per month, prophylactic therapy with daily TMP-SMX has been shown to decrease infections by 95%. Drinking cranberry juice daily can decrease recurrence rates by 50%. Postcoital prophylaxis with TMP/SMX is another effective option for women who get frequent UTIs associated with sexual activity.

What treatment is appropriate for community-acquired pyelonephritis?

The major treatment decision is whether to hospitalize. Admit when vomiting prevents oral medication usage and makes IV fluids necessary, and when noncompliance is likely. For uncomplicated pyelonephritis, choose antibiotics with good gram-negative activity such as aminoglycosides, third generation cephalosporins, or quinolones. Amoxicillin is a poor choice, as 25%–35% of community-acquired *E. coli* are resistant. Increasing *E. coli* resistance to TMP-SMX is occurring, now reported to be about 15%–20%. TMP/SMX is a good treatment option to switch to if results of urine cultures confirm sensitivity. Duration of therapy is controversial; most physicians treat acute uncomplicated pyelonephritis for two weeks. Initial bacteremia and fevers that persist for several days into therapy are common and should not change treatment.

K E Y   P O I N T S

▶ **Cystitis does not cause fever.**

▶ **In young women with UTI, three day TMP/SMX is the preferred treatment.**

▶ **Patients with Foley catheters or recent instrumentation of the urinary tract are at high risk for resistant gram-negative rods or enterococcal infection.**

▶ **Obtain urine culture for recurrent UTIs and pyelonephritis.**

CASE 30–9. A 67-year-old woman presents with dysuria and frequency but is otherwise healthy. Her past medical history includes breast cancer and hypertension. She is sexually active with her husband. Her vital signs are stable. Urinalysis reveals LE+, RBCs, and WBCs.

    A. Is any further evaluation necessary?

    B. What prescription will you write for her?

REFERENCES

Gupta K, Hooton TM, Stamm WE: Increasing antimicrobial resistance and the management of uncomplicated community-acquired urinary tract infections. Ann Intern Med 135:41, 2001.

Hooton TM, Stamm WE: Diagnosis and treatment of uncomplicated urinary tract infection. Infect Dis Clin North Am 11:551, 1997.

31

Nephrology

ACID-BASE DISTURBANCES

▶ ETIOLOGY

What causes acid-base disturbances?

The body normally keeps arterial blood pH at 7.4. Respiratory or metabolic derangements can alter pH. Hyperventilation removes CO_2 and hydrogen ions, creating a respiratory alkalosis. Hypoventilation or airway obstruction raises pCO_2 and creates a respiratory acidosis. Metabolic derangements altering pH include ingestion of particular substances, changes in renal bicarbonate processing, or production of endogenous acids such as ketones or lactate (Table 31–1).

TABLE 31–1			
Causes of Acid-Base Derangements			
Respiratory		**Metabolic**	
Acidosis $pCO_2 > 40$	*Alkalosis* $pCO_2 < 40$	*Acidosis* $HCO_3^- < 24$	*Alkalosis* $HCO_3^- > 24$
Hypoventilation	Pulmonary embolus	Anion gap acidosis	Chloride sensitive
Asthma	Pneumonia	lactic acid (sepsis)	vomiting
COPD	Pulmonary edema	uremia	volume contraction
	Aspirin	aspirin	diuretics
	Hepatic insufficiency	ketoacidosis	Chloride resistant
	Fever	with osmolar gap	Cushing's
	Anxiety	methanol	hyperaldosteronism
	Pregnancy	ethylene glycol	Bartter's syndrome
		paraldehyde	
		Nongap acidosis	
		diarrhea	
		acetazolamide	
		renal tubular acidosis	

What do the terms acidemia and alkalemia mean?

These terms refer to arterial blood pH. Patients with pH less than 7.4 are acidemic; those with pH greater than 7.4 are alkalemic. In contrast, the terms acidosis and alkalosis refer to processes that cause excess accumulation of acid or alkali. Multiple processes can coexist, each affecting pH (Table 31–2).

What are the causes of metabolic acidosis?

Metabolic acidosis is divided into anion gap and nonanion gap acidosis. *Anion gap* acidosis occurs when an unmeasured anion lowers pH. The mnemonic MULE PAK may help you remember the causes of anion gap acidoses: *M*ethanol, *U*remia, *L*actic acidosis, *E*thylene glycol, *P*araldehyde, *A*spirin, *K*etoacidosis. Most common on this list are lactic acidosis (i.e., sepsis) or ketoacidosis, which can be from uncontrolled type 1 diabetes, starvation, or alcohol ingestion. *Nonanion gap acidosis* is caused by loss of bicarbonate through the gut or kidney (see Table 31–1).

What is renal tubular acidosis (RTA)?

Renal tubular acidosis occurs when kidneys waste bicarbonate owing to malfunctioning tubules. RTA is proximal, type 2, or distal, types 1 and 4, depending on which tubules are affected. Type 4 is most common and is seen with diabetes. Type 1 is often associated with nephrolithiasis.

What causes metabolic alkalosis?

Metabolic alkalosis is either sodium chloride responsive or sodium chloride resistant, depending on whether it corrects with sodium chloride volume infusion. Sodium chloride responsive alkalosis is common and occurs with vomiting, NG suction, or diuretic-induced volume contraction. In these conditions, urine chloride is low. Sodium chloride–resistant metabolic alkalosis is

TABLE 31–2

Interpretation of Key Lab Tests in Patients with Acid-Base Disorders

Value	Normal	Interpretation if High	Interpretation if Low
pH	7.4	Alkalemia	Acidemia
HCO_3^-	24 mEq/L	Metabolic alkalosis	Metabolic acidosis
pCO_2	40 mm Hg	Respiratory acidosis	Respiratory alkalosis

rare and causes elevated urine chloride. Examples of this hormonally driven chloride wasting include hyperaldosteronism and Cushing's and Bartter's syndromes.

What are primary and compensatory acid-base processes?

The primary process is the main alteration in pH. The term acidemia implies a primary acidosis; alkalemia implies a primary alkalosis. Compensatory processes occur when the kidney or respiratory system reacts to correct an altered pH. Respiratory compensation is immediate, whereas renal compensation takes twelve to twenty-four hours to kick in.

▶ EVALUATION

Is there a systematic way to approach acid-base problems?

Absolutely (Box 31–1). Routinely calculate anion gap in all hospitalized patients. Suspect an acid-base derangement when you see an abnormal respiratory rate, altered bicarbonate, elevated anion gap, poor oxygenation, suspected CO_2 retention, or unexplained altered mental status. If any of these are present, draw an arterial blood gas for pH and pCO_2. This, combined with chemistry panel (sodium chloride and bicarbonate, HCO_3^-), allows you to calculate anion gap and identify primary, compensatory, and other concurrent acid-base processes.

BOX 31–1

Systematic Steps to Interpret Acid-Base Problems
(see text for details)

1) Identify the primary process.
2) Identify the compensatory process.
3) Calculate anion gap correcting for low albumin (even if pH is normal or high).
4) If anion gap is elevated, calculate osmolar gap.
5) If anion gap is elevated, use delta-delta to find simultaneous metabolic derangements.
6) Use clues in history and physical to determine specific conditions causing alterations.

My patient's pH = 7.3, pCO$_2$ = 60, and HCO$_3^-$ = 30. How do I identify the primary process?

Here are some key principles:

- Patients never overcompensate for the primary acid-base derangement.
- Respiratory processes alter pCO$_2$ (pCO$_2$ greater than 40 = acidosis; less than 40 = alkalosis).
- 3) Metabolic processes alter HCO$_3^-$ (HCO$_3^-$ greater than 24 = alkalosis; less than 24 = acidosis).
- Change in pH is inversely related to CO$_2$, and directly related to HCO$_3^-$.

The pH of 7.3 reveals an acidemia so the primary process is an acidosis. Now you are ready to decide whether the source of the low pH is respiratory (true if pCO$_2$ is high) or metabolic (true if HCO$_3^-$ is low). In this case, the high pCO$_2$ of 60 reveals the primary respiratory acidosis.

I found the primary process. How do I identify a compensatory process?

Using the same example, look next at the HCO$_3^-$. The high bicarbonate reveals a metabolic alkalosis, which is compensating for the respiratory acidosis. Here's another example: pH = 7.2, pCO$_2$ = 20, HCO$_3^-$ = 15. The pH reveals acidemia, low HCO$_3^-$ reveals a primary metabolic acidosis. The low pCO$_2$ reveals the compensatory respiratory alkalosis.

How can I tell if a patient has compensated or uncompensated respiratory acidosis?

With sudden onset respiratory acidosis, pH falls before the kidney has time to compensate. In uncompensated respiratory acidosis, pH falls 0.08 for each CO$_2$ rise of 10. In compensated respiratory acidosis, the kidney will make extra bicarbonate so the drop in pH will be less.

How do I calculate the anion gap?

To calculate the anion gap, subtract anions from cations: anion gap = sodium − (chloride + bicarbonate). The normal anion gap is 8 to 12. This number represents unmeasured negative charges, mostly on albumin. If albumin is abnormally low, then the baseline normal anion gap will also be smaller (see later for correction). When unmeasured anions appear, such as lactate or ketones, they displace chloride and bicarbonate and the anion gap increases. It is significant when anion gap rises by greater than eight points.

What does a low anion gap mean and why is this important?

Multiple myeloma, hypoalbuminemia, and lithium provide positively charged, unmeasured cations, which lower the baseline anion gap. This can mask a significant anion gap acidosis. To avoid this, correct the expected anion gap for albumin: if albumin is low, estimate baseline anion gap as three times the albumin level. For example, a calculated anion gap of 14 may look normal; however, when albumin = 2, the baseline anion gap should be expected to be $2 \times 3 = 6$. Thus, the change from a baseline expected anion gap of 6 to a measured anion gap of 14 represents a significant anion gap acidosis.

When and how do I calculate the osmolal gap?

When your patient has an anion gap acidosis, calculate the osmolar gap:

Osmolar gap = (measured Osms) – (calculated Osms)

where calculated Osms = 2(sodium) + BUN ÷ 2.8 + glucose ÷ 18.

If the osmolar gap is greater than 10, suspect methanol or ethylene glycol ingestion. Look for oxalate crystals in the urine, seen with ethylene glycol ingestion. Blood levels of these agents can be measured but won't be available soon enough to be useful.

What is a "triple ripple" and how do I use the "delta-delta"?

A triple ripple occurs when multiple acid-base disorders coexist. Use the delta-delta when an anion gap acidosis is present to find a concurrent metabolic alkalosis or nongap acidosis. In an isolated anion gap acidosis, the anion gap should rise from baseline (delta-AG) by the same amount that the HCO_3^- falls (delta HCO_3^-). If delta-AG is not the same as delta-HCO_3^- then another metabolic process is present. This concept may be put to use in various ways. One way is to add the change in anion gap (= measured gap – normal gap) to the measured HCO_3^- to see if you get a number esti-

TABLE 31–3

Finding Concurrent Metabolic Processes Using the Delta-Delta Concept

When:	Then the Patient Has:
Change in anion gap* + HCO_3^- = 24	Isolated anion gap acidosis†
Change in anion gap + HCO_3^- > 24	Anion gap acidosis plus metabolic alkalosis
Change in anion gap + HCO_3^- < 24	Anion gap acidosis plus nongap acidosis

*Change in anion gap = measured anion gap – normal baseline anion gap.
†Change in anion gap should equal change in bicarbonate if there are no other concurrent metabolic processes.

mating a normal HCO_3^-. If the result is greater than 24, there is a concurrent metabolic alkalosis. If the result is less than 24 there is a concurrent nongap acidosis (Table 31–3). Practice this on Case 31–2. Be sure to correct the normal anion gap for low albumin levels.

What are pertinent history and exam clues in my patient with a low pH?

You must use clues from history and exam to decide what specific conditions are causing the acid-base disturbances. Alcoholism increases the likelihood of alcoholic ketoacidosis. Alcoholics are more likely to ingest methanol and ethylene glycol as alternatives to alcohol and ethanol. Elderly patients are at increased risk for lactic acidosis (sepsis, bowel necrosis) or inadvertent aspirin overdosage. Patients with a history of suicide attempts are at risk for aspirin, methanol, or ethylene glycol ingestion.

▶ TREATMENT

Treat the underlying disorder.

K E Y   P O I N T S

▶ When pH is less than 7.4 there is a primary acidosis; when pH is greater than 7.4 there is a primary alkalosis.

▶ A low baseline anion gap from low albumin or myeloma may mask significant gap acidosis.

▶ If you find a patient breathing deeply and rapidly with no immediately apparent cause, suspect respiratory compensation for sepsis or other metabolic acidosis.

▶ If a significant anion gap is present check for an osmolal gap.

CASE 31–1. A 45-year-old man with a long history of chronic low back pain presents with several days of melena and the following labs: Na = 140, Cl = 103, HCO_3^- = 15, glucose = 108, BUN = 20, Osm = 295, pH = 7.5, pCO_2 = 20, pO_2 = 90. He asks for morphine for his pain.

A. What is his primary acid-base derangement?
B. Is there a compensatory acid-base adjustment and, if so, what is it?

Continued

CASE 31–1. *Continued*

C. Are there any other acid-base derangements present?
D. What do you think is going on clinically to cause his acid-base derangements?

CASE 31–2. A 21-year-old woman is found unresponsive. Her friends report that she was going to the bathroom all the time and was vomiting profusely earlier in the day. Na = 130, Cl = 88, HCO_3^- = 10, pH = 7.1, pCO_2 = 32, pO_2 = 88, BUN = 28, glucose = 720, Osm = 315.

A. What is her primary acid-base derangement?
B. Is there a compensatory acid-base adjustment and, if so, what is it?
C. Are there any other acid-base derangements present?
D. What do you think is going on clinically to cause her acid-base derangements?

ACUTE RENAL FAILURE

▶ ETIOLOGY

What causes acute renal failure (ARF)?

Acute renal failure is rapid deterioration of renal function resulting in azotemia (elevated BUN and creatinine) and possibly oliguria (less than 400 mL urine output/24 hours). Causes are divided into prerenal (40%–80%), intrinsic renal, and postrenal, based on the site of injury (Table 31–4).

What causes prerenal ARF?

Prerenal azotemia occurs with inadequate blood supply to glomeruli. This can be due to decreased cardiac output (CHF), hypovolemia (bleeding, diarrhea, burns, diuretics), or changes in renal vessels from stenosis or medications. Whereas ACEIs dilate efferent arterioles, NSAIDs block prostaglandins, resulting in afferent arteriolar narrowing. Severe prerenal status can cause renal ischemia, leading to acute tubular necrosis (ATN).

TABLE 31-4

Common Causes of Acute Renal Failure (% of Total ARF Cases)	
Location of Injury	**Common Causes**
Prenal (40%–80%)	Hypovolemia: bleeding, diarrhea, sepsis, drugs
	Poor perfusion: renal artery stenosis, thrombosis, drugs
	Poor cardiac output: CHF
Postrenal (10%)	Bladder outlet obstruction: BPH, cancer
	Medications: anticholinergics, narcotics
Intrinsic renal (30%–50%)	Immune: IgA nephropathy, lupus, Wegener's, Goodpasture's
Glomeruli	Infectious: hepatitis B/C, poststrep, HIV, endocarditis
	Toxic: heroin
Interstitial nephritis	Drugs: NSAIDs, penicillins, sulfonamides
	Infection: pyelonephritis
Acute tubular necrosis	Toxins: radiocontrast, aminoglycosides, myoglobin
	Tubular obstruction: myoglobin, myeloma
	Tubular ischemia: sepsis, hypotension

What causes glomerulonephritis and interstitial nephritis?

Intrinsic renal failure can occur in the glomeruli (glomerulonephritis), the interstitium (interstitial nephritis), or the tubules (acute tubular necrosis). Glomerulonephritis, or injury to the glomeruli from any cause, is most commonly immune mediated. Examples include systemic lupus erythematosus, poststreptococcal glomerulonephritis, Goodpasture's disease, and hepatitis C. Interstitial nephritis is inflammation in the interstitial space and is caused by NSAIDs, antibiotics (e.g., penicillins and cephalosporins), and infectious diseases. Patients are often asymptomatic or may present with fever, rash, and joint pain. Some toxins such as NSAIDs are important mediators of renal injury by both prerenal and intrarenal mechanisms.

What is acute tubular necrosis (ATN)?

This common cause of ARF occurs with tubular ischemia from any severe prerenal state, such as septic shock. Nephrotoxins such as radiocontrast dye and aminoglycosides are the second major cause. Prehydration, nonionic contrast, and possibly N-acetylcysteine minimize dye toxicity. Once-daily dosing decreases aminoglycoside toxicity. Other causes of ATN include tubular deposition of myoglobin from rhabdomyolysis or paraproteins from multiple myeloma. Renal function frequently recovers after ATN.

What postrenal cause of acute renal failure is most common?

Postrenal azotemia is caused by obstruction of the bladder or of both ureters. Bladder outlet obstruction is most common, due to

BPH or prostate cancer. Once a Foley catheter is placed, postob-structive diuresis can produce severe volume and electrolyte deple-tion. Other causes include neurogenic bladder dysfunction or obstruction due to papillary sloughing, stones, or abdominal tumor.

What toxins damage the kidneys?

Toxins can injure the kidney at various sites. NSAIDs cause acute interstitial nephritis and nephrotic syndrome. NSAIDs also decrease renal blood flow by blocking the dilating effect of prostaglandins on the afferent arterioles, a particular problem in patients with low intravascular volumes such as in CHF, cirrhosis, or nephrotic syndrome.

What is nephrotic syndrome?

Nephrotic syndrome is a common final pathway of many intrinsic renal diseases including diabetes and hepatitis B. Massive protein loss, greater than 3.5 gm/24 hours, leads to hypoalbuminemia, edema, hyperlipidemia, and hypercoagulability due to loss of antithrombin III in the urine.

Why are patients with diabetes at particular risk for acute renal failure?

Diabetic nephropathy is common in patients with diabetes (50% in type 1, less than 50% in type 2) and increases risk for ARF from other causes, especially toxins. High rates of atherosclerosis in patients with diabetes also increase the likelihood of renal artery stenosis. Diabetic neuropathy may result in atonic bladder, urinary retention, and postrenal azotemia.

▶ EVALUATION

What signs and symptoms should I look for to detect renal failure?

Symptoms are nonspecific and are due to accumulation of nitroge-nous wastes or volume overload. Patients may have nausea, vomit-ing, anorexia, or cardiopulmonary symptoms, such as chest pain from pericarditis or dyspnea from pulmonary edema. Patients may also report fatigue, confusion, or pruritus. Look for signs of volume overload such as elevated jugular venous pressure, cardiac gallop, or pulmonary crackles. Bladder obstruction can sometimes be detected by abdominal mass or suprapubic dullness from a dis-tended bladder. Chronic renal failure may cause pallor from anemia and skin excoriations due to pruritus.

What are the first steps in diagnosing the cause of acute renal failure?

For acute oliguric renal failure, rule-out obstruction by placing a Foley catheter and obtaining ultrasound to detect hydronephrosis (dilation of ureters or calyces). Then, use fluid challenge (or diuretics if volume-overloaded) to establish urine output. Review medications and remove nephrotoxins. Collect a fresh urine sample for urine sediment evaluation. Send BUN and creatinine. A ratio greater than 20:1 suggests a prerenal state.

What is an "active" urine sediment?

An active urine sediment refers to the presence of dysmorphic red cells or cellular casts in a fresh, centrifuged urine specimen and indicates intrinsic renal disease. Prerenal sediment usually shows only hyaline or granular casts. ATN is associated with muddy brown casts. Obstruction may lead to infection with white cells. Specific laboratory tests may be useful when intrinsic renal disease is suspected (Table 31–5), but renal biopsy may be required.

What is a "FeNa" and how does it help diagnose prerenal states?

FeNa is the fractional excretion of sodium from serum (s) into the urine (u). If, on the one hand, the FeNa is less than 1, the nephron

TABLE 31–5			
Characteristic Urine Findings and Special Labs for Major Types of ARF			
Location of Injury	**Urine Dipstick**	**Urinalysis**	**Other Labs**
Prerenal	Negative*	Hyaline casts	FeNa <1, UNa < 20 BUN:Cr ratio > 20:1
Postrenal	Negative	Negative	BUN:Cr ratio < 20:1
Intrinsic renal			FeNa > 2
Glomerulonephritis	3+ Blood 3+ Protein	Red cell casts Dysmorphic red cells	Consider: antistrep Ab, ANA, ANCA, SPEP, ESR, HIV, uric acid, hepatitis serology, renal biopsy
Interstitial nephritis	1+ Blood 1+ Protein†	Eosinophils White blood cell casts	Serum eosinophils
Tubular injury	Negative‡	Muddy brown casts Tubular cells	Myoglobin

*Persistent prerenal azotemia can cause ATN, so the urinalysis findings will be those of ATN.
†Proteinuria <1.5 g/day = interstitial nephritis; >3.5 g/day = nephrotic syndrome.
‡If ATN is due to rhabdomyolysis, the urine dipstick will be positive for blood because of cross-reacting myoglobin, but microscopic urinalysis will be negative for red blood cells.

is working hard to retain salt and water, so the cause of acute renal failure is likely prerenal. If, on the other hand, the FeNa is greater than 2, the nephron is not able to retain sodium, indicating an intrinsic renal process.

$$FeNa = \frac{Cr^S \times Na^U}{Cr^U \times Na^S} \times 100$$

FeNa < 1 = prerenal cause
FeNa > 2 = intrinsic renal cause

Diuretics may falsely increase the FeNa. If the FeNa is equivocal, or the patient is on diuretics, a urine sodium less than 20 indicates prerenal disease.

What lab tests can help me distinguish chronic from acute renal failure?

Patients with chronic renal failure usually have anemia (decreased erythropoietin), low calcium, and small kidneys on ultrasound. With ARF, anemia is less likely and kidneys are not small.

▶ TREATMENT

How is ARF managed?

Most patients require hospitalization for diagnosis and volume management. Decide whether volume depletion or overload exists. Then use daily weights, "ins and outs" including free water losses (~10 mL/kg for adults), and exam to guide volume repletion or diuresis. Watch for infection, an increased risk in patients with renal failure. Nutrition is a priority since anorexia is common. Renal-dose all medications based on calculated creatinine clearance.

$$\text{Creatinine clearance} = \frac{(140 - \text{age}) \times \text{body weight (kg)}^*}{72 \times \text{serum creatinine}}$$

*Multiply by 0.85 for women to correct for lean body mass.

Remember that with ARF the creatinine clearance changes rapidly.

What labs should I follow?

In oliguric ARF, expect daily increases in creatinine of 0.5–1.0 mg/dL and BUN of 10–20 mg/dL. Acidemia and hyperkalemia are common, so follow electrolytes at least daily. Obtain CBC, uric acid, calcium, magnesium, and phosphate at admission. If renal failure persists, consider rechecking these levels periodically. Check arterial blood gas as needed to monitor pH and acidosis.

When is dialysis required?

When symptomatic renal failure is present, dialysis may be needed, especially in oliguric patients. The indications for emergent dialysis are listed (Box 31–2).

BOX 31-2

Indications for Dialysis

Severe volume overload with CHF
Life-threatening acidosis
Severe electrolyte abnormalities, especially hyperkalemia
Pericarditis
Toxins that can be removed by dialysis

K E Y   P O I N T S

▶ With the work-up for ARF consider prerenal, intrarenal, and postrenal causes.

▶ Acidemia, hyperkalemia, and CHF are common and may necessitate dialysis.

▶ Treatment involves careful volume and electrolyte management; all medications must be dosed based on creatinine clearance.

CASE 31–3. A 79-year-old man presents with three days of nausea, vomiting, and anorexia. He has a history of BPH with a normal PSA one year ago. His BP is 86/palpable, P is 104. He has clear lungs, heart is normal, no edema, stool is Hemoccult negative. He is able to pass only 30 mL of dark urine. HCT = 46, K^+ = 5.1 mEq/L, HCO_3^- 31 mg/dL, BUN = 46 mg/dL, Cr = 1.9 mg/dL, uNa = 4 mm/L, uCr = 97 mm/L, Na = 144 mg/dL.

A. What is the most likely diagnosis and what work-up would confirm your diagnosis?
B. Calculate the FeNa for this patient.
C. What problems might develop over the next few days and how will you monitor them?

CASE 31–4. A 75-year-old man recently started diphenhydramine for sleep. He reports increasing grogginess, fatigue, and mild nausea. On exam you palpate a suprapubic mass, and his prostate is enlarged. BUN is 65, CR is 3.6, and CBC is normal.

A. What is your first diagnostic step?

B. What subsequent complications may he develop?

CASE 31–5. A 39-year-old woman with a single kidney and a long-term Foley catheter is hospitalized for pseudomonas pneumonia and treated with piperacillin-tazobactam. Her baseline creatinine is 1.2 mg/dL. On hospital day seven she becomes febrile to 38.3°C, with BP 140/82, P 100, her BUN is 36 mg/dL, creatinine 2.8 mg/dL, urinalysis: moderate proteinuria, rare red blood cells, and moderate eosinophils.

A. What is the differential diagnosis for her renal failure?

B. What is appropriate management?

CASE 31–6. A 54-year-old man seeks a second opinion from you about his chronic sinusitis. He has had multiple sinus infections, two sinus drainage procedures, and two episodes of "pneumonia." He is currently on TMP-SMX, pseudoephedrine, and nasal beclomethasone spray. His BP is 150/94. Exam is unremarkable except for poor maxillary sinus transillumination and crackles at his left lung base. His WBC is normal, his HCT is 35, and his creatinine is 1.9 mg/dL.

A. What is the differential for his elevated creatinine?

B. What additional history, exam, and tests would you like?

C. Predict what his urinalysis will show.

CASE 31-7. A 30-year-old man reports increasing edema. He used heroin until three months ago. His PMH is otherwise negative and he takes occasional ibuprofen for headaches. BP is 160/100; P is 80. His exam shows old needle track marks, bibasilar crackles, and 3+ pitting edema to the knees. He has 4+ protein on UA, a creatinine of 2.4 mg/dL, and a BUN of 20 mg/dL. His cholesterol is 346. A twenty-four-hour urine shows six grams of protein.

A. What is his diagnosis and what are the possible causes?
B. What work-up should he have?
C. List two findings you expect to see on his sediment exam.

ELECTROLYTE DISTURBANCES: CALCIUM

► ETIOLOGY

What causes hypercalcemia and hypocalcemia?

The causes of hypercalcemia and hypocalcemia are listed in Boxes 31-3 and 31-4. Apparent hypocalcemia may result from hypoalbuminemia because most serum calcium is bound to albumin. Total calcium drops by 0.8 mg/dL for every 1 mg/dL fall in albumin.

BOX 31-3

Causes of Hypercalcemia (From Most to Least Common)

Primary hyperparathyroidism
Drug induced
   Thiazide diuretics
   Vitamin D excess
Malignancy
   Osteolytic metastasis (breast cancer)
   PTH-like hormone production (lung cancer)
   Direct bone invasion (lymphoma)
Granulomatous disease (TB, sarcoid)
Immobilization

BOX 31-4

Causes of Hypocalcemia
Hypoalbuminemia (apparent hypocalcemia)
Renal failure
Hypoparathyroidism
Low magnesium
Pancreatitis
Multiple blood transfusions (citrate binds calcium)

▶ **EVALUATION**

When should I suspect hypercalcemia or hypocalcemia?

Hypercalcemia causes nonspecific symptoms or may be discovered inadvertently. Check calcium in any older patient with confusion, recalcitrant constipation, or polyuria. Other nonspecific signs include lethargy, nausea, vomiting, anorexia, and abdominal pain (from renal stones, pancreatitis). Severe hypercalcemia causes dehydration by diuresis and/or vomiting. Severe or rapidly acquired *hypocalcemia* causes painful tetany (muscle spasms). Classic findings are Trousseau's sign (carpal spasm with a blood pressure cuff inflated just above systolic pressure) and Chvostek's sign (facial twitching elicited by tapping just anterior to the ear). Lethargy, confusion, or seizures may also occur.

What evaluation is warranted in patients with calcium abnormalities?

With hypercalcemia, obtain H & P for signs of malignancy; pursue focal findings with further evaluation. When no signs of cancer are present, check complete blood count, renal function, and intact PTH. Look carefully at the medication list, as thiazide diuretics are a common cause of hypercalcemia. For hypocalcemia, ask about neck surgery (inadvertent parathyroid removal) and other autoimmune disorders, which may be associated with hypoparathyroidism. Obtain albumin, magnesium, phosphorous, PTH, vitamin D, and creatinine. PTH is low with primary hypoparathyroidism and hypomagnesemia, but elevated with other causes of hypocalcemia.

What ECG findings suggest calcium abnormalities?

The QT interval is shortened with hypercalcemia and prolonged with hypocalcemia. Hypocalcemia also worsens ECG findings of digoxin toxicity.

▶ **TREATMENT**

How do I treat hypercalcemia?

Treat the underlying cause. For severe hypercalcemia (greater than 13 mg/dL) or symptoms, start with normal saline hydration. After volume repletion, add furosemide, then a bisphosphonate or calcitonin if needed.

How do I replace calcium in patients with hypocalcemia?

Give intravenous calcium gluconate to acutely symptomatic patients. Replace low magnesium. Find and treat underlying causes. Give oral vitamin D and calcium carbonate for hypoparathyroidism.

K E Y   P O I N T S

- ▶ Patients with hypercalcemia present nonspecifically; check for it in any confused older patient.
- ▶ Hypocalcemia potentiates digoxin toxicity.

ELECTROLYTE DISTURBANCES: POTASSIUM

▶ **ETIOLOGY**

What causes elevated potassium?

Pseudohyperkalemia commonly occurs when red blood cells lyse during sample collection, releasing intracellular potassium. Redraw blood with a larger gauge needle and make sure the tourniquet is not on too long. True hyperkalemia occurs with renal failure, rhabdomyolysis (muscle cell injury releases intracellular potassium), extracellular shift of potassium with acidosis, potassium-sparing diuretics (e.g., spironolactone), ACEIs, and TMP-SMX.

What causes hypokalemia?

Most hypokalemia is due to diuretics. Vomiting and diarrhea are also common causes. Magnesium depletion can cause hypokalemia, especially in patients with excessive alcohol use.

Medications causing potassium depletion include diuretics, cis-platinum, theophylline, aminoglycosides, and amphotericin.

▶ **EVALUATION**

What evaluation is warranted in patients with hypokalemia?

Patients on diuretics may not need further tests. Check magnesium when patients use heavy alcohol or when hypokalemia resists aggressive replacement. With hypertension and hypokalemia, consider an adrenal hormone excess.

What clues on ECG suggest a potassium abnormality?

Hyperkalemia causes peaked T waves, progressing to widened QRS complexes and sine waves as potassium continues to rise. Hypokalemia causes T wave flattening and U waves.

▶ **TREATMENT**

How should I treat a patient with hyperkalemia?

ECG changes mandate emergent treatment. Give intravenous calcium gluconate to stabilize cardiac membranes, then intravenous glucose, insulin, and bicarbonate to drive potassium into the cells. If the patient can make urine, give intravenous furosemide. Kayexalate, a sodium/potassium exchange resin, is given orally or as an enema but acts slowly. In extremely urgent situations use dialysis.

How do I replace potassium?

Replace orally with KCl or K_3PO_4. If intravenous replacement is required, give no faster than 10 mEq/hr.

K E Y   P O I N T S

▶ Hyperkalemia is due to excess intake, shift from the intracellular compartment (acidosis, cell injury), or inability to excrete potassium (renal failure, drugs).

▶ Refractory hypokalemia may be due to coexistent hypomagnesemia.

ELECTROLYTE DISTURBANCES: SODIUM

▶ ETIOLOGY

What leads to hypernatremia?

Hypernatremia is commonly caused by lack of water. Patients unable to get to water become hypernatremic (e.g., from acute CVA when home alone and coma). Occasionally, fluid requirements are too great to sustain enough intake (e.g., diabetes insipidus).

What causes hyponatremia?

Causes are categorized by volume status as hypo-, eu-, or hypervolemic. In hypovolemic hyponatremia, both water and sodium are depleted and sodium losses exceed volume losses. With hypervolemic hyponatremia, patients actually have total body excess sodium with even greater excess water in edematous states such as CHF, cirrhosis, or severe hypoalbuminemia from nephrotic syndrome. Euvolemic hyponatremia is most often from a syndrome of inappropriate antidiuretic hormone (SIADH) release (Table 31–6). Patients with hyponatremia due to SIADH usually have low BUN and uric acid levels. Thiazide diuretics are a common cause of euvolemic hyponatremia, with the exact pathogenesis unclear. Pseudohyponatremia occurs with severe hyperlipidemia, hypergammaglobulinemia, or hyperglycemia. For each increase of glucose by 100 mg/dL over a normal glucose level of 100, the serum sodium decreases by 1.6 mEq/L.

▶ EVALUATION

When should I suspect sodium disturbances?

Patients with hypernatremia are often volume depleted and may have altered consciousness preventing them from fluid intake.

TABLE 31–6

Cause of SIADH

Cause of SIADH	Examples
Severe pulmonary disease	Lung abscess, severe pneumonia, mechanical ventilation with PEEP
Tumor	Small cell lung carcinoma
CNS disorders	Meningitis, encephalitis, tumor
Drugs	Morphine, tricyclic antidepressants, sulfonylureas, tegretol
Endocrine disorders	Hypothyroidism, primary adrenal failure

Symptoms of hyponatremia include confusion, disorientation, and anorexia. Seizures or coma may occur with severe or rapidly developing hyponatremia. For patients with any sodium derangement, first establish volume status.

What evaluation is helpful in patients with hyponatremia?

Find out about medications and a recent history of GI losses, pulmonary or CNS disease, or malignancy. Examine vital signs, neck veins, mucus membranes, and skin turgor with an eye to determining volume status, but remember that none of these signs are particularly sensitive or specific for hypovolemia. Measure urine sodium. A urine sodium less than 20 suggests poor renal perfusion but a normal kidney, as with CHF or hypovolemia. A urine sodium above 40 suggests SIADH, renal failure, or other inappropriate wasting of sodium. A concurrent alkalosis may suggest volume contraction from diuretics or emesis. A metabolic acidosis may suggest renal or adrenal failure as the source of hyponatremia. Normal pH would be expected with SIADH and edematous states.

▶ TREATMENT

How do I treat hypernatremia?

Replace volume deficit with normal saline, then replace free water deficit with D5W over thirty-six hours, reducing sodium by 0.5 to 1 mEq/hr. Calculate the free water deficit:

Free water deficit = (serum sodium/140 − 1) × 0.6 × weight in kg

For central diabetes insipidus, replace ADH.

How do I treat hyponatremia?

Use water restriction for mild euvolemic hyponatremia. For seizures or coma, correct more rapidly with normal (0.9%) or hypertonic saline (3%) and furosemide. Treat hypovolemic hyponatremia with intravenous normal saline. Treat hypervolemic hyponatremia with both salt and water restriction along with diuretics as needed. Bring the serum sodium level up slowly. Different recommendations exist for exactly how slowly to normalize the low sodium, ranging from 8–12 mEq/24 hours maximum, to avoid central pontine myelinolysis. No cases of central pontine myelinolysis have been seen with rates of 8 or less mEq/24 hours, so this is probably the safest choice of correction rate. If patients have ongoing seizures, some recommend more rapid initial correction of the sodium by 1–2 mmol/hour for the first few hours, then return to a slower rate. In the acute setting of sodium correction, sodium levels require monitoring every one to three hours to avoid too rapid a correction.

How do I estimate the change in serum sodium that will occur with IV fluids I give to patients with hyponatremia?

You'll need to know the sodium content of your fluid: 154 mEq are in a liter of normal saline, and 513 mEq are in a liter of 3% saline. Then use the following formula to calculate the effect of each liter of fluid used:

$$\text{Change in serum sodium} = \frac{\text{infusate Na} - \text{serum Na}}{\text{total body water} + 1}$$

Total body water, in kilograms, is estimated at 60% of total weight for men, 50% for women and elderly men, and 45% for elderly women. Once you calculate the change in serum sodium with each liter, you can then see how fast to give the fluid to obtain the rate of change you desire. For example, a man weighing 60 kilograms has a serum sodium of 110. Each liter of 3% normal saline will raise the sodium $(513 - 113)/((0.6 \times 60) + 1)$, or 10.81 mEq. If you wish to raise the serum sodium by only 8 mEq over twenty-four hours, you would need to use only about 800mL out of a liter bag of 3% saline.

K E Y   P O I N T S

▶ Categorize hyponatremia by volume status.

▶ Treat most mild to moderate euvolemic hyponatremia with volume restriction.

▶ Correct sodium imbalances slowly by no more than 1 mEq/hour.

FLUID MANAGEMENT

▶ ETIOLOGY

In which situations do patients need fluid administration?

Hospitalized patients unable to drink owing to illness or procedures need maintenance fluid, electrolytes, and glucose replacement. Volume-depleted patients need volume resuscitation.

▶ **EVALUATION**

How do I evaluate volume status?

Look for volume depletion by weight loss, postural hypotension, poor skin turgor, dry mucous membranes, oliguria, and tachycardia. An increased BUN/creatinine ratio of greater than 20 is also a clue. Look for fluid overload (often a preventable iatrogenic occurrence) by weight gain, jugular venous distention, edema, and rales. Evaluate volume status daily in hospitalized patients.

▶ **TREATMENT**

How do I design maintenance fluid and electrolyte therapy?

Patients unable to eat need approximately 2 liters of fluid per day, as 1/4 or 1/2 normal saline with glucose for calories. Standard basal requirements for electrolytes are about 1 mEq/kg/day of Na, K, Cl, with adjustments as needed for excess losses.

How do I choose appropriate resuscitation fluid for a dehydrated patient?

Fluid therapy is an exercise in balancing input and output of electrolytes and water. Know the electrolyte content of various solutions (Table 31–7). For volume resuscitation in patients with dehydration or low blood pressure, choose a fluid with high saline content that will stay in the intravascular space (normal saline or lactated Ringer's). Remember that lactated Ringer's has potassium, so don't give large volumes to anuric patients. Giving fluid in boluses is preferable to running fluids at a high rate and forgetting about the continuous infusion.

TABLE 31–7

Electrolyte Concentrations in Various Intravenous Solutions (in mEq/L)

Fluid	Sodium	Potassium	Chloride	Bicarbonate	Lactate
1/2 normal saline (0.45%)	77		77		
Normal saline (0.9%)	154		154		
Hypertonic saline (0.3%)	513		513		
Ringer's lactate*	130	4	110		28
Sodium bicarbonate (per amp)	44.5			44.5	
5% dextrose in water (D5W)†					

*Also contains 3 mEq calcium/L.
†Has 50 g of dextrose per liter of water and no other electrolytes.

This method lowers the risk of iatrogenic volume overload. Frequent exams of fluid status are mandatory in patients receiving volume resuscitation to evaluate their response and plan further fluid therapy.

K E Y   P O I N T S

▶ Assess fluid status at least once daily in all hospitalized patients.

▶ Use 1/2 normal saline with glucose and potassium for maintenance fluids.

▶ Fluid resuscitate with normal saline boluses and reassess fluid status between boluses.

CASE 31–8.
A 50-year-old man with history of poorly controlled hypertension and renal failure requiring dialysis three times a week comes to the ED because he feels weak and short of breath. He has missed his last three dialysis appointments. Exam shows HR = 90, BP = 180/100, RR = 22, T = 98.4°F, O_2 sat = 93%, JVP elevated to 10 cm, bibasilar rales, an S3, and 1+ leg edema. Na = 130, K = 8.0, $HCO_3^- = 18$, Cl = 100, BUN = 60, creatinine = 8.5. Chest film shows prominent vessels in the upper lung fields.

  A. What is this patient's most life-threatening problem and why?
  B. What would this man's ECG show?
  C. Name the interventions you could use to manage his hyperkalemia and state how each works.

CASE 31–9.
A 67-year-old woman with a long history of heavy smoking, hypertension, and alcohol use is brought to clinic. She lives in a nursing home and has become more disoriented over the last week. She always has a rattly cough but her sputum has increased. Today, she is breathing hard and not making sense. Her only medication is hydrochlorothiazide. Labs show WBC = 15, HCT = 37, Na = 118, K = 3.5, Cl = 85, $HCO_3^- = 23$.

  A. List possible causes of hyponatremia in this patient.
  B. What aspects of exam will help you categorize this patient's hyponatremia?
  C. On exam she is euvolemic with bronchial breath sounds and dullness to percussion over the left lower lung field. What is the likely cause of her hyponatremia?
  D. How do you want to treat it?

REFERENCES

Adrogue HJ, Madias NE: Hyponatremia. N Engl J Med 25;342(21): 1581–1589, 2000.

Kapoor M, Chan GZ: Fluid and electrolyte abnormalities. Review. Crit Care Clin 17(3):503–529, 2001.

HYPERTENSION

▶ ETIOLOGY

How prevalent is hypertension?

Hypertension is present in 23% of whites and in 32% of non-Hispanic African Americans. In patients older than age 65, more than 50% have either isolated systolic or systolic *and* diastolic hypertension.

What are the consequences of hypertension?

Hypertension is a major risk factor for stroke, intracerebral hemorrhage, coronary artery disease, left ventricular hypertrophy, chronic renal insufficiency, and end stage renal disease. Other sequelae include erectile dysfunction, decreased visual acuity, and dementia as a consequence of multiple infarcts. Acute, markedly elevated blood pressure is life-threatening.

What proportion of patients are adequately treated for their hypertension?

In the NHANES III study of 16,000 patients, 75% of white patients were either unaware of having hypertension or were inadequately treated. These numbers were even higher in African Americans and Mexican Americans. In the latter group, only 15% had controlled blood pressure and slightly over half were even aware that they had high blood pressure.

What blood pressure reading is considered "hypertension"?

The Joint National Consensus Panel on Hypertension VI (JNC VI) categorizes levels of blood pressure elevation. As the blood pressure levels increase, so does the risk of adverse outcomes (Table 31–8).

TABLE 31–8

JNC VI Categorization of Blood Pressure

	Systolic (mm Hg)	Diastolic (mm Hg)
Optimal	<120	<80
Normal	<130	<85
High normal	<130–139	85–89
Hypertension		
Stage 1	140–159	90–99
Stage 2	160–179	100–109
Stage 3	>180	>110

What are the risk factors for primary hypertension?

The cause of primary or "essential" hypertension is not known, although it is correlated with several risk factors. These include family history of hypertension, personal history of obesity, excessive alcohol use, and African-American descent. Increased salt intake may contribute to, but is not causative of, hypertension.

What are secondary causes of hypertension?

Secondary hypertension accounts for about 5% of hypertension and is caused by an identifiable, treatable structural or endocrine abnormality. Younger patients with hypertension or patients poorly responsive to three or more antihypertensive medications should be considered for screening for secondary causes, including renal artery stenosis, acute and chronic renal insufficiency, pheochromocytoma, sleep apnea, coarctation of the aorta, Cushing's syndrome, and primary hyperaldosteronism.

What factors are important in risk-stratifying patients with hypertension?

JNC VI recommends risk stratifying patients to determine how aggressively to begin antihypertensive therapy. Patients with no risk factors, Risk Group A, are at low immediate risk for adverse cardiovascular events. Patients with one or more risk factors, Risk Group B, are at intermediate risk of adverse outcome, and those with proven end organ disease or diabetes, Risk Group C, are at highest risk (Table 31–9). This risk stratification then assists in determining how rapidly to intervene with medications (Table 31–10).

TABLE 31–9

Risk Factors and Target Organ Damage in Hypertension

Risk Factors	Target Organ Damage
Smoking	Retinopathy
Hyperlipidemia	Peripheral artery disease
Diabetes	Nephropathy
Age > 60	Heart disease (LVH, CAD, CHF)
Men and postmenopausal women	Stroke
Family history	

*High number of risk factors or the presence of targer organ damage increases risk of adverse outcome from hypertension and warrants more aggressive intervention.

TABLE 31–10

JNC VI Recommendations for Antihypertensive Medication Initiation

Blood Pressure Stage	Risk A (none)	Risk B (1 risk or greater)	Risk C (DM or TOD)*
High Normal	Lifestyle	Lifestyle	Drug
Stage 1	Lifestyle	Lifestyle	Drug
Stage 2, 3	Drug	Drug	Drug

*Diabetes mellitus (DM) and target organ damage (TOD)

Is systolic hypertension as important a risk factor as diastolic hypertension?

Yes. Several large studies have clearly established that systolic hypertension is a strong risk factor for cardiovascular disease. Recent clinical trials have demonstrated that treatment of systolic hypertension prevents cardiovascular events.

What is "white coat" hypertension?

For roughly 25% of patients with mildly elevated blood pressure in clinic, their outside readings will be normal. Long-term studies in these patients have shown mild increases in left ventricular mass, but the consequence of white coat hypertension is not known.

► EVALUATION

How do I measure blood pressure?

Patients should be sitting down for five minutes, in a calm environment. They should not have had caffeine within the past hour or cigarettes within the past half hour. For accurate measurement, their arm should be at the level of their heart. The height of the cuff should be as wide as the patient's arm. The shirt should be removed so there is no restrictive clothing, and the patient should not be talking.

How is hypertension diagnosed?

A single reading does not constitute hypertension. Blood pressure varies from visit to visit, and studies have shown that readings drop by 10 to 15 mm Hg between visits one and three for newly diagnosed patients, not yet on medications. The JNC VI recommends measuring blood pressure twice on two separate occasions. In the absence of target organ damage, the patient should not be labeled as hypertensive unless the averaged blood pressure is persistently elevated on at least two visits.   *Need to measure @ least 2x*

What is the role of ambulatory monitoring?

This device measures a patient's blood pressure over a twenty-four-hour period. The automatic cuff inflates every fifteen minutes while the patient is awake and every thirty to sixty minutes while the patient is asleep, thus obtaining "real world" measures of blood pressure. This tool is particularly useful when office and outside blood pressure readings do not match (e.g., white coat hypertension), when patient education with closer monitoring may help adherence, and when patient symptoms suggest the blood pressure is overtreated or there is autonomic dysfunction present (lightheadedness, presyncope).

What history should I obtain in patients with hypertension?

Ask about symptoms or sequelae of hypertension: headache, visual changes, chest pain. Review exacerbants of hypertension: alcohol, stimulant (especially cocaine) and salt intake, hormone or nonsteroidal use, level of exercise. Screen for causes of secondary hypertension: daytime somnolence, morning headache, or snoring at night (sleep apnea); young age at diagnosis, claudication (coarctation of the aorta); flushing, anxiety, episodic hypertension (pheochromocytoma); diabetes, proximal leg weakness, depression (Cushing's); cold/heat intolerance, hair or skin changes, diarrhea or constipation (thyroid disease); young age at diagnosis of hypertension or presence of peripheral vascular disease, or rapid onset of severe hypertension in an elderly patient (renal artery stenosis).

What examination is important in patients with hypertension?

BP: check the measurement in both arms. If elevated, particularly in a young person, check lower extremity blood pressure and if it is lower, suspect coarctation of the aorta

Weight/height: obesity is a major risk factor for hypertension

Pulse: tachycardia may suggest hyperthyroidism, hypoxemia, or CHF

Skin: abdominal striae, hirsutism, or purpuric bruises of Cushing's

HEENT: funduscopic exam for hypertensive changes of AV nicking, arterial narrowing, hemorrhages, exudates, or papilledema

Neck: carotid bruit of atherosclerosis, goiter of hyperthyroidism

Lungs: rales of congestive heart failure from prolonged hypertension

Heart: S3/4, heave, indicating left ventricular hypertrophy or enlargement

Abd: bruit of renal artery stenosis, mass of polycystic kidney disease

Ext: edema from congestive heart failure or medication side effect, proximal muscle weakness from Cushing's

What tests are useful in the initial evaluation of patients with new hypertension?

The initial evaluation includes ECG, urinalysis, glucose, electrolytes, BUN and creatinine, and lipid panel. ECG screens for signs of prior infarct and for left ventricular hypertrophy (LVH) associated with increased mortality, and serves as comparison for future ischemia. Urinalysis showing casts, RBCs, or protein suggests kidney disease, either the cause or result of hypertension. Glucose screens for diabetes. Low potassium suggests hyperaldosteronism or Cushing's and may worsen BP control. Elevated creatinine suggests renal disease. Lipid panel provides additional information about cardiovascular risk.

▶ TREATMENT

What benefit will my patient receive from blood pressure treatment?

A meta-analysis of clinical trials with 37,000 patients showed a 42% reduction in stroke and a 14% reduction in CAD. In African-American women, the number needed to treat to prevent one cardiovascular event is 21. The findings are also striking in diabetes where tight control of BP, less than 144/82, vs. less tight (154/87), resulted in a 44% reduction in stroke and a 47% reduction in visual acuity decline. In renal insufficiency, progression of disease and increasing proteinuria directly relate to inadequate blood pressure control, as well as proteinuria.

What degree of BP improvement occurs with each type of intervention?

The reduction in BP is roughly the same for lifestyle modifications and starting medications doses: 5–10 mm Hg.

What lifestyle modifications can make a difference?

Obesity is a major risk factor for hypertension and weight loss results in a decrease of 0.3–1 mm Hg for every 1 kg lost. For a patient who loses 10 pounds, the blood pressure may decrease by 5 mm Hg. Salt restriction to 2–2.5 g may reduce blood pressure an average of 2–5 mm Hg. Alcohol intake of more than two drinks a day increases blood pressure and this appears dose-dependent—greater than five drinks a day has the most impact on blood pressure. Thirty to forty-five minutes of aerobic exercise most days of the week has also been shown to reduce blood pressure.

Is it worth treating hypertension in elderly patients?

Because the elderly have a higher baseline risk of cardiovascular events, the benefit of even short-term treatment is higher than in younger patients. In patients older than age 80, the number needed to treat is just 21 to prevent a cardiovascular event, and 30 to prevent a stroke. While treating hypertension aggressively in these patients, keep a close eye on side effects of multiple medications. It is recommended to keep the diastolic blood pressure above 65.

How soon should I start medications in patients?

Start medication at the time of diagnosis for patients with high normal blood pressure and target organ damage, i.e., retinopathy on fundoscopic exam or diabetes (Table 31–10). Start medications without waiting for a lifestyle modification trial in any patient with a confirmed systolic pressure greater than 160 and/or diastolic pressure greater than 100. In all patients, diet and exercise are an important part of therapy.

What is the goal blood pressure?

For low-risk patients, a target of less than 140/90 is adequate. For higher risk patients, the target level is lower. In diabetes, according to the JCN VI, the goal is less than 130/85 mm Hg. In patients with proteinuria, the goal is less than 125/75 mm Hg.

Which antihypertensive is the most effective?

When starting a blood pressure medication, take into consideration the established efficacy, cost, quality of life, and any comorbid conditions. Thiazide diuretics and β-blockers have the longest history of improving morbidity and mortality in hypertension, are inexpensive, and well tolerated at low doses. These factors have combined to make these the starting medications of choice for many patients with hypertension. ACEIs are increasingly used for first line therapy as a result of clinical trials demonstrating reduction in cardiovascular end points and effects that are equivalent to β-blockers and diuretics.

What if the initial medication is ineffective?

Antihypertensives are approximately equivalent in their initial efficacy—about 40%–60% of patients respond to the first medication. There are two approaches for what to do next. Either start one medication and increase the dose to maximum, or keep the dose relatively low and combine with other agents for an additive effect and minimization of side effects. Diuretics enhance the effects of all other classes of antihypertensives.

What comorbidities affect antihypertensive choice?

For a number of conditions, data support using specific medications in addition to, or instead of, a diuretic or β-blocker. These include ACEIs in CHF; ACEIs in diabetes and renal disease to slow progression of kidney damage; and calcium channel blockers in angina that is inadequately controlled by β-blocker.

Are the calcium channel blockers safe?

Although studies of short-acting calcium channel blockers suggest an increased risk of myocardial infarction, these findings have not replicated with long-acting CCBs. In fact, long-acting CCBs are considered safe but less effective than diuretics, β-lockers, and ACEIs. They are most appropriate as fourth line therapy. One exception is that long-acting CCBs are equally effective to thiazide diuretics in treating isolated systolic hypertension in the elderly and in this circumstance can be used as an alternative to diuretics. Never use sublingual nifedipine to acutely control a patient's blood pressure. This is an outdated and potentially dangerous practice.

How often should I monitor BP short- and long-term?

For stage 3 disease (systolic greater than 180, diastolic greater than 110), the patient should be seen again within a week to determine whether therapy is effective and control is improving. While adjusting medications, monitoring response, and side effects, it is useful to see the patient every four to six weeks. Check electrolytes, BUN, and creatinine one week after changing an ACEI or diuretic dose. Once stable, patients can be seen annually.

What are possible reasons that my patient's blood pressure is not improving?

Adherence is frequently challenging for patients with hypertension. To help patients, attend to their reported side effects and change medications where possible. Remind them that with better blood pressure control they will often feel better. Simplify medication regimens by limiting the number of medications and the frequency of dosing. Investigate how patients pay for their medications and work with the pharmacist to devise the most cost-effective and health-effective dose. In a patient with poorly controlled hypertension, the medication may be ineffective. Switch to or add another agent. Another major factor in poorly controlled hypertension is volume expansion in part due to high levels of salt intake. Reinforce low salt diet, refer to a nutritionist, and add a diuretic if not already prescribed. For persistently poor control in an adherent patient on multiple medications, evaluate for secondary causes, of which renal artery stenosis is the most common (Table 31–11).

Are there specific side effects or unwanted sequelae of these medications?

The cough accompanying ACEIs can be quite severe and affects 10% of whites and 40% of Asians (Table 31–12).

When should I admit someone for hypertension?

Admit the patient with elevated BP and acute symptoms or signs of end-organ strain: confusion, chest pain, papilledema, hematuria/proteinuria, or pulmonary edema. A BP reading greater than 240/130 is associated with significant mortality, so even asymptomatic patients with this level of hypertension should be admitted.

TABLE 31-11

Reversible Causes of Hypertension and Their Evaluation

Condition	Test
Alcohol use	CAGE questions, serum GGT
Hyperthyroidism	TSH
Sleep apnea	Nocturnal pulse oximetry or sleep study
Cushing's	24-hour urine cortisol
Hyperaldosteronism	Serum renin/aldosterone ratio
Renovascular disease	Spiral CT or MRA
Pheochromocytoma	24-hour urine catecholamines

TABLE 31-12

Once Daily Dosed Antihypertensive Medications, Relative Cost, and Side Effects

Drug	Cost	Important Side Effects	Also Treats
Diuretic Hydrochlorothiazide Chlorthalidone	$	Frequent urination Decreased potassium Increased lipids at doses >25 mg Increased uric acid	Volume overload Leg edema
β-Blocker Atenolol Nadolol Propanolol SR	$	Fatigue Decreased exercise tolerance Impotence Asthma Bradycardia	Prevents MI recurrence Migraine (prophylaxis) Angina
ACE inhibitor Benazepril Lisinopril	$$$	Renal insufficiency Teratogen Hyperkalemia Cough (10%–20%) Life-threatening angioedema	CHF Diabetic nephropathy
α-Blocker Doxazosin Terazosin	$$	Postural hypotension Headache Weakness	Benign prostatic hypertrophy

**Calcium
   channel blocker**
 	
Amlodipine
Nifedipine SR
Diltiazem CD
	$$$$	Bradycardia, and negative
		   inotropy (only with
		   diltiazem)
		Constipation
		Leg edema
		Reflux
			Angina

Angiotensin receptor blocker Losartan Valsartan Irbesartan	$$$	Hyperkalemia	CHF Diabetic nephropathy

K E Y   P O I N T S

► Blood treatment reduces risk of stroke and heart disease.

► Goal blood pressure depends on comorbidities: 130/85 for diabetes and other target organ damage and 140/90 for patients without other risk factors.

► Diet, exercise, salt reduction can all reduce blood pressure.

▶ Treat other risk factors for cardiovascular disease (smoking cessation, lipid management). Prescribe aspirin as an additional method to prevent cardiovascular disease.

▶ In uncomplicated hypertension, start a diuretic or β-blocker. ACEIs have an increasing role in first line treatment.

▶ In hypertension complicated by diabetes and CHF, an ACEI is first line therapy.

▶ Elderly patients and minorities are less likely to be well controlled.

▶ Treat hypertension in the elderly, including isolated systolic hypertension, but keep diastolic above 65.

CASE 31–10. A 27-year-old woman presents with a recent ankle sprain with no personal or family history of hypertension. She uses ibuprofen since the injury and oral contraceptives. She drinks four beers a night. On exam, her BP is 146/92.

A. What could be elevating her blood pressure?
B. How soon would you like to see her again?
C. What changes would you like to ask her to make before her next visit?

CASE 31–11. A 72-year-old woman comes to see you for the first time. Aside from chronic constipation and occasional gout, she is remarkably healthy. Her only real medical problem is high blood pressure that has been present "for years and years." Her medications are Metamucil, milk of magnesia, and nifedipine 20 mg tid. From time to time she takes a "water pill" for her swollen legs. Her BP is 150/84 and her P is 59.

A. Would you recommend a change in her BP medication and why/why not?
B. What evaluation will you do?
C. What medication would you choose for her?

CASE 31–12. A 57-year-old woman with obesity, diabetes, and depression sits in your office crying because you have just told her she has hypertension. When she is depressed, she eats potato chips and has gained 30 pounds over the past year. She is extremely tired all the time; in fact she fell asleep while driving over to see you. In her family, all her siblings have hypertension and diabetes. On exam, her blood pressure is 166/117. She has stretch marks on her stomach, and has lower extremity swelling. Her ECG and UA are normal. Her labs show low potassium.

A. Name at least five possible causes of, or contributors to, hypertension in this patient.
B. Would you order any further tests and if so, why?
C. How would you start to treat her?

REFERENCES

The Sixth Report of the Joint National Committee on Detention, Evaluation, and Treatment of High Blood Pressure. Arch Intern Med 157:2413, 1997.
Pavlik VN: Hyman DJ: Characteristics of patients with uncontrolled hypertension in the United States. N Engl J Med 16;345:479–486, 2001.

32

Neurology

NEUROLOGIC EXAM

What should I cover with the neurologic exam?

Perform a screening neurologic exam on all new inpatients and on clinic patients who request a "full physical." This includes assessment of mental status, cranial nerves, strength, sensation, reflexes, and coordination. A sample normal screening exam is provided in Box 32–1. This should take no more than three to five minutes to perform on an alert, cooperative patient. To facilitate the exam, tell your patient why you are doing each step. For example you can say, "I'm going to test your coordination now. Touch my finger, now touch your nose, now go back and forth." When you record motor strength, use a scale from 0 to 5 (Box 32–2).

BOX 32–1

Sample Normal Screening Neurologic Exam

Mental status: alert and oriented to person, place, and time

Cranial nerves: pupils equal, round, reactive to light, and accommodation (PERRLA), extraocular movements intact (EOMI), facial sensation and movement normal, palate elevation symmetric, tongue midline and strong (or cranial nerves 2 through 12 intact)

Sensation: intact to vibration in the toes and light touch in all four extremities

Motor: 5 out of 5 strength in all four extremity muscle groups

Coordination: intact to finger-nose-finger; gait normal

Reflexes: symmetric and 2/4 at the biceps, triceps, knees, and ankles; 1/4 at the brachioradialis; toes downgoing

---

BOX 32–2

Grading Motor Strength

0 = no movement
1 = trace movement
2 = movement when the force of gravity removed
3 = able to move against gravity but not resistance
4 = able to move against resistance but weaker than expected for age and size
5 = full strength against resistance

When do I need to perform a more detailed neurologic exam?

If the screening neurologic exam is abnormal, or if the patient presents with a neurologic problem, a more detailed exam is warranted and can be tailored to fit the circumstances (Table 32–1).

K E Y   P O I N T S

▶ Master a five minute screening neurologic exam for inpatients and outpatient physicals.

▶ Focus the neurologic exam depending on the clinical situation.

ALTERED MENTAL STATUS

▶ ETIOLOGY

What causes altered mental status?

Altered mental status is a spectrum ranging from normal to coma. Avoid imprecise terms such as lethargic, stuporous, or obtunded. Instead, describe the level of stimulus required to arouse the patient (e.g., wakens to voice, unarousable to noxious stimuli) and the degree of drowsiness (e.g., falls asleep after several minutes of conversation). Coma means that there is no purposeful response

TABLE 32-1

Additional Neurologic Examinations for Specific Conditions

Condition	Neurologic Exam	Observe and Record
Stupor or coma	Responsiveness	Level of stimulus required to rouse patient: voice, shaking, noxious stimuli
	Motor response	Appropriate withdrawal or posturing to noxious stimuli
	Pupil size, response	Size in mm; direct and consensual response to light
	Eye movements	Centered, disconjugate or conjugate gaze deviation, doll's eyes or cold water calorics. Clear cervical-spine first before doing doll's eyes maneuvers
	Corneal reflexes	Blink elicited when cornea touched with Q-tip
	Breathing	Cheyne-Stokes respirations, neurogenic hyperventilation, apneustic or ataxic respirations
Stroke	Simultaneous double stimuli	Left hemi-neglect is found in patients with right parietal lesions
	Language	Normal, dysarthric, or aphasic
	Carotid auscultation	Listen for carotid bruits
	Romberg	Stand up straight with eyes closed
	Pronator drift	Keep arms extended out at shoulder height with palms up; abnormal if one palm or arm turns downward
	Gait	Symmetry, stride, arm swing, stance (wide or narrow)
Memory loss	MMSE	30-Point Mini-Mental Status Exam
Decreased sensation	Pain/temperature	Sharp toothpick, cold metal
	Proprioception	Toe up or down
	Light touch	Identify pattern: dermatomal, stocking-glove-Monofilament testing

to the environment and signifies lesions in both cerebral hemispheres or in the reticular activating system (RAS) in the brain stem. Lesser degrees of altered mental status can arise from metabolic/toxic derangements or structural problems (Table 32–2).

▶ EVALUATION

What historical clues are helpful in determining the cause of confusion?

Ask family, friends, and emergency medical staff for clues. Abrupt onset suggests a discrete event such as stroke or seizure, whereas more gradual onset suggests a diffuse metabolic process. Onset with a "worst-ever headache" suggests subarachnoid hemorrhage (SAH). Progression from an initial focal deficit is a clue to the loca-

TABLE 32–2

Causes of Altered Mental Status

	Common Causes	Less Common Causes
Metabolic or toxic	Anoxia (hypoperfusion, hypoxia) Drugs (Rx, non-Rx, illicit) Electrolytes (Ca^{++}, Na^+, glucose) Epilepsy Infection (UTI, pneumonia) Liver failure Myocardial infarction	Adrenal insufficiency Hypertensive encephalopathy Hypothyroidism Vitamin B_{12} deficiency
Structural	CNS trauma Infection (meningitis, encephalitis) Stroke, hemorrhagic or ischemic	CNS tumor CNS abscess

tion of a structural problem. Ask about potential precipitating factors such as trauma, alcohol withdrawal, or drug overdose. Obtain pill bottles from the patient's home if possible. Medical history such as a recent fall or trauma, diabetes, seizures, drug overdose, and heroin or alcohol use are also clues to possible causes of altered mental status. For elderly patients, confusion is often the final common presenting pathway for a number of conditions including MI, urosepsis, and pneumonia. Even if the history is atypical for these common ailments, maintain a high suspicion and rule them out routinely.

How do I recognize the difference between delirium, psychosis, and dementia?

Delirium is transient, fluctuating confusion and loss of attentiveness, often accompanied by agitation and adrenergic signs such as tachycardia and diaphoresis. In the elderly, delirium is frequently caused by infection. Delirium usually resolves with treatment of the causal metabolic derangement. *Psychosis* may look like delirium but has no underlying metabolic derangement. In contrast, *dementia* is a confusional state in which patients remain attentive. It is chronic, persistent, and slowly progressive with memory loss as a prominent feature (Table 32–3).

What studies should I order in a confused patient?

Order ECG, O_2 saturation, CBC, electrolytes, renal and liver function, glucose, and urinalysis to detect a metabolic cause for altered mental status. If no abnormality is found, order the following only

TABLE 32–3

Features Distinguishing Delirium from Dementia

	Delirium	Dementia
Level of consciousness	Impaired	Normal*
Clinical course	Acute, fluctuates over hours	Slowly progresses over years
Autonomic hyperactivity	Present	Absent
Prognosis	Usually reversible	Usually irreversible

*Patients usually retain normal level of consciousness until very late in the course of dementia.

TABLE 32–4

Evaluation and Management of the Comatose Patient

Immediate Issues for Stabilization	Urgent Issues After Stabilization	Later Issues
Stabilize airway, breathing, and circulation	History	Correct electrolytes
Vital signs including pulse oximetry	Thorough neurologic exam	Correct acid-base imbalances
Cervical spine films to clear neck	ABG, CBC, renal and liver function, electrolytes, urinalysis, and toxicology screen	CXR
Naloxone 0.4–1.2 mg IV	Head CT ± contrast	Other labs if indicated
Thiamine 100 mg IV*	LP if indicated	EEG if indicated
Glucose 25 gm IV*	ECG and rule out MI with cardiac enzymes, especially in the elderly	
Rapid exam for trauma, neurologic deficits	Antibiotics if meningitis suspected	

*Always give thiamine before glucose.

as indicated by the specific case: alcohol or drug levels, toxicology screening, ABG, carboxyhemoglobin levels, and head CT. Most mass lesions or bleeds in the cerebral hemispheres are easy to detect on CT; however, 5% of SAHs can be missed on an early CT scan. A negative CT in a patient thought to have SAH requires an LP to look for bloody CSF. Perform LP in any patient with fever and altered mental status unless a good explanation for both is quickly found.

How do I evaluate a comatose patient?

Prioritize your approach to address urgent issues first (Table 32–4). Focus your neurologic exam on level of consciousness, breathing pattern, motor response to central noxious stimuli (finger in the stylomastoid foramen), pupillary responses, and eye movement with doll's eyes maneuver and cold water caloric testing. Cheyne-Stokes respiration is a rhythmic waxing and waning of respiratory rate and volume seen with bilateral hemispheric damage, although it can occur in normal subjects, at high altitudes, and in patients with heart failure. Central neurogenic hyperventilation, apneustic breathing (prominent pauses), or ataxic breathing (random, irregular, deep, and shallow breathing) suggests injury in focal parts of the brain stem. Eyes may deviate conjugately toward an ipsilateral hemispheric structural lesion. The doll's eyes maneuver is performed on comatose patients with intact cervical spines, by watching eye movements when the head is rotated rapidly to one side. A positive test occurs when the eyes move in their sockets to remain fixed on a point on the ceiling even though the head is turned. An intact brain stem is required for this reflex response. In awake patients, the doll's reflex is suppressed by the cortex. With cerebral dysfunction but an intact brainstem, doll's eyes testing is positive. With a low brain stem lesion involving the pontine gaze center, doll's eyes maneuver is negative, meaning the eyes stay fixed in their sockets and point wherever the head is turned.

Cold water caloric testing is performed by injecting cold water in one ear. The normal awake response to cold caloric stimulation is nystagmus, with the fast beating component generated by the cortex going opposite the stimulated ear, and the slow component generated by the brain stem headed toward the stimulated ear. With cerebral dysfunction, only the slow deviation toward the cold stimulus remains. With a low brain stem lesion affecting the pontine gaze center, there is neither slow nor fast beats of nystagmus. Further evaluation should include ECG and the standard labs listed previously.

What information helps determine likely outcome in a comatose patient?

Use prognostic information to counsel families. Good prognosis is associated with drug intoxication (90% survival), intact pupillary and oculomotor reflexes, and rapid initial clinical improvement. Poor prognosis is associated with loss of pupillary, corneal, and oculovestibular reflexes for greater than six hours after onset of insult (95% mortality), unwitnessed cardiac arrest, prolonged resuscitation, nontraumatic coma with failure to improve after four days, and traumatic coma in the elderly. Mortality in a comatose patient is 75% with subarachnoid hemorrhage, 50% with head injury, and 40%–50% from cardiac arrest, tumor, infection, or metabolic insult. Permanent, severe impairment occurs in 15%–25% of coma survivors.

▶ TREATMENT

How do I treat a patient with altered mental status?

For patients with severe mental status alterations, often you must make therapeutic interventions urgently even before diagnostic work-up is complete. The first priorities are airway, breathing, and cardiac function (ABCs). Intubate if necessary to protect the airway. For severe alterations in mental status, begin rapid empiric treatment with naloxone to reverse potential respiratory depression from opiates, then sequentially give thiamine and glucose to reverse Wernicke's encephalopathy and hypoglycemia, respectively. Do not give glucose before thiamine in a chronic alcohol user, as this can precipitate Wernicke's encephalopathy. After these urgent interventions, treat the underlying cause. If meningitis is suspected, give immediate IV antibiotics even before the LP is completed, to optimize outcome.

K E Y P O I N T S

▶ Patients with coma need rapid, prioritized evaluation and management.

▶ Altered mental status with fever suggests meningitis, unless pneumonia or UTI is obvious.

▶ Delirium is an acute alteration in mental status that may fluctuate and is usually caused by a reversible metabolic or toxic abnormality.

STROKE

▶ ETIOLOGY

How important is stroke as a disease?

The age-dependent incidence of stroke is 1–2/1000 population per year. In mortality rates, stroke ranks third after heart disease and cancer. In disability rates, stroke ranks first.

What causes ischemic stroke?

Stroke can be either ischemic or hemorrhagic. *Ischemic stroke* is a disruption of blood flow, food (glucose), or oxygen to the brain resulting in cerebral dysfunction. Transient ischemic attack (TIA) is a variant of stroke in which the neurological deficit lasts less than twenty-four hours and on imaging there is no infarct. Ischemic strokes can be caused by emboli, thrombosis, hypoperfusion, or a myriad of other rarer causes (vasculitis, hypoxia, others). *Emboli* can originate from arteries or veins, often in the setting of a hypercoagulable state. *Thrombosis* can occur in vessels of different sizes. Closure of larger vessels usually is due to rupture of atherosclerotic plaque, although trauma, radiation, arterial dissection, fibromuscular dysplasia, inflammation, and other etiologies can play a role.

Lacunes are deep, small vessel strokes that likely result from closure of deep penetrating arteries. This closure is precipitated by local thrombosis superimposed on lipohyalinosis, a progressive thickening of the vessel wall that occurs over years. Lacunes are also caused by emboli, carotid disease, and other etiologies up to 25% of the time. The biggest risk factors for lacunar disease are hypertension, diabetes mellitus, and smoking. Hypoperfusion leads to damage primarily in vascular border zones, which is the region where two different blood vessels cross/anastomose, and where perfusion pressure is the lowest. *Hypoperfusion* can occur in the anterior or posterior circulation, between the anterior and middle, or posterior and middle cerebral artery circulations. Stroke can occur more slowly in this situation. Carotid atherosclerosis deserves special mention because it can lead to stroke by any of the three mechanisms described (thrombosis, emboli, hypoperfusion) and effective prevention of recurrence is possible by carotid endarterectomy.

What causes hemorrhagic stroke?

Hemorrhagic stroke is caused by a disruption of blood vessel integrity and is classified as either subarachnoid or intracranial depending on the location of bleeding. Hemorrhagic stroke should be distinguished from hemorrhagic conversion, which refers to bleeding into an area of ischemic stroke. In approximately 30% of patients with stroke, no etiology is found.

What other diseases can look like stroke?

Stroke must be distinguished from other diseases such as subdural or epidural hematoma, migraine, seizure, tumor, toxic/metabolic encephalopathy, infection, spinal stenosis, and peripheral neuromuscular disease.

What are the risk factors for stroke?

The most important risk factor is age. The most modifiable risk factor is hypertension. Other common and important risk factors are atrial fibrillation, smoking, diabetes, congestive heart failure, and heavy alcohol use.

▶ EVALUATION

What is the primary goal of stroke evaluation?

The primary goal is to prevent future strokes through logical treatment. Treatment means both risk factor modification and medication. The only way to accomplish this goal is to understand the mechanism or cause of the stroke. Admittedly, this can be very difficult and even stroke experts disagree about stroke mechanism and appropriate treatment when given the same information. Nonetheless, start with trying to understand the underlying mechanism, whether embolic, thrombotic, hypoperfusion hemorrhagic, or other.

How is timing of onset helpful?

Timing of onset lends important clues. Most stroke patients present with acute, maximal symptoms at onset. "Stroke in evolution" and "stuttering stroke" are less common and refer to deficits worsening or fluctuating over hours to days. Such presentations suggest a propagating arterial or venous thrombus, recurrent emboli, vasculitis, edema, enlarging hematoma, or hypoperfusion. Deficits lasting less than twenty-four hours are called transient ischemic attacks (TIAs) and are considered warning signs of potential future stroke.

How does the pattern of deficits give clues about the location of a stroke?

Patterns of deficits are helpful in predicting the type, size, and location of stroke (Table 32–5). Strokes deep in the brain or brain stem are usually lacunar or hemorrhagic and, although they involve small areas of brain, they cause very significant deficits because all the nerve tracks are compact. For example, a pure motor stroke involving the left face, arm, and leg is usually due to a small vessel stroke in the right internal capsule or right basis pontis. Strokes that occur in a more cortical location are usually embolic or thrombotic and, although they involve larger vessels and larger areas of brain, they may cause more focal deficits. For example, occlusion of a branch of the right MCA (middle cerebral artery) may cause weakness only in the left hand. Strokes of other branches of the MCA can affect different functions depending on which hemisphere is involved. Most people are left-brain dominant, which means that language and handedness are controlled by the left brain, and visual-spatial processing is controlled by the right brain. Thus, a left MCA branch stroke can affect language, either as an expressive or a receptive aphasia. A right brain MCA branch stroke may affect visual or spatial functions, causing neglect of a limb or difficulty recognizing objects by feel. Dysarthria, in contrast to aphasias, is a motor deficit in speech, which can occur with either

TABLE 32–5

Classic Patterns of Stroke Deficits

Deficit	Brain Distribution Involved
Strength	
Ipsilateral face, arm, leg weakness	Deep lacune in internal capsule or basis pontis
Focal hand/arm weakness	Cortical stroke, contralateral MCA branch
Speech	
Expressive aphasia	Cortical stroke, left brain Broca's area
Receptive aphasia	Cortical stroke, left brain Wernicke's area
Dysarthria	Deep motor tract, or cortical motor area stroke
Vision	
Visual field deficits	Cortical stroke, occipital lobes, or MCA and optic tract
Combined	
Weakness and sensory loss of arm and face with contralateral visual field cut	Proximal MCA stroke
Other	
Altered consciousness	Large hemispheric strokes, brainstem strokes
Vomiting, vertigo, ataxia, CN palsies	Posterior circulation stroke (vertebrobasilar artery)
Stroke mimickers	
Worst headache ever with meningismus	Subarachnoid bleed from ruptured aneurysm
Unilateral vision loss (amaurosis fugax)	Not brain, but retina from retinal artery embolism from carotid stenosis
Variable	Migraines

deep motor tract or cortical motor area stroke on either side of the brain.

How does headache play a role in patients with stroke?

"The worst headache of my life" is often a presenting symptom of subarachnoid bleeding from a ruptured berry aneurysm, usually in the circle of Willis. This subarachnoid hemorrhage may be accompanied by vomiting, meningismus (stiff neck, Kernig's and Brudzinski's signs), focal neurologic deficits, or rapid loss of consciousness. Headache may also be prominent in hemorrhage deeper within the brain. In contrast, in ischemic stroke, headache is present in only 20%, is typically mild, and is not the primary symptom. In cerebral venous thrombosis headache is a major feature.

What work-up should be accomplished in the emergency room?

As with any medical problem, the history and physical are most important. The history should focus on time of onset, symptoms, course, risk factors, medications, and past medical problems. Rapidly review head CT results and consult a neurologist regarding the clinical criteria for thrombolysis, as tPA may be of benefit in some stroke patients if used within three hours of symptom onset. Assess vital signs. Most patients will be hypertensive to some degree even if that is not a baseline issue. Perform a thorough but rapid neurologic examination including mental status, language, visual fields, cranial nerves, strength, sensory function, reflexes, cerebellar function, gait, and cardiac function. Listen for carotid bruits and cardiac abnormalities. Order ECG, head CT, and labs (Table 32–6). Controversy exists regarding which patients to admit to expedite further work-up. Strongly consider admitting any person with stroke, including TIA, if the onset was within the last forty-eight hours. If stroke onset was more than forty-eight hours ago, admission will depend on the ED work-up, suspected or known cause, deficits, and social support.

What secondary work-up should be considered?

After an initial evaluation in the ED, try to categorize the stroke and then limit the secondary work-up appropriately, usually with the assistance of a neurologist. One of the most useful studies is a diffusion-weighted MRI because it can distinguish new from old stroke and help predict a cause. Carotid duplex is important because carotid disease can be involved in many stroke categories, and there is treatment available for high-grade stenosis. Consider a check for antiphospholipid antibodies including PTT, lupus anticoagulant, cardiolipin antibodies, and anti-beta 2 glycoprotein. Other tests used are cardiac echo, transcranial doppler, Holter monitor, angiography, rheumatologic labs (ESR, ANA, ANCA), syphilis serologies, and lumbar puncture, especially to rule out SAH.

TABLE 32-6

Common Studies in Acute Stroke

Study	Potential Findings
ECG	Atrial fibrillation, myocardial ischemia, or infarction
Noncontrast head CT	Ischemia or hemorrhage, deep vs. cortical distribution May be normal in first 6–24 hours
Labs	
Lytes, glucose, mag	Metabolic cause
CBC	Infection
CBC, platelets	Hyperviscosity Bleeding problem (PT/PTT if tPA or heparin are being considered)

▶ TREATMENT

How do I treat stroke in the acute setting?

The most immediate decision concerns tPA. The major drawback of using tPA is the 10-fold greater risk of intracerebral hemorrhage (6.4% with tPA, compared with 0.6% in those treated more traditionally). A second drawback to tPA application is that patients often don't meet the within-three-hours-of-onset criteria. Other acute stroke management principles are listed (Box 32–3). Do not lower arterial pressure too aggressively. Higher blood pressures are required to perfuse brain tissues near areas of injury in the days following a stroke. Gently lower systolic pressures above 210 with labetalol. Do not use diuretics as these will lower intravascular volume. Use isotonic maintenance fluids such as normal saline to avoid dehydration. Keep glucose below 150 mg/dL (using an insulin drip, if necessary), magnesium above 2.0 mg/dL, and temperature normal (with Tylenol) for the first forty-eight hours because abnormalities in any of these areas worsen outcome.

Monitor for and treat complications such as pneumonia, urinary tract infection, and DVT. Heparin is only indicated in specific situations (consult a neurologist). Its use is debated because it carries a higher risk of hemorrhagic conversion, especially in strokes involving large distributions. Heparin should not be given as a bolus in neurology patients and the PTT goal is 50–80, lower than for other medical problems. Start aspirin early if not beginning thrombolysis or anticoagulation. For all stroke patients, perform frequent vital signs and neurologic exams in the first hours to days to monitor for extension or complications of the initial stroke.

How can I prevent stroke?

Primary prevention (i.e., avoiding the patient's first stroke) is addressed through treatment of risk factors such as hypertension, diabetes, and hyperlipidemia. Where indicated, e.g., known hyper-

---

BOX 32–3

General Principles in the Treatment of Acute Stroke

Avoid hypotension.
Treat hypertension with labetalol only if BP greater than 210/120.
Keep SaO_2 greater than 92%.
Maintain glucose control less than 150 mg/dL with insulin drip.
Treat fever with Tylenol.
Correct volume depletion with normal saline.
Keep Mg^{2+} greater than 2.0 mg/dL.
Prevent DVT.
Prevent aspiration if at risk (NPO).

coagulable state, begin antiplatelet therapy or anticoagulation. Once a patient has had a stroke, begin secondary prevention. Stroke risk in these patients is at least 5% per year. If possible, identify the cause of the stroke and treat appropriately (Table 32–7). In patients for whom a cause is not identified, it is reasonable to start a daily aspirin regimen. Aspirin is generally the antiplatelet therapy of first choice due to its ease of administration, low cost, low risk, and universal access, despite evidence that the other three available antiplatelet drugs are a little better. The optimal dose (range 81–1300 mg) remains controversial, but lower doses are generally prescribed. When stroke recurs on aspirin (an "aspirin failure"), alternate antiplatelet therapy includes clopidogrel (Plavix) in combination with aspirin or Aggrenox. Ticlopidine (Ticlid) is a third choice. Coumadin is indicated for stroke despite antiplatelet therapy, and for atrial fibrillation, where stroke risk is reduced by 64% over placebo in certain groups. Keep in mind the bleeding risks. Although not covered in this chapter, rehabilitation is a very important component in the treatment of stroke.

When is surgery indicated?

Refer patients with vascular malformations to a surgeon. An important finding is carotid stenosis of greater than or equal to 70% *in combination with* symptoms referable to that artery's vascular distribution. In two-year follow-up, such patients managed medically have a 26% risk of stroke, whereas those managed surgically have a 9% risk of stroke. Hospitals and surgeons have varying

TABLE 32–7

Secondary Prevention of Stroke

Etiology	Treatment
Embolic stroke	
Atrial fibrillation	Anticoagulation
CHF	Anticoagulation
Septic embolus	Antibiotics
Antiphospholipid Ab syndrome	Anticoagulation (INR 3-4)
Carotid stenosis	
<70%	Antiplatelet
>70% and symptomatic	Endarterectomy
Thrombotic stroke	
Large vessel stroke	Antiplatelet or anticoagulation
Small vessel lacunar stroke	Antiplatelet
Hemorrhagic stroke	
Amyloid angiopathy	BP control, avoid aspirin and coumadin
Hypertension	BP control long term

complication rates, and this fact may significantly alter the risk/benefit profile. In asymptomatic patients with carotid stenosis, benefit is less clear. Another situation in which surgical intervention has a potential role is in the evacuation of intraparenchymal blood in severe hemorrhage. If the volume of blood is greater than 60 mL and the patient is comatose, however, surgical evacuation is unlikely to change the outcome of death or disability.

K E Y   P O I N T S

▶ **Hypertension is the most modifiable risk factor for stroke.**

▶ **Categorizing stroke can help limit the work-up and lead to appropriate treatment.**

▶ **Aspirin therapy is often the correct choice for secondary stroke prevention.**

▶ **Do not aggressively lower blood pressure in patients presenting with stroke.**

SEIZURE

What causes seizure?

Seizures are paroxysmal, transient electrical discharges of groups of neurons within the brain. Approximately 10% of the population will experience one or a few provoked seizures within their lifetimes, often related to a structural or metabolic derangement such as CNS infection, childhood fever, hypoglycemia, electrolyte disturbance, CNS hypoperfusion, alcohol or benzodiazepine withdrawal, illicit drug use, medication overdose or side effect, or closed head injury.

Epilepsy is defined as recurrent seizures without an easily reversible cause. Epilepsy affects approximately 1% of the population. Epilepsy may have a genetic or idiopathic etiology or may be caused by stroke, tumor, trauma, or degenerative diseases. Patients can present with epilepsy at any age.

What types of seizures are there?

Seizures are broadly classified as primarily generalized or partial as determined by a history and EEG. *Primarily generalized seizures* result from a synchronized discharge of the whole brain at the same time. Onset is almost invariably before the age of 18 and current wisdom is that they often have a genetic basis. Seizure types include tonic-clonic, absence, myotonic, and atonic. The classic tonic-clonic seizure begins with a stiff phase of tonic muscle contraction lasting several seconds, followed by generalized rhythmic jerking movements, clonus, during which consciousness is lost. Incontinence of bowel or bladder, or tongue trauma may occur, although these are nonspecific features of loss of consciousness from any cause. With absence seizures, patients stare blankly without loss of posture or shaking. With atonic seizures, also known as drop attacks, patients abruptly lose postural tone. A prolonged postictal period of extreme sleepiness and confusion is typical for tonic-clonic seizures. In contrast, there is no postictal state after absence or atonic seizures and patients are able to return to normal function immediately.

Partial seizures result from a focal cortical discharge. The spread of this focal discharge and the area of brain involved predict the symptoms and signs associated with the seizure. If full consciousness is maintained, the seizure is referred to as simple partial. An abnormal sense of smell is a classic example of a simple partial seizure when the temporal smell centers are involved. If consciousness is reduced, the seizure is referred to as complex partial and reflects a larger area of brain involvement. When partial seizures secondarily generalize, the result is a tonic-clonic seizure, which can be indistinguishable from a primarily generalized tonic-clonic seizure. Patients with partial complex seizures often present with staring episodes, which can be confused with absence seizures. Distinguishing primarily generalized from partial seizures is very important because many treatments are specific for one and not for the other.

What else can look like a seizure?

The differential diagnosis for seizure includes migraine, sleep disorders, syncope, stroke, movement disorders, and psychological causes.

▶ EVALUATION

What work-up is warranted in patients presenting with their first seizure?

Individualize your work-up, with a focus on looking for a treatable cause. As usual, the H & P are most important, both to rule-in a seizure and to rule-out disorders that mimic epilepsy. Determine the exact sequence of events, especially whether the first movements were generalized or focal. Both seizure and syncope can be associated with loss of consciousness, but seizure and not syncope will have a postictal period longer than a few minutes. Ask about possible precipitants such as alcohol or benzodiazepine withdrawal, drug overdose, or cocaine use. Look for signs of trauma, tongue laceration, or incontinence. Note vital signs. Order labs and tests only to investigate your clinical suspicions (Table 32–8). Hospitalize the patient if there is an underlying illness, slow recovery, or poor social situation or no one able to look after the patient.

When a patient with known epilepsy has a seizure, what work-up is warranted?

Obtain drug levels and compare with the patient's known therapeutic level. Correct low levels. Most new anticonvulsants do not have helpful drug levels; doses are raised until the desired effect is obtained or side effects are intolerable. The history dictates if other work-up is needed, but this is generally not the case.

▶ TREATMENT

What is a rational approach to treating seizures?

Designing rational seizure therapy requires that you address three questions: 1) Are the seizures provoked and reversible? 2) If this

TABLE 32–8

First Seizure Evaluation

Test	Looking for
Labs	
CBC	Infection
Glucose	Hypoglycemia
Electrolytes, calcium, magnesium	Abnormal levels
Toxicology screen	Intoxication
Imaging	
Urgent: CT with and without contrast	Bleeding, trauma, tumor, stroke, signs of infection
Nonurgent: MRI	Better for all of the above, plus vascular malformations
Lumbar puncture*	Cancer
	Infection
	Rare: Beçhet's syndrome, CNS sarcoidosis
	Limitation: postictal CSF pleocytosis <80 may occur for days
EEG*	Seizure confirmation and classification
	Information to guide drug therapy and prognosis
	Limitations: sensitivity of 50%-70%, 2% have a false-positive (sensitivity increased by sleep EEG or repeating EEG; 24-hour CCTV-EEG monitoring may be helpful)

*Not always required.

is the first seizure, what are the chances more will occur? 3) If more seizures are likely, is there a rational therapy? A single tonic-clonic seizure provoked by an identifiable reversible cause should be managed with correction of the underlying problem and does not warrant anticonvulsant medication. Seizures likely to recur owing to slow resolution of the underlying derangement warrant phenytoin, which can be given initially as an intravenous loading dose of 18 mg/kg. Side effects include hypotension with rapid loading, rash, and rare but potentially life-threatening leukopenia or hepatitis. Continuous seizing, status epilepticus, requires a more rapid-acting drug such as diazepam in 5 mg intravenous boluses.

Predicting a second seizure must take multiple factors into account. If no cause is found and the EEG is normal, the risk of a second seizure in the next two years is about 25%. If there is an identifiable cause or the EEG is positive, the risk is 50%–80%. When the decision is made to use medication, issues to consider include type of seizure, ease of use, side effects, drug monitoring, drug interactions, and cost. Multiple medications are available for the different classes of seizures (Table 32–9). Except for ethosuximide, most of the drugs in the three lists are somewhat interchangeable. For instance, although valproic acid is the best drug for many generalized seizure disorders, it does have efficacy in partial seizures. Likewise, phenytoin is an excellent drug for partial seizures and can be used for generalized onset tonic-clonic seizures, although not for myoclonic or absence seizures. Surgical options are occasionally warranted but are beyond the scope of this chapter.

K E Y   P O I N T S

▶ Obtain a history and EEG to classify a seizure as partial or primarily generalized.

▶ First time seizures require evaluation for cause.

MOTOR WEAKNESS

See Table 32–10 for the presentation and diagnosis of some diseases causing motor weakness.

TABLE 32–9

Treatment of Seizures

	First Line Therapy	Second Line Therapy
Partial seizures		
Simple complex	Phenytoin, carbamazepine	Lamotrigine
Tonic-clonic, secondary	Phenytoin, carbamazepine	Lamotrigine
Primarily generalized seizures		
Tonic-clonic, primary	Valproic acid, lamotrigine	Phenytoin, topiramate
Myoclonic	Valproic acid	Lamotrigine, benzodiazepines
Atonic	Valproic acid	
Absence	Ethosuximide	Valproic acid

TABLE 32–10

Motor Deficit Syndromes

Syndrome	Presentation	Diagnosis
Amyotrophic lateral sclerosis (ALS)	Mixed upper and lower motor neuron deficits cause progressive weakness, twitching, wasting, and muscle cramps; may involve tongue, palate, gag reflex; spares extraocular muscles, death after 3–5 years	Clinical picture Electrodiagnostic testing
Botulism	Fulminating weakness 12–72 hours after ingestion of contaminated food (usually home-canned food); begins with diplopia, ptosis, facial weakness, dysphagia; progresses to respiratory difficulty; no sensory deficits	Test food and stool for *Clostridium botulinum* Repetitive nerve stimulation increases motor response
Multiple sclerosis	Focal episodes of weakness, numbness, unsteadiness, visual change hyperreflexia; episodes relapse and remit over days to months, or may be progressive with persistent deficits	MRI shows focal, scattered demyelinating plaques in the brain, spinal cord, and optic nerves. CSF for oligoclonal bands. Prolonged evoked potential latencies.
Guillain-Barré Syndrome	Symmetric ascending weakness beginning in legs and progressing upward at varying rates; usually accompanied by sensory complaints, autonomic disturbances, and respiratory muscle involvement	CSF shows increased protein, normal cell count Electrodiagnostic testing shows conduction slowing of sensory and motor nerves

Table 32–10. Motor Deficit Syndromes *continued*

Syndrome	Presentation	Diagnosis
Myasthenia gravis	Weakness that occurs with activity and abates with rest. Diplopia and ptosis are almost invariable. Sensory is normal.	Repetitive nerve stimulation decreases motor response Acetylcholine receptor antibodies
Poliomyelitis	Prodromal flulike illness followed by focal, asymmetric, rapid onset weakness, aseptic meningitis, myalgias	RNA virus can be isolated from nasal cultures, stool, CSF

CASE 32–1. A 75-year-old woman is sent to the ED by her nursing home for worsening confusion over the last week. She is unable to give a history. On exam, she is only oriented to her name and falls asleep several times during the interview and exam. Her mucus membranes are dry and vital signs show orthostatic changes with a sitting pulse of 110, BP of 95/60, T of 36°C. Neurologic exam shows intact reactive pupils at 2 mm, cranial nerves appear intact, although she cannot comply with testing. She is moving all four extremities symmetrically, but appears to be weak. She has difficulty standing for measurement of orthostatic vital signs.

A. Is this delirium or dementia and why do you think so?
B. What could be causing her altered mental status?
C. What evaluation do you wish to pursue (see answer for results)?
D. From results of tests, what is causing altered mental status?
E. What further tests and treatment does she need?

CASE 32–2. A 27-year-old man is brought to the ED after seizing. His girlfriend reports he cried out, went stiff, and then began shaking all over for about a minute or two. As far as she knows, he has never done this before. On exam he is dazed, drooling, and breathing heavily. HR 120, BP 150/100, RR 24. Fundi show no papilledema and reflexes are brisk but symmetric. No focal deficits are apparent, although he is not awake enough to actively participate in the neurologic exam.

Continued

CASE 32–2. *Continued*

A. What is the differential diagnosis for his presentation?
B. What more do you want to ask his girlfriend?
C. What other tests are warranted?
D. What treatment do you want to give him?

33

Psychiatry

DEPRESSION

▶ ETIOLOGY

How common is depression?

Of all causes of death and disability worldwide, depression ranks fourth. Lifetime risk for major depression is 7%–12% in men and 20%–25% in women. Only one third to one half of patients with major depression are properly recognized by primary care providers. Further, in one study, 30% of patients presenting with a physical symptom had either depression or anxiety.

Do medications or other substances cause depression?

Many medications have been associated with depression, but a clear causal relationship is rare. Medications that are causal should be stopped when treating depression (Box 33–1). Alcoholism is no more frequent in depressed patients than in the general population; however, patients with alcoholism have much higher rates of depression, as high as 30% at time of presentation. This suggests that

---

BOX 33–1

Medications That Are Associated with Depression

Causal
Centrally acting antihypertensives: reserpine, methyldopa clonidine
CNS depressants: alcohol, sedatives, opiates, and psychedelics
Corticosteroids

Possibly causal
Propranolol
Oral contraceptives, progesterone
L-Dopa

---

alcoholism is not the result of a patient's attempt to medicate depression with alcohol, but rather the ongoing alcohol abuse results in depression.

What is the interaction of grief and depression?

Acute grief, such as over the death of a spouse, has similar symptoms to depression: sorrow, tearfulness, depressed mood, lack of interest, trouble sleeping. Patients with normal grief usually maintain self-esteem and their grief reaction resolves within several months, whereas those with grief-related depression may have feelings of worthlessness and their symptoms can persist for prolonged periods if untreated. In the year after a loss, 15%–35% of grievers will develop depression, with resolution in 94%. Of interest, when grief-related depression is treated with an SSRI, the symptoms of depression resolve whereas the intensity of the grief does not. This may reassure patients who do not wish to "medicate" their loss.

What are some subtypes of depression?

Major depressive disorder is a serious illness with presence of multiple severe symptoms (see later). A subtype, depression with atypical features, includes symptoms of hypersomnia, overeating, lethargy, and rejection sensitivity. One example of this subtype is seasonal affective disorder, which occurs during the short days of winter in far northern and southern hemisphere climates. Another subtype is postpartum depression, occurring two weeks to six months after delivery. Adjustment disorder with depressed mood occurs in reaction to some identifiable stressor or loss and is usually accompanied by anger and guilt. Dysthymia is a chronic, persistent depressed mood lasting two years or more, with fewer and milder symptoms than major depression.

What medical conditions are associated with depression?

Hypothyroidism, Cushing's syndrome, and vitamin B_{12} deficiency are clearly associated with depression. Treatment of these conditions results in improvement or resolution of depression. Many chronic medical conditions are associated with increased rate of depression, although no causative role has been established (Box 33–2).

▶ EVALUATION

What are the criteria for diagnosis of depression?

Depression is common but frequently missed. To make the diagnosis of depression, either depressed mood or loss of interest

BOX 33–2

Medical Conditions and Their Associated Risk of Depression

Stroke	50%
Diabetes with end organ damage	50%
Myocardial infarction	40%–65%
Cancer	Varies with type and severity
Pancreatic disorders	50%
Acute leukemia awaiting transplant	Less than 2%

must be present. Be certain to include one of these as a question in your review of symptoms. In addition, five of the listed criteria should be present for two weeks or more (Box 33–3). In the elderly, irritability, agitation, diminished cognitive function, and sleep disruption are more likely than frank depressed mood. This is also true in adolescents, where irritability may be the predominant mood state. Ask about suicidality as well as symptoms suggesting a history of mania or psychosis.

How can I ask my patients about depression without making them defensive?

It is helpful to question patients about the more physiologic symptoms of depression, such as sleep, food intake, and energy. For example, "How are you sleeping?" investigates the classic pattern of early morning awakening. You can then define depression as a physiologic state that causes the physical symptoms the patient is experiencing before entering into discussion of mood. This helps patients understand depression as a physiologic condition, rather than something that is "all in their head."

BOX 33–3

Criteria for Major Depression

Five out of nine required for over two weeks for a diagnosis of major depression
Depressed mood
Anhedonia (loss of interest in most, if not all, activities)
Weight loss or gain (5% of body weight in one month) or appetite loss/gain
Insomnia or hypersomnia
Psychomotor agitation/retardation
Fatigue or loss of energy nearly every day
Feelings of worthlessness or inappropriate guilt
Trouble concentrating, indecision
Recurrent thoughts of death or suicide

When should I be concerned about bipolar disorder?

Screen any patient with depressive symptoms for bipolar disorder by asking about any prior or current episodes of symptoms suggesting mania: hyperactivity, irritability, flight of ideas, hypersexual behavior, impulsivity, spending large amounts of money, sleeplessness, or grandiosity. It is important to rule out bipolar disorder before treating patients for depression because antidepressants may trigger an acute manic episode. Refer patients with a personal history suggesting manic episodes to a psychiatrist to confirm a diagnosis and start treatment.

Should I get any lab tests on patients with depression?

Because of the potentially causative role, it is reasonable to check TSH and to consider a metabolic panel including glucose. For patients with elevated glucose, elevated bicarbonate, and cushingoid body habitus, also consider twenty-four-hour urine cortisol testing to look for Cushing's syndrome.

If I ask about suicidal thoughts, will this make my patient more likely to try suicide?

There is no evidence that asking patients about suicidality makes them more likely to commit suicide. Although these thoughts are not uncommon in depression, ask about specific plans and access to means (e.g., guns). If a patient is suicidal with a plan, contact a social worker or psychiatrist right away so they can assist in admitting the patient for acute inpatient care.

▶ TREATMENT

Why is depression important to treat?

In addition to the death and disability from depression itself, evidence is mounting that depression has a significant impact on other medical conditions. In one study of patients with myocardial infarction, concurrent depression was an independent risk factor for mortality equivalent to left ventricular dysfunction. Whether this is due to decreased compliance with medications or other factors is not known. Further, although depression may spontaneously remit, untreated depression may also wax and wane, resulting in dysthymia and depression that is more resistant to therapy.

What are treatment options other than traditional allopathic medications?

Evidence exists that psychotherapy and medications achieve approximately equivalent response rates of 50%–70%. There appears to be a synergistic effect with psychotherapy and medications. Some data suggest that relapse rates are decreased when a patient receives cognitive therapy. Aerobic exercise, half an hour three to five times a week, has been effective in several studies, although increased social activity may have confounded the results. St. John's wort may be effective for mild depression but is clearly not effective for major depression based on a randomized controlled trial. SAMe (S-adeno-syl-L-methionine) has limited data and so is controversial.

Can I prescribe medications for depression without a psychiatrist's help?

Internists can and should treat uncomplicated cases of depression. In more severe cases with suicidality, poor response to medicine, or complicating psychiatric conditions such as personality disorder, mania, or delusions, refer the patient to a psychiatrist.

What medication should I use?

The most common medications currently used to treat depression are the serotonin reuptake inhibitors (SSRIs). A study of SSRIs (sertraline, fluoxetine, and paroxetine) in nearly 600 depressed patients in the general medicine outpatient setting showed two thirds of patients recovered by nine months. If the patient did not respond to the first SSRI tried, there was a high likelihood of success with switching to a second agent. All three medications had similar rates of side effects. Tricyclic antidepressant medications are equally effective for depression. Their side effects include sedation, dry mouth, constipation, and orthostatic hypotension as well as potential for cardiac arrhythmia. SSRIs are relatively safe in overdose, in contrast to the tricyclic antidepressants. Sexual side effects including difficulty with orgasm are fairly common in patients on SSRIs.

How shall I counsel my patient about starting medications?

Counsel patients at the outset that side effects will often precede symptom improvement. Ask patients to commit to a four-week medication trial. Compliance is improved if you have the patient return for a visit in one to two weeks. Counsel patients that if the first medication is not effective by two to four weeks, or isn't tolerated, there are many other options for treatment.

How long will medications be required?

First-episode depression should be treated for six to nine months or until symptoms have completely resolved, whichever is longer. When stopping an antidepressant, taper the dose to the lowest possible dosage before cessation. Tapering the medication is important for paroxetine in particular; abrupt cessation may result in a self-limited but unpleasant withdrawal syndrome of dysequilibrium. If depression recurs shortly after cessation, longer-term therapy is necessary. With a third recurrence of depression, lifelong medication is recommended.

When should I combine medications?

For marked sleep disturbance, add a low dose of a sedating antidepressant at bedtime, such as 10–25 mg of doxepin or 50 mg of nefazodone. Use caution with benzodiazepines for insomnia, even briefly, because of their addictive potential. Do not try to combine high dose antidepressants. Monoamine oxidase inhibitors with SSRIs can be lethal (see serotonin syndrome later). Refer the patient to a psychiatrist for refractory depression.

When should I should start an antidepressant other than an SSRI?

In patients with chronic pain, start with a tricyclic antidepressant. This class of medication is slightly more effective for neuropathic pain than the serotonin reuptake inhibitors. SSRIs will treat the depression that often accompanies chronic pain, but are less effective than TCAs for the pain itself. If there is a history of significant sexual dysfunction, consider selecting another class of drug rather than an SSRI, such as bupropion or nefazodone. Note that depression itself often manifests with decreased libido. For smokers interested in cessation, data support bupropion as an aid.

When should I prescribe benzodiazepines for my anxious patients?

Generalized anxiety disorder is a relatively uncommon condition. By contrast, depression manifesting as anxiety is quite common. A patient who seems anxious or overly concerned about his or her medical condition needs an evaluation for anxiety and/or depression. Benzodiazepines can be used to treat a patient's insomnia and agitation for the short term until the antidepressant begins to take effect. Because of the addiction risk with benzodiazepines, this approach should be taken cautiously.

What is my depressed patient's prognosis?

Most depression resolves at one year without any intervention. Antidepressants or psychotherapy shortens this interval to one to two months. Fifty percent of patients are cured with first-time therapy and depression never recurs. In 50% of patients, depression does return when medications are stopped. Of those patients whose depression recurs, another 50% will never have another episode. Ten percent of patients with depression will suffer from chronic symptoms.

What will happen if my patient stops medication abruptly?

With some antidepressants, there will be a withdrawal syndrome. This is most profound in the shorter-acting SSRIs such as paroxetine. In this medication, withdrawal can precipitate sudden episodes of disequilibrium and imbalance. This resolves within a week or so of discontinuation of the medication.

What is the serotonin syndrome?

This syndrome occurs when serotonin-producing or -sparing medications are combined. Although there have been case reports of numerous medications, the most common culprits are SSRIs with MAO inhibitors or high dose TCAs. Of note, cocaine, reserpine, and nefazodone are also implicated. Patients experience agitation, mental status changes, diarrhea, and autonomic changes such as hypertension and fever.

K E Y   P O I N T S

▶ Depression is common and responds to medications, counseling, and exercise.

▶ Most patients can be managed in the primary care setting.

▶ Suicidality, symptoms of mania, and poor response to therapy require referral to psychiatry.

CASE 33–1. A 78-year-old woman with diabetes and hypertension is brought to clinic by her son who is concerned about her memory and her lack of interest in her life. She is agitated with him and vehemently denies she is depressed and states that she is just "tired." Her MMSE score is 27/30 and her neurological exam is grossly normal.

  A. What is your differential diagnosis?
  B. What further questions do you want to ask?
  C. What further testing will you order?
  D. If her laboratories and exam are normal, what medication might you recommend?

CASE 33–2. A 24-year-old man comes in to clinic after breaking up with his girlfriend. He reports several weeks of sleeplessness, agitation, poor appetite, and trouble concentrating on his graduate studies. He feels he is depressed and in fact, his father has been depressed. When questioned, he acknowledges feeling suicidal once, a few weeks ago. He adamantly refuses any medication.

A. Does he meet criteria for depression?
B. What further questions do you want to ask to assess his suicide risk?
C. What questions can you ask him about his concern about medications?
D. What options can you provide him for treatment for his depression?

REFERENCES

Depression Guideline Panel. Depression in primary care: Treatment of major depression: Clinical practice guideline. US Department of Health and Human Services, Public Health Service, Agency for Health Care Policy and Research. AHCPR publication 93–0551, Rockville, MD, 1993.

Kroenke K, West SL, Swindle R, et al: Similar effectiveness of paroxetine, fluoxetine, and sertraline in primary care: A randomized trial. JAMA 286(23):2947, 2001.

Snow V, Lascher S, Mottur-Pilson C: Pharmacologic treatment of acute depression and dysthymia. Ann Intern Med 132:738, 2000.

34

Pulmonary

ASTHMA

▶ ETIOLOGY

What is asthma?

Asthma is defined as a chronic inflammatory disorder of the airways that leads to reversible bronchoconstriction, the hallmark of asthma, as well as airway hyperresponsiveness, airflow limitations, respiratory symptoms, and disease chronicity. In the early stages, reversible bronchoconstriction is the rule. If left untreated, however, chronic remodeling occurs and leads to irreversible airway narrowing. Most asthmatics fluctuate between good days with minimal symptoms and bad days with aggravation of symptoms. Hospitalization is often necessary for acute exacerbations because patients can unpredictably and rapidly progress to respiratory failure and death. Currently between 14 and 15 million people in the U.S. suffer from asthma; 5 million of these are children. The highest asthma mortality rates are among African Americans aged 15 to 24 years.

What are the common forms of asthma?

Asthma subtypes have important implications for treatment (Table 34–1). Any given person may have more than one form. Aspirin-induced asthma often occurs as a triad of nasal polyps, chronic rhinitis, and wheezing (Samter's syndrome) and results from an increase in leukotriene activity. Occupational asthma can be due to low-level intermittent exposure to precipitants at work, such as plastic resin and wood. Often symptoms resolve when the worker is removed from the location. In some patients, the exposure causes a more generalized and protracted airway hyperresponsiveness that persists despite precipitant removal. Exercise-induced asthma precipitates bronchoconstriction by cooling and drying of the airways and is usually worst five to ten minutes after exercise ceases.

TABLE 34–1

Precipitants and Special Interventions for Different Types of Asthma

Asthma subtype	Precipitant	Special Interventions Beyond Usual Asthma Therapies
Allergen-induced asthma*	Animal dander, cockroaches, dust mites, molds, pollen	Allergen avoidance Immunotherapy
Aspirin-intolerant asthma	Aspirin and NSAIDs	Avoid aspirin and NSAIDs
Cold-air intolerant asthma	Cold air	Pre-exposure bronchodilator
Exercise-induced asthma	Exertion	Pre-exercise bronchodilator
GERD-induced asthma	Gastroesophageal reflux	Antacids, GERD prevention measures (see Dyspepsia section)
Occupational asthma	Occupational irritant	Respirator at work, or reassignment
Stress-induced asthma	Stressful situations	Pre-exposure bronchodilator
URI-related wheezing	Viral respiratory infection	Bronchodilator for URI

*Formerly termed "extrinsic" asthma and associated with elevations in serum IgE; now characterized by asthma induction by a wide range of allergens without elevations in serum IgE or serum eosinophils.

What other diseases can cause reversible bronchoconstriction?

Nonasthmatics may present with transient wheezing for six to eight weeks after a viral upper respiratory infection. Lung diseases such as chronic bronchitis and emphysema may have a significant component of bronchospasm, which responds to the same treatment as classic asthma. Congestive heart failure can cause cardiogenic wheezing ("cardiac asthma"), which reverses with treatment of the pulmonary edema. Less common causes of bronchospasm include endobronchial neoplasms, cystic fibrosis, upper airway obstruction, allergic bronchopulmonary aspergillosis (ABPA), and pulmonary lymphangitic spread of some tumors, such as breast cancer.

What is cough-variant asthma?

In this form, bronchospasm causes coughing more than wheezing or chest tightness, even with severe exacerbations. Precipitants, classification of severity, and treatment are the same.

Why is asthma classified by severity?

To guide therapy, the National Asthma Education Project Program suggests categorizing asthma severity as mild-intermittent, mild-persistent, moderate-persistent, or severe-persistent (Table 34–2). Although these categories describe the chronic condition, even patients with mild-intermittent disease can have exacerbations severe enough to warrant hospitalization.

TABLE 34-2

NAEPP* Classification of Asthma

Classification	Symptoms	Nighttime Symptoms	Lung Function
Mild Intermittent	Less than 2 times per week Asymptomatic between exacerbations Exacerbations brief	Less than 2 times a month	FEV_1 > 80% predicted PEF variability < 20%
Mild Persistent	Symptoms > 2 times per week but less than daily Exacerbations may limit activity	More than 2 times a month	FEV_1 > 80% predicted PEF variability 20%-30%
Moderate Persistent	Daily symptoms Daily use of β-agonist Exacerbations limit activity Exacerbations more than two times per week, may last days	More than 1 time a week	FEV < 80% > 60% predicted PEF variability > 30%
Severe Persistent	Continual symptoms Limited physical activity Frequent exacerbations	Frequent	FEV_1 < 60% predicted PEF variability > 30%

Note: Top severity within any category determines classification. All four classifications may have severe and life-threatening exacerbations.
*National Asthma Education and Prevention Project

▶ **EVALUATION**

What are the common symptoms of asthma?

The clinical presentation of asthma varies, but common symptoms include chest tightness, wheezing, cough, and exercise intolerance. Sputum production is common with acute exacerbations, even in the absence of infection. Symptoms can wax and wane and may be difficult to distinguish from respiratory infections, congestive heart failure, and COPD exacerbations. Some patients have other symptoms of allergic disease (allergic rhinitis, atopic dermatitis, urticaria).

How do I document reversible airway constriction?

Document reversible airway constriction with office spirometry. People with asthma commonly have an obstructive pattern such that FEV_1/FVC ratio is less than 80%. Significant reversibility of airflow obstruction is defined by an increase of greater than or equal to 12% and 200 mL in FEV_1 or greater than or equal to 15% and 200 mL in FVC after inhaling a short-acting bronchodilator. Commonly, even asthmatics with an FEV_1 considered normal demonstrate significant increases in FEV_1 with albuterol.

What if a patient has a history suggestive of asthma but spirometry is normal?

This is not uncommon. For cases like this, reversible bronchoconstriction can be documented in other ways. One approach is to have patients come to see you at "their worst." Often morning bronchoconstriction is missed at afternoon office appointments. Or have patients keep a diary of peak expiratory flow rates (PEFR, also called "peak flow") and symptoms. Variability of morning and evening PEFRs can often be diagnostic findings. Methacholine challenge, in which patients are given increasing concentrations of a histamine-like substance, can show increased sensitivity to low concentrations in asthmatics, but this test is not usually necessary to make a diagnosis and risks significant bronchoconstriction.

What key questions should I ask a patient with asthma?

- **Description of symptoms:** symptoms, when they occur (day or night, season of the year, during final exams), how long they last, what triggers them, what makes them better, and where they occur (at work, at home, on the softball field); symptoms at nighttime, with exercise intolerance, cough, or symptoms suggestive of GERD. (Acid reflux can exacerbate asthma.)
- **Past asthma history:** prior ER visits, hospitalizations, intubations, childhood symptoms

- **Other allergy history:** allergic rhinitis, eczema, urticaria, previous skin testing, or allergies to aspirin or NSAIDs
- **Family medical history:** asthma or other allergy-like syndromes in parents and siblings
- **Home environment:** carpets, dust collectors (books, stuffed animals), plants, pets
- **Work environment:** chemical exposures, animal exposures, workday symptoms improved when off from work or on vacation
- **Medication use:** current and past prescriptions, over-the-counter and alternative therapies
- **Use of tobacco or inhaled street drugs** often make asthma more difficult to treat.

What are the key features of an outpatient evaluation for asthma?

Perform history as described to gauge severity of symptoms. Physical exam usually shows normal vital signs and breath sounds that range from normal to diffuse end-expiratory wheezing. The expiratory phase time may be prolonged. There may be signs of other allergic disease, such as conjunctival irritation, or atopy with eczema. Use the exam to rule-out cardiac disease or other significant lung disease. Office spirometry is essential; many patients with seemingly mild symptoms can have alarmingly compromised lung function. A WBC differential may show elevated eosinophils, although it is neither sensitive nor specific. Ask the patient to keep an asthma diary, including PEFR monitoring, to assist with diagnosis and guide treatment. Allergy skin testing may help identify specific allergens to avoid or may guide immunotherapy.

▶ TREATMENT

What are the goals of asthma therapy?

The goals of asthma therapy are to give patients more symptom-free days, better quality of life, and fewer days of missed productivity, and to prevent the chronic remodeling of the airways that permanently impairs pulmonary function. There is no cure for asthma. Even an asthmatic with excellent control of symptoms has occasional exacerbations.

What is the best therapy for chronic asthma?

Asthma requires a three-pronged approach: 1) control precipitants, 2) relieve acute bronchoconstriction, and 3) control inflammation (Table 34–3). For all but the mildest intermittent asthma, you must address all three components. Add medications one at a time and monitor for response to minimize the number required. Repeat patient education about these three components and how to use medications to help patients successfully manage their asthma. To control precipitants (see Table 34–3), refer to allergist for skin testing and subsequent recommendations for environmental modifications or immunotherapy, aggressively pursue smoking cessation, vaccinate against influenza, consider Pneumovax, and consider a trial of medications for GERD. To relieve acute bronchoconstriction (Table 34–4), use β2-agonists such as albuterol, salmeterol, and metaproterenol to relax airway smooth muscles and reduce bronchoconstriction. Salmeterol is long-acting and so is particularly useful in preventing nocturnal wheezing.

For patients intolerant of β2-agonists, inhaled anticholinergics such as atrovent can provide short-term relief. Theophylline is an oral smooth muscle relaxant that is second-line because it has a narrow therapeutic window and is much less potent. When these bronchodilators are required daily, the asthma is no longer mild-intermittent; therefore, for longer-term control, it is important to reduce inflammation (Tables 34–5 and 34–6). Corticosteroids are the mainstay of anti-inflammatory therapy. They are the only agents proved to decrease chronic airway remodeling. Inhaled steroids have fewer systemic side effects than do oral steroids and are available in a range of potencies. Mast cell stabilizers are particularly helpful in mild persistent and allergen-induced asthma and have very low toxicity; for this reason, they are considered for adjunctive therapy. There is less long-term experience with leukotriene antagonists, but studies thus far have shown some benefit in asthma of all types. A four to six week trial of either of these last two agents may be useful for patients whose symptoms are inadequately controlled with standard therapy.

TABLE 34–3

The Three Fundamental Components of Asthma Therapy

Component	Examples	When to Use
Control precipitants	Environmental modifications such as carpet removal, cockroach extermination, pet removal, polyurethanemattress covers for dust mites, or job change or reassignment GERD therapy Immunotherapy Influenza vaccine Intranasal steroids for rhinitis Smoking cessation	In all cases, as dictated by exposures, allergies and comorbidities
Relieve broncho-constriction	β_2- Agonist inhaler Anticholinergic inhalers Theophylline tablets	As needed for bronchospasm
Control inflammation	Corticosteroids: inhaled, oral, or IV Mast cell stabilizers Leukotriene antagonists	Daily for all but mild to intermittent asthma

TABLE 34–4

Long-Term Control Treatments for Asthma

Classification	Long-term Control Treatments

All forms	Patient education in
	    Self-monitoring
	    Inhaler use technique
	    Treatment action plan
	Group education if available
	Control precipitants (see Table 34–3)

Mild Intermittent	No long-term control medication needed
Mild Persistent	Inhaled steroid 200–500 μg/day *or* cromolyn *or* nedocromil
Moderate Persistent	Inhaled steroid 800–2000 μcg/day *and* Long-acting inhaled β_2-agonist
Severe Persistent	Inhaled steroid 800–2000 μg *and* Long-acting inhaled β_2-agonist *and* Oral corticosteroid therapy

Note: Daily use of short-acting bronchodilators warrants long-term control measures. In addition to those outlined below, consider leukotriene antagonist and theophylline as alternative or adjunctive treatment. These agents are second line because with the leukotriene antagonist there is less long-term experience and with theophylline, toxicity is a concern.

TABLE 34–5

Medications That Relieve Symptomatic Bronchoconstriction in Asthma

Short-acting β2-agonists	
Albuterol (Proventil, Ventolin)	2–4 puffs q4–6h prn sx or before exercise
Terbutaline (Brethine, Brethaire)	2–4 puffs q4–6h prn sx; 5 mg po tid (in adults)
Pirbuterol (Maxair)	1–2 puffs q4–6h prn-asthma sx
Metaproterenol (Alupent)	2–3 puffs q3–4h prn-asthma sx
Long-acting β2-agonists	
Salmeterol (Serevent)	2 puffs qd – bid (NEVER exceed 4 puffs/24 hr)
Methylxanthines	
Theophylline (Theodur and others)	100–400 mg po bid; follow serum levels

How do you treat acute asthma exacerbations?

Each patient should have a written action plan that guides initial self-management based on peak flow measurements. Mild exacerbations are treated with increases in inhaled β2-agonist frequency and in inhaled steroids, control/avoidance of precipitants,

TABLE 34-6	
Medications That Control Inflammation in Asthma	
Inhaled Corticosteroids*	
Beclomethasone (Vanceril, Beclovent)	2–4 puffs bid-qid (42, 84 μg)
Triamcinolone(Azmacort)	2 puffs tid-qid or 4 puffs bid (100 μg)
Flunisolide (Aerobid)	2–4 puffs bid (250 μg)
Budesonide (Pulmicort)	1–2 puffs bid (200 μg)
Fluticasone (Flovent)	2–4 puffs bid (44, 110, 220 μg)
Mast Cell Stabilizers	
Cromolyn (Intal)	2–4 puffs tid-qid
Nedocromil (Tilade)	2–4 puffs bid-qid
Leukotriene Antagonists†	
Zileuton (Zyflo)	600 mg PO qid (check LFTs for the first 3 months)
Zafirlukast (Accolate)	20 mg PO bid one hour before or two hours after meals
Montelukast (Singulair)	10 mg PO qd

*Listed from minimum to maximum potency.
†Rare cases of eosinophilic vasculitis (Churg-Strauss syndrome) have occurred among patients withdrawn from oral steroids after beginning a leukotriene receptor.

antibiotic therapy if indicated, oral steroid therapy, and a plan for when to go to the ED. For severe acute asthma exacerbation, ED-based management is warranted and the cornerstone of treatment is systemic corticosteroids. Give oral prednisone 60 mg PO (or 1 mg/kg) or IV methylprednisolone 120 mg immediately. This approach usually takes effect in four to eight hours. In the meantime, give repeated nebulized albuterol treatments. Epinephrine can be given to patients in status asthmaticus. The use of IV aminophylline and magnesium has fallen out of favor. Observe the patient for signs of improvement before discharging. If clinically improved and stable, discharge the patient on oral steroids at 40–60 mg daily and rapidly taper over the ensuing week.

What medications should I avoid in patients with asthma?

Aspirin, NSAIDs, and β-blockers can worsen bronchospasm to varying degrees in patients with asthma. Inquire about use of these agents and don't forget eyedrops, as they are a source of β-blockers.

What can be done for a severe asthmatic who does not respond to usual therapy?

Observe the patient's metered-dose inhaler technique and review medication adherence. Review the known asthma precipitants and try to identify others. Send for allergy testing. GERD may aggravate asthma symptoms, so try H$_2$-blockers or proton-pump inhibitors. Reconsider the diagnosis; other less common diseases such as cardiac ischemia or undiagnosed endobronchial lesions may be the causes. Refer the patient to a pulmonary specialist for further treatment recommendations and evaluation. Bronchoscopy is often useful in this setting. There are rare asthmatics who are insensitive to corticosteroids. These patients can be treated with other immunosuppressives, but this should be a last resort when other diagnoses have been ruled out.

What are the side effects of steroids?

Oral steroids in the short term can cause psychosis, hypertension, hypokalemia, and glucose intolerance. Long-term use of oral steroids or of high-dose inhaled steroids (usually greater than 1000 mcg/day) can cause osteoporosis, immunosuppression, elevated intraocular pressure, altered bone homeostasis, and cataract formation. Systemic absorption can be minimized by mouthrinsing after each administration and by use of spacer devices.

When should an asthmatic with an acute exacerbation be hospitalized?

There are no clear guidelines but signs of concern include prior hospitalizations or intubations, inability to speak in full sentences, use of accessory muscles for breathing, loss of wheezes due to absent air movement, hypercarbia or hypoxemia on ABG, and sluggish response to initial treatment. Decisions are also based on such considerations as duration and severity of symptoms, severity of airflow obstruction (measurements of FEV$_1$ or PEF), course and severity of prior exacerbations, medication use at the time of the exacerbation, access to medical care, adequacy of support, and presence of comorbidities. When deciding whether to hospitalize, always err on the side of patient safety.

K E Y   P O I N T S

▶ **Asthma is a disease of chronic airway inflammation triggered by a wide array of precipitants.**

▶ **Treatment for asthma should always include modification of the precipitants, an inhaled corticosteroid or other anti-inflammatory, and symptom relief with bronchodilators.**

▶ **Treat asthma exacerbations with systemic steroids and increased bronchodilators.**

CASE 34–1. A 30-year-old woman presents to your office with increasing difficulty controlling her asthma since moving to a new house. She has had asthma since childhood and has managed well with occasional use of her albuterol inhaler until recently, when she has used it almost daily. She reports frequent coughing and occasional chest tightness, with nighttime awakenings due to asthma symptoms.

A. What further history would be helpful?
B. What are your next steps in therapy?
C. What information do you share regarding the risks and benefits of treatment?

CASE 34–2. A 52-year-old grandmother with asthma calls you stating that for the last three days she has been feeling wheezy and short of breath. About one week ago she had URI symptoms after visiting her grandchild. You try to ask her some questions on the phone, but she is only able to answer you in short two-to three-word answers.

A. What do you do?
B. How should she be evaluated?
C. Should this patient be hospitalized?

REFERENCES

Clinical practice feature beginning with a case vignette focusing on mild asthma, followed by evidence supporting treatment strategies, a review of guidelines, and clinical recommendations.
Expert panel report II: guidelines for the diagnosis and management of asthma. Bethesda, Md.: National Asthma Education and Prevention Program, 1997. (NIH publication no. 97-4051.)
Naureckas ET, Solway J: Mild asthma. N Engl J Med 345:1257–1262, 2001.

USEFUL WEBSITES

http://www.nhlbi.nih.gov/guidelines/asthma/asthgdln.pdf
New Guidelines for the Diagnosis and Management of Asthma from the National Asthma Education and Prevention Program updating the 1991 Expert Panel Report of the National Heart, Lung, and Blood Institute. July 1997. (NIH Pub. No. 97-4051.)

http://www.nlm.nih.gov/medlineplus/asthma.html
Comprehensive summary of links to resources for the diagnosis and management of asthma provided by the National Library of Medicine.

CHRONIC OBSTRUCTIVE PULMONARY DISEASE

▶ ETIOLOGY

What is COPD?

Chronic obstructive pulmonary disease, or COPD, is a chronic disorder characterized by persistent respiratory symptoms in the presence of partially irreversible airflow obstruction. Chronic bronchitis and emphysema are the two primary disease processes that account for the cough and dyspnea experienced by patients with COPD. Chronic bronchitis is diagnosed clinically and is defined as the presence of a productive cough on most days for a minimum of three months per year for at least two consecutive years in the absence of another discernible cause. Emphysema is characterized by permanent enlargement and destruction of the alveolar air spaces and respiratory bronchioles with loss of the surrounding pulmonary capillaries. These pathologic changes have a characteristic appearance on chest CT scan that allows the diagnosis to be made radiographically rather than using lung biopsy. Most patients with COPD have varying degrees of both chronic bronchitis and emphysema. Although an "asthmatic" or reversible component is often present, some degree of irreversible airflow obstruction persists. Individuals with episodic, completely reversible airflow limitation have asthma rather than COPD. As asthma progresses, an irreversible airflow obstruction may develop, blurring the lines between asthma and COPD. Sputum production can occur with both asthma and COPD and is not a helpful discriminator.

What are the risk factors for COPD?

Between 80% and 90% of the risk of developing COPD comes from cigarette smoking. Pipe and cigar smokers have a risk intermediate between cigarette smokers and nonsmokers. Only 10% to 15% of smokers develop clinically significant COPD, so genetic factors clearly play an important role. Other risk factors for COPD include α_1-antitrypsin deficiency, air pollution, exposure to occupational dusts and chemicals, intravenous methylphenidate use, and possibly, childhood respiratory infections.

What causes COPD exacerbations?

COPD exacerbations are characterized by increases in cough, sputum production, sputum purulence, and dyspnea. Respiratory tract infections are a known trigger, but the relative importance of viral and bacterial pathogens is controversial. Noncompliance with medications, along with environmental factors such as exposure to dusts, fumes, pollens, tobacco smoke, and weather changes also play a role. In about a third of patients, the cause remains unknown.

▶ EVALUATION

How do patients with COPD present?

The presence of chronic cough, sputum production, and dyspnea in the setting of chronic tobacco use is highly suggestive of COPD. Cough is the most common symptom and may precede airflow limitation by many years. Patients tend to present with exertional dyspnea, at which point extensive, irreversible airway destruction may be present. To diagnose COPD earlier in the course of disease, obtain spirometry in all patients with chronic cough and exposure to risk factors, regardless of whether dyspnea is present. Differential diagnosis for the presentation of cough and dyspnea includes asthma, congestive heart failure, bronchiectasis, pneumonia, malignancy, and pulmonary embolism.

What exam findings suggest COPD?

Exam findings of COPD include decreased breath sounds, wheezes, rhonchi, and prolonged expiration. Look for tobacco staining of the fingertips or teeth. In advanced disease, look for barrel-shaped chest, pursed-lip breathing, emaciation, and accessory muscle use. Cor pulmonale is defined as right ventricular enlargement caused by lung disease. This often accompanies late COPD in which destruction of the lung parenchyma and vascular bed increases pulmonary artery pressures and therefore right ventricular afterload. The resulting right ventricular hypertrophy and pulmonary hypertension manifest as a loud second heart sound and a right-sided gallop and/or murmur. Sustained cor pulmonale results in right heart failure with elevated neck veins, hepatic congestion manifesting as an enlarged tender liver, and lower extremity edema.

What tests are appropriate for the evaluation of COPD?

Postbronchodilator spirometry reveals an FEV_1/FVC ratio less than 70% indicating airflow obstruction which, in the proper clinical setting, confirms the diagnosis of COPD. The American Thoracic Society has suggested the following staging system using postbronchodilator FEV_1: FEV_1 greater than 80% = mild; 30%–80% =

moderate; less than 30% = severe. In patients with advanced disease, obtain an ABG to assess hypoxemia and to establish baseline degrees of CO_2 retention. CXRs may reveal flattened diaphragms and bullae, but these findings are nondiagnostic and radiographs are primarily useful for excluding competing diagnoses.

What are common complications of COPD?

Anorexia and weight loss are common in advanced disease. Poor nutrition, steroid use, and smoking all increase the risk of osteoporosis. Depression and anxiety frequently accompany COPD but often go unrecognized, despite significant effect on quality of life. Polycythemia may develop in response to chronic hypoxemia. Advanced COPD is almost invariably accompanied by cor pulmonale. Structural changes of the right heart, along with hypoxemia and high doses of β-agonist bronchodilators trigger a variety of arrhythmias (e.g., multifocal atrial tachycardia, atrial fibrillation, ventricular tachycardia, and premature beats). Pneumothorax is more common in COPD; even small pneumothoraces can cause life-threatening respiratory failure in patients with limited ventilatory reserve. Leaks are often slow to heal and may require surgical management.

▶ TREATMENT

What nonpharmacologic interventions are available for stable COPD?

Smoking cessation is the most effective means of slowing the progression of disease and should be pursued aggressively in all smokers. Reduction or elimination of occupational exposures is important in patients with work-related disease. Yearly influenza vaccination reduces COPD morbidity and mortality. Less compelling evidence is available for pneumococcal vaccine, but it is recommended for patients with COPD by the Advisory Committee on Immunization Practice (ACIP). Long-term continuous oxygen therapy improves survival in patients with severe hypoxemia (PaO_2 less than or equal to 55 mm Hg or oxygen saturation less than 88%) and in patients with PaO_2 less than or equal to 59 mm Hg and cor pulmonale or polycythemia. Intermittent oxygen is appropriate for patients who experience desaturation exclusively during exercise or sleep. Pulmonary rehabilitation, a comprehensive program to address deconditioning, weight loss, medication compliance, and psychosocial well-being, improves exercise tolerance and decreases symptoms at all stages of disease. Surgery is being studied as an option in patients with severe, debilitating disease, but at this juncture it is difficult to predict which patients will likely benefit from bullectomy, lung volume reduction surgery, and/or lung transplantation.

What pharmacologic options are available for stable COPD?

Pharmacotherapy improves symptoms and reduces the frequency of exacerbations, but it does not alter the progressive decline in lung function. Inhaled bronchodilators are first line therapy for all symptomatic patients. Availability and patient response dictate whether a β-agonist such as albuterol, or an anticholinergic, such as ipratropium bromide, is used initially. Combining drugs from each class has an additive effect. Long-acting β-agonists such as salmeterol are good options for patients requiring frequent use of short-acting bronchodilators. Because of potential toxicity, methylxanthines, such as theophylline, generally are used as second line bronchodilators. The use of inhaled corticosteroids in stable COPD is controversial. Symptomatic patients with a combination of severe disease and frequent exacerbations, or an objective response to a six-week trial of therapy (FEV_1 improvement of 15% and at least 200 mL), are most likely to benefit. It is important to periodically review proper inhaler technique and encourage the use of spacer devices.

What therapies are appropriate for exacerbations of COPD?

The initial management of a COPD exacerbation consists of a rapid assessment for an alternative diagnosis while providing treatment that will decrease the need for intubation (Table 34–7). Hypoxemia typically corrects easily with low levels of supplemental oxygen. Saturations around 90% are adequate. Steroids reduce the need for hospitalization and shorten hospital stays. Antibiotics are frequently used for the triad of increased dyspnea, sputum production, and sputum purulence, although data supporting this is limited.

What is the role of noninvasive ventilation?

The most important development in the management of COPD exacerbations is the use of "mask" or noninvasive positive pressure ventilation (NIPPV). Early initiation of NIPPV in patients with moderate to severe respiratory distress improves gas exchange and reduces the need for mechanical ventilation and mortality. NIPPV is labor intensive and requires close monitoring by experienced personnel. The decision to proceed to intubation is complex and multifactorial. In general, patients with progressive respiratory failure and distress despite maximal medical therapy and a trial of NIPPV should be intubated unless their preference is to forego mechanical ventilation.

TABLE 34–7

Management of Acute COPD Exacerbations

Initial

Assess Severity
 VS, RR, ABG, WOB, LOC
Consider intubation
 Review patient preferences
Consider alternative diagnoses
 Exam, CXR, ECG, laboratories
 DDx: CHF, pneumonia, pneumothorax,
  MI, arrhythmias, pulmonary embolism
Supplemental O_2 to keep sat >90%
 Consider repeat ABG to eval ↑CO_2
High dose β_2 agonist
 e.g., albuterol 4–6 puffs
  via spacer or nebulizer q 20 min

Subsequent

Add IV or oral steroids
 Methylprednisolone or prednisone dose variable (e.g., 60 mg q6h with a rapid taper over 2 wks)
Add anticholinergic*
 e.g., ipratropium bromide 4–6 puffs via spacer or nebulizer q 20 min
Consider NIPPV
 Contraindications: ↓LOC, ↑secretions, respiratory arrest, facial deformity, CV instability,
  morbid obesity
Consider antibiotics*
Consider intravenous methylxanthine*
 e.g., aminophylline, watch for toxicity

*Unclear efficacy.
 Abbreviations: ABG=arterial blood gas, CHF=congestive heart failure, CV=cardiovascular, CXR=chest x-ray, DDx=differential diagnosis, ECG=electrocardiogram, LOC=level of consciousness, MI = myocardial infarction, NPPV = non-invasive positive pressure ventilation, RR=respiratory rate, VS=vital signs, WOB = work of breathing.

K E Y   P O I N T S

▶ COPD is a chronic, progressive disease characterized by largely fixed airflow obstruction.

▶ Smoking cessation is the most important intervention in slowing progression of COPD.

▶ A variety of medications can ameliorate symptoms, but none alters the decline in lung function.

▶ Supplemental oxygen reduces mortality in patients with COPD and severe hypoxia.

▶ NIPPV reduces the need for intubation and improves mortality in selected patients.

CASE 34-3.

A 48-year-old woman presents to your clinic for the first time reporting she has had asthma for the past four years. She walks three or four blocks before dyspnea forces her to stop. She is a former smoker with a 30 pack-year history. Her symptoms persist despite prednisone 10 mg/day and albuterol MDI 14 puffs/day. She is lean, alert, with normal vital signs, and oxygen saturation. Breath sounds are clear but decreased, and the ratio of expiratory to inspiratory time is increased to 3:1. Heart sounds are distant, JVP is 7 cm H_2O, and extremities are without edema or clubbing. CXR findings include a flattened diaphragm and hyperlucency in the lower lung fields consistent with bullous disease. Spirometry reveals moderate obstruction with FEV_1/FVC of 60% and FEV_1 of 1.2 L (55% of predicted). There is no improvement following bronchodilator.

A. Is the patient more likely to have COPD or asthma?
B. What risk factors for COPD besides tobacco use should be considered in this patient?
C. What changes, if any, in her medications would you recommend?

CASE 34-4.

A 68-year-old man with 50 pack-years of tobacco use has an FEV_1 that is 25% predicted and was diagnosed with COPD twelve years ago. On exam, he is barrel-chested, using accessory muscles at rest, and has markedly prolonged expiration with diffusely decreased breath sounds. Heart sounds are distant and his JVP is about 12 cm H_2O. He has hepatomegaly and bilateral lower extremity edema. His ABG is pH 7.37, $PaCO_2$ 55 mm Hg, PaO_2 56, with serum bicarbonate of 35 mEq/L. He is on inhaled bronchodilators and has infrequent exacerbations.

A. What would you expect the remainder of his pulmonary functions tests to show: FEV_1/FVC, TLC, DLCO?
B. Is long-term oxygen therapy indicated in this patient?
C. What intervention will slow progression of his COPD most effectively?

REFERENCES

Pauwels RA, Buist AS, Calverley PM et al: Global strategy for the diagnosis, management, and prevention of chronic obstructive pulmonary disease. Am J Respir Crit Care Med 163:1256-1276, 2001.

Pierson DJ: Clinical approach to the patient with obstructive lung disease. In Pierson DJ, Kacmarek RM: Foundations of Respiratory Care. New York, Churchill Livingstone, 1992, pp 679-688.

PULMONARY EMBOLISM

▶ ETIOLOGY

What causes pulmonary embolism (PE)?

Pulmonary embolism is an under-recognized and potentially fatal condition. The majority of PEs are not identified before death. The major origin of PE, accounting for 90% of cases, is deep venous thrombosis (DVT) of the lower extremities. Untreated, 50% of proximal lower extremity DVTs embolize to the lungs. Risk factors for DVT and PE include Virchow's triad of hypercoagulability, immobility, and endothelial injury (Box 34–1).

BOX 34-1

Risk Factors for Pulmonary Embolus

Venous stasis

> Prolonged immobilization
> Recent surgery
> Obesity
> CHF, MI

Hypercoagulability

> Malignancy
> Inherited abnormality of clotting factors
> Oral contraceptives, pregnancy
> Nephrotic syndrome

Blood vessel intimal damage

> Lower extremity surgery, trauma
> Age older than 60

▶ EVALUATION

How do patients with PE present?

Symptoms and signs of PE are nonspecific: chest pain (may be pleuritic), dyspnea, cough, hemoptysis, sweating or syncope, sudden onset fatigue. Up to 40% of patients are asymptomatic. Ask patients with any of these symptoms about risk factors for PE. Findings on exam may include tachypnea, tachycardia, fever, cyanosis, diaphoresis, accentuated second heart sound, S_3 or S_4 gallop, right ventricular heave, or pulmonary friction rub if a PE has infarcted lung tissue at the pleural surface. Massive PE may cause hemodynamic collapse with critically low blood pressure or cardiac arrest. Unilateral lower extremity edema can be a clue to the original DVT. (Measure calf diameters to compare.)

What initial tests should I order when I suspect PE?

Initially obtain standard tests for dyspnea including CBC, chemistry panel, ABG, CXR, pulse oximetry, and ECG. ABG may be normal with PE but usually shows a significant A-a gradient (Box 34–2) and respiratory alkalosis. (Hypoxia causes patients to breathe faster, drops CO_2 and raises pH.) CXR may be normal or may show atelectasis, pleural effusion, or infiltrates. It may also identify another disorder such as pneumonia or CHF. Occasionally on CXR with PE, there is a triangular infarct from occlusion of a pulmonary artery (Hampton's hump) or focal oligemia (Westermark's sign). ECG may show an alternate diagnosis such as MI. PE commonly causes sinus tachycardia or nonspecific ST/T wave changes but may also cause atrial arrhythmia, right heart strain, right axis deviation, right bundle branch block, or "S1, Q3 and T3" pattern (S wave in lead I, Q wave and flipped T wave in lead III). Consider drawing blood for a hypercoagulability work-up.

BOX 34–2

Calculating the Alveolar-Arterial Oxygen Gradient (A-a gradient)

A-a gradient = $PAO_2 - PaO_2$

where

PaO_2 = Alveolar oxygen concentration = FiO_2 (PB − 47) − $PaCO_2/0.8$ (approximately 100 at sea level with normal $PaCO_2$)
PaO_2 = Arterial oxygen concentration = blood gas PaO_2
FiO_2 = Fraction of oxygen in inspired air (0.21 for sea level)
PB = Atmospheric pressure (760 mm Hg at sea level)

A-a gradient on room air = 150 − p PaO_2 − $PaCO_2/0.8$

Normal A-a gradient is < 10 if younger, < 20 if older

When should I pursue further testing for PE and what tests should I order?

Your level of clinical suspicion based on risk factors, history, exam, and initial tests is key in guiding further work-up. Doppler ultrasound of the lower extremities detects 95% of proximal leg clots and obviates the need for further tests if positive. A ventilation/perfusion (V/Q) scan is a nuclear medicine test that identifies perfusion defects due to PE that are not matched by lung ventilation defects. V/Q scans are read as normal, nondiagnostic (formerly called low and intermediate probability), and high probability for PE. The likelihood of PE based on V/Q scan results depends on clinical suspicion for PE. Data from the Prospective Investigation of Pulmonary Embolus Diagnosis (PIOPED) study provide estimates of PE likelihood combining the clinical suspicion and V/Q result (Table 34–8). A high probability scan establishes the diagnosis of PE, and a normal scan rules it out. Most commonly, the scan is nondiagnostic, especially when the CXR is abnormal, necessitating more testing.

Helical (spiral) CT scan is a newer, minimally invasive option for diagnosing PE, particularly large central emboli. Helical CT is typically ordered instead of V/Q scan in patients with underlying cardiopulmonary disease, in whom V/Q scans are usually nondiagnostic (unhelpful). A D-dimer ELISA blood test, if normal, is helpful in *ruling out* PE, but it is not available in all labs. If the D-dimer result is elevated, it suggests DVT or PE but is nonspecific and should be used with another imaging study to confirm the diagnosis. Pulmonary angiogram is the standard for diagnosing PE. It is not a first line test, but is an important tool when clinical suspicion is high and results of other studies are nondiagnostic.

TABLE 34–8

Likelihood of PE Based on Level of Clinical Suspicion and V/Q Scan Results

	Normal V/Q, %	Indeterminant VQ, %	High Probability V/Q, %
Clinical suspicion (pretest probability)		(formerly "low probability")	(formerly "intermediate probability")
Low	2	4	16	56
Intermediate	6	16	28	88
High	0	40	66	96

► **TREATMENT**

How do I treat PE?

Stabilize the airway, breathing, and circulation. Administer oxygen. Start IV heparin if there are no contraindications (Box 34–3). If clinical suspicion for PE is high, treatment is started even before definitive diagnosis is made. Start warfarin once PE is confirmed and continue heparin until the INR is 2.0–3.0 (usually five days). Treatment usually lasts six months, although warfarin may be continued indefinitely if risk is not modifiable (e.g., cancer, inherited hypercoagulable state).

What other treatment options exist?

For patients with massive PE and hypotension, thrombolytic therapy is recommended to lyse the clot and improve hemodynamics. These patients have a very high mortality rate. Inferior vena caval filters can be placed when patients have absolute contraindications to anticoagulation (see Box 34–3) or recurrent PE on appropriate anticoagulation. The filter is a wire barrier that is placed under angiographic guidance into the IVC. It allows blood flow but stops larger clots from proceeding to the lungs.

BOX 34–3

Contraindications to the Use of Heparin

Absolute contraindications

Active internal bleeding
Intracranial bleeding
Intracranial lesions likely to bleed
Severe heparin-induced thrombocytopenia
Malignant hypertension

Relative contraindications

Hemorrhagic diathesis
Recent stroke
Recent major surgery
Severe hypertension
Bacterial endocarditis
Thrombocytopenia
Peptic ulcer disease

KEY POINTS

▶ The clinical presentation of PE and initial diagnostic tests are nonspecific; you must have a high index of suspicion, especially in patients with risk factors.

▶ Use risk factors, H & P and noninvasive tests to guide your clinical suspicion for PE.

▶ Anticoagulate with heparin when clinical suspicion is high and there are no contraindications as you pursue PE work-up.

▶ Use clinical suspicion and PIOPED data to interpret likelihood of PE from V/Q scan.

CASE 34–5. A 48-year-old woman presents with progressive difficulty walking up hills on her usual morning exercise walk for the past several days. She has a mild cough but no fever, chest pain, or abdominal pain. She recalls that two to three weeks ago she slammed her left lower leg into a car door as she was closing it, and she has had mild leg pain and bruising since. Past medical history includes cholecystectomy, mild asthma, and menometrorrhagia due to uterine fibroids, for which she was recently prescribed oral contraceptive pills. In addition to her oral contraceptives, she uses an albuterol inhaler approximately twice per month. On physical examination, she is a well-appearing woman in no acute distress. T is 37.2°C, HR 100, BP 110/70, RR 22, oxygen saturation 94% on room air. Chest is clear to auscultation. Cardiac exam reveals a regular rate and rhythm with no murmurs, rubs, or gallops, and abdomen is benign. Extremity exam reveals left calf ecchymoses and edema. WBC 10, HCT 37, platelet 350,000, PT 12, INR 1.0, PTT 30.

A. What is your differential diagnosis for this patient's shortness of breath?

B. What are her risk factors for pulmonary embolism?

C. What further evaluation do you perform?

D. You diagnose a pulmonary embolism. How do you treat her?

CASE 34–6.

A 75-year-old man with metastatic non–small-cell lung cancer is brought to the ED by ambulance with shortness of breath and altered mental status. One week prior to admission, his family noted cough with purulent sputum and increased work of breathing. His family doctor prescribed azithromycin, but symptoms progressed. The patient had fever and chills, no URI symptoms, headache, neck pain, or abdominal complaints. On exam, the patient is in respiratory distress with accessory muscle use. Temperature is 38.5°C, BP 110/65, HR 120, RR 36, oxygen saturation 90% on room air. Chest examination reveals coarse breath sounds bilaterally with expiratory wheezes. Cardiac exam shows a normal PMI, distant heart sounds, no extra sounds or murmurs. Abdomen is benign. Extremities show no cyanosis, clubbing, or edema.

A. What is your differential diagnosis?

WBC count is 17,000, HCT 35%. CXR shows bilateral pulmonary infiltrates. The patient is treated with broad spectrum antibiotics and oxygen with improvement in his cough. Several days later, the patient suddenly desaturates to 80% on room air, 85% on 6 L oxygen by nasal cannula. Temperature is 37.5°C, BP 90/50, HR 130. Chest is clear. Jugular venous pressure is 12 cm (normal is 5–8), and there is a loud P_2. CXR shows improvement in bilateral infiltrates. ECG shows sinus tachycardia with nonspecific ST segment changes.

B. What is your differential diagnosis now?
C. What diagnostic studies will you perform?
D. What treatment would you recommend?

REFERENCE

Hyers TM, Agnelli G, Hull RD, et al: Antithrombotic therapy for venous thromboembolic disease. Review. Chest 119(1 Suppl):176S–193S, 2001.

USEFUL WEBSITE

www.americanheart.org/presenter.jhtml?identifier=1200000 and search on "pulmonary embolism" for a consensus statement on Management of Deep Vein Thrombosis and Pulmonary Embolism.

35

Rheumatology

GOUT

▶ ETIOLOGY

What causes gout?

Gout is an inflammatory arthritis caused by the deposition of monosodium urate crystals in a joint. Crystals form because of under-excretion (90%) or overproduction of uric acid. Risk factors for gout include medications, alcohol use, obesity, hereditary predisposition (extremely common in individuals from Samoa and the Philippines), and hyperuricemia—although not all of these patients develop gout. Less common precipitants of gout include lead poisoning and tumor lysis syndrome seen during chemotherapy for various cancers.

What medications cause increases in uric acid?

Diuretics are the most commonly used medications that trigger gout. Low-dose aspirin, cyclosporine, and niacin are also important precipitants of gout.

What are common triggers for an attack in patients with a history of gout?

Rapid changes in urate level can trigger gout. Decreased uric acid secretion and fluid shifts are contributing factors associated with physiologic stresses, such as surgery, trauma, medical illness, and new medications that decrease uric acid secretion. Hospitalization triggers acute gout attacks in up to 85% of those with a history of gout. Physical activities such as running and long walks may precede gouty attacks in the first metatarsophalangeal (MTP) joint. Occasionally, starting therapy with allopurinol precipitates or worsen a gouty attack. For this reason, allopurinol is not started during an acute attack.

▶ EVALUATION

What is the typical presentation of gout?

Men are much more commonly afflicted with gout than are women. The most common first site of involvement is the MTP joint of the great toe (greater than 50% of initial gout attacks). In greater than 80% of cases, the first episode of gout is monarticular. The pain is great and is exacerbated by even minimal pressure of bed sheets on the joint. Erythema and warmth of the affected joint are typical. The onset of pain is usually sudden and often involves only one joint. In older patients it is common for gout to occur in joints with osteoarthritis. The ankle, foot, or knee can be the site of acute gout. Hips and shoulders are hardly ever affected.

What symptoms and signs do you see with a severe attack of gout?

Common findings are fever, multiple joint involvement, tachycardia, and high WBC. The patients are frequently misdiagnosed as having an infection.

How do I diagnose gout?

WBCs and ESRs are usually elevated during acute attacks, but are nonspecific. The diagnosis is made by aspirating the involved joint and examining the fluid under polarized microscopy. Urate crystals are needle-shaped or rod-shaped and are both intracellular in neutrophils and extracellular. They are strongly negatively birefringent when examined under compensated polarized microscopy. Most patients with gout have a high uric acid level (greater than 7 mg/dL). Occasionally, uric acid levels are depressed during an acute attack. Recheck the uric acid level in those patients once the attack subsides. In patients with an established diagnosis of gout and recurrent episodes, there is no need to tap the joint again unless clinical features suggest the possibility of a septic joint (fever, chills, lack of response to gout therapy).

What happens to patients with long-standing gout?

Patients may have acute attacks separated by long symptom-free periods. Gouty arthritis can also become chronic, with urate deposition in joints and periarticular tissues that can lead to chronic, destructive, deforming arthritis. With chronic joint destruction, x-rays may show classic "rat-bite" erosions that look like punched-out areas of bone loss with an associated overhanging rim of cortical bone. Gout crystals can precipitate in the subcutaneous tissues causing deforming tophi. The digits and ears are the most common sites for tophi.

▶ TREATMENT

How should I treat an acute attack of gout?

The mainstay for treatment is nonsteroidal anti-inflammatory medication, e.g., indomethacin 50 mg three times a day. Be extremely careful to avoid using NSAIDs in patients with contraindications such as congestive heart failure, renal insufficiency, history of gastric or peptic ulcer disease, or allergy to aspirin/NSAIDs. The alternatives for treatment of acute gout are prednisone (5–7 day course) or joint injection with corticosteroids. Treatment-dose colchicine should not be used in patients with renal insufficiency. Colchicine causes severe diarrhea at treatment doses and is the least attractive option for treating gout. It should not be given in treatment doses to patients with renal insufficiency.

Who should receive chronic medication to prevent gouty attacks?

Patients who have had more than two attacks of gout within a year are reasonable candidates. After a first attack, 75% of patients will have a second attack within two years. Patients with more than two attacks are likely to have more recurrences.

What therapy should be used for preventing attacks?

Allopurinol and probenecid are both effective in preventing recurrent acute attacks and in resorbing chronic tophaceous deposits. Allopurinol decreases production of uric acid, whereas probenecid decreases renal reabsorption of filtered urate. Probenecid only works with intact renal function. Do not start either drug during an acute attack because they can prolong or worsen the attack. Allopurinol is the preferred drug in patients with overproducing of urate, urate stones, or renal insufficiency. Allopurinol can infrequently cause rash, vasculitis, and hepatitis. Low-dose colchicine (0.6 mg a day) is an effective therapy to bridge the gap between acute treatment and prophylactic drug treatment.

KEY POINTS

▶ Common medications that trigger gout are diuretics and niacin.

▶ Do not start allopurinol during an acute attack.

▶ Treat acute gout with NSAIDs except in patients with renal insufficiency or PUD.

CASE 35–1. A 39-year-old man with type 1 diabetes presents with severe pain in his left foot. On exam he has erythema over the first MTP joint of the left foot. Labs: BUN 39, creatinine 3.3, glucose 350, HCT 35, WBC 4.6. Joint fluid—crystals consistent with urate. Uric acid 8.8, Hgb$_{alc}$ 10.0.

    A. What therapy would you use?

CASE 35–2. A 61-year-old man is evaluated for an acute episode of gout involving his right knee. Three months ago and one year ago, he had gouty attacks involving his left great toe. Medical problems include hypertension and renal insufficiency (creatinine 2.4).

    A. What therapy would you recommend?
    B. What would be an appropriate plan to help prevent future attacks of gout?

REFERENCES

Agudelo CA, Wise CM: Gout: Diagnosis, pathogenesis, and clinical manifestations. Curr Opin Rheumatol 13(3):234–239, 2001.

Simpkin PA: Gout and hyperuricemia. Curr Opin Rheumatol 9(3):268–273, 1997.

RHEUMATOID ARTHRITIS

▶ ETIOLOGY

What is rheumatoid arthritis?

Rheumatoid arthritis (RA) is a chronic autoimmune disease of unclear etiology that causes synovial inflammation with erosion of articular cartilage and bone. Worldwide prevalence is 1%, with women developing RA three times as frequently as men. It occurs in all age groups, although generally increases with age. The course of RA is highly variable, but it usually causes significant morbidity and decreased longevity.

▶ **EVALUATION**

What are the most common symptoms of RA?

RA is usually a symmetric polyarthritis involving characteristic peripheral joints, especially the metacarpophalangeal (MCP) and MTP joints (Figure 35–1). Lumbosacral and distal interphalangeal joints are hardly ever involved. The inflamed joints produce a deep, aching discomfort. Stiffness is most severe in the morning or after periods of inactivity and characteristically lasts one hour or longer. Constitutional symptoms may precede overt arthritis and include weight loss, low-grade fever, and fatigue. Twenty percent of patients develop extra-articular manifestations (Figure 35–2).

What should I look for on the musculoskeletal examination?

Palpate each joint for effusions, synovial swelling, and tenderness. Presence of synovial proliferation gives the joint a boggy consistency and diffuse tenderness. In comparison, tendonitis and bursitis cause

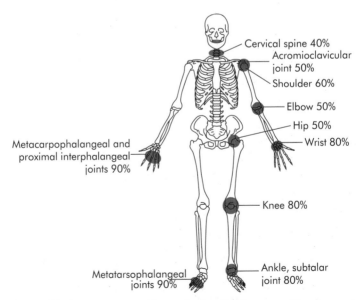

Figure 35–1. Joints commonly involved in RA (pattern of involvement is usually symmetrical and involves the MCP, MTP, and PIP joints).

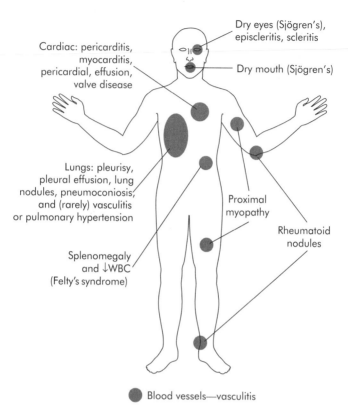

Figure 35–2. Extraarticular manifestations of RA.

focal pain without boggy synovial swelling. Check active and passive range of motion (ROM). In tendinitis only active ROM is painful, whereas with joint involvement both passive *and* active ROM are painful. Detailed measurements of ROM are rarely necessary. Describe ROM as normal; slightly, moderately, markedly limited; or fused. Rheumatoid nodules may be found at sites of pressure such as the posterior elbow and over the Achilles tendon. Watch for common deformities including ulnar deviation of fingers, subluxation of MCP joints, swan neck, boutonniere deformities of the fingers, and cock-up deformities of the toes (Figure 35–3). Asymptomatic flexion contractures (easily noticed in superficial joints such as the elbow) suggest active synovitis.

What might I see on neurologic exam of a patient with RA?

Check for paresthesias of the hands and feet because compressive neuropathies are common due to active synovitis (e.g., carpal

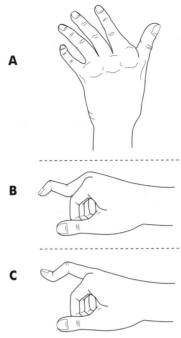

Figure 35–3. Characteristic joint deformities seen in RA. **A,** Ulnar deviation; **B,** Swan neck deformity; **C,** boutonnière deformity.

tunnel syndrome). The cervical spine can become unstable owing to erosive synovitis, particularly at the atlantoaxial junction (C1-C2). If localized pain and x-ray findings suggest this is the case, perform a careful neurologic exam at every visit. Patients with significant C1-C2 subluxation can have chronic, progressive pyramidal tract (upper motor neuron) compression leading to weakness, spasticity, and pathologic reflexes. Sudden, acute cervical cord compression can also occur after only minor trauma or as a complication of intubation for surgery.

How do I diagnose RA?

RA is a clinical diagnosis requiring presence of at least four of seven criteria (Box 35–1).

What lab tests should I order if I suspect RA?

Order rheumatoid factor, an IgM antibody specifically active against IgG. Although RF is present in 80% of adults with RA, it is nonspecific (found in many other inflammatory conditions) and suggests RA only if other clinical criteria are present

BOX 35-1

Revised Criteria (1987) for the Diagnosis of RA
- Four criteria are required for diagnosis.
- Criteria numbers 1–4 must be present for six weeks or more
  1. Morning stiffness lasting at least one hour
  2. Arthritis in at least three joints
  3. Arthritis of the hand joints
  4. Symmetrical arthritis
  5. Rheumatoid nodules
  6. Positive serum rheumatoid factors (RF)
  7. X-ray changes typical of RA

(see Box 35–1). High titers are associated with worse joint disease and extra-articular manifestations (see Figure 35–2). Once rheumatoid factor is positive, you never need to check it again, because it does not correlate with disease activity or response to treatment. ESR and C-reactive protein (CRP) are typically elevated and roughly correlate with disease activity, although normal values do not rule out RA. Other helpful labs to monitor include hematocrit because anemia of chronic disease is common in active RA.

What will I see on a joint aspiration with RA?

Joint aspirations in patients with RA show inflammation (WBC 3–35,000 with predominately PMNs). Tap a joint if you are uncertain of the diagnosis of RA and are looking for evidence of another disease process such as gout or if you think the joint might be infected. Strongly consider tapping a joint that is persistently or excessively inflamed compared with the patient's other joints because patients with RA are at risk for joint infections.

Are x-rays helpful in diagnosis of RA?

X-rays early in the disease usually are normal or show juxta-articular osteopenia and are not helpful for diagnosis. It may take months to years for erosive changes, including joint space narrowing and joint margin erosions, to develop on x-ray, although x-rays have an important role in monitoring disease progression.

What are potential extra-articular manifestations of rheumatoid arthritis?

Extra-articular manifestations include interstitial lung disease, rheumatoid nodules (lung, cardiac, subcutaneous tissue), pleuropericarditis, myocarditis, neuropathy either from compression (cervical spine instability, carpal tunnel syndrome) or vasculitis (skin ulcers, mononeuritis multiplex, vessel changes), scleritis, episcleritis, splenomegaly, Sjögren's syndrome, osteoporosis, myositis, neutropenia, thrombocytopenia, anemia, and cricoarytenoid abnormalities, leading to hoarseness and upper airway obstructions.

What evaluation is warranted on routine follow-up of patients with known RA?

Assess disease activity and severity by asking about the number of joints involved, the severity of pain and fatigue, and the time it takes for morning stiffness to resolve. Compare level of function between visits by identifying an activity that the patient can perform only marginally well (e.g., combing hair, slicing bread, walking more than two blocks) and have them describe their level of function with this activity at each visit. Ask about onset of any new extra-articular manifestations. Elevations in C-reactive protein and sedimentation rate levels, as well as drops in albumin and hemoglobin levels all correlate with disease activity. A high rheumatoid factor portends a worse prognosis overall but does not fluctuate with disease activity. At least three joints involved without extra-articular manifestations indicates mild disease. Moderate disease is characterized by 6–20 joints with signs of early inflammation on x-rays (periarticular osteopenia and swelling). Severe disease involves any one or more of the following: more than 20 joints affected, anemia, hypoalbuminemia, erosions on x-rays and/or extraarticular disease.

▶ TREATMENT

Are there any nonpharmacologic therapies recommended for patients with RA?

Patient education and counseling are key to ensure a good therapeutic alliance as treatments often require adjustment and can cause toxicities. Advise periods of rest for symptoms of severe fatigue or to decrease joint wear and tear during periods of joint inflammation. Regular exercise and range of motion improves function, maintains joint mobility, and prevents muscle and bone loss. Physical therapy maneuvers with ultrasound, heat or cold applications, ROM exercises, and splinting painful joints can reduce pain and increase function. Weight loss is advised for obese patients to decrease joint stress. Bone loss is common from the effects of RA directly, as well as from steroids used to decrease inflammation and treat complications. Calcium, 1000–1500 mg/day, and vitamin D, 400–800 IU/day, are essential. Bisphosphonates may also be used to protect against further bone loss.

What medicines are used to treat RA?

There is no cure for RA, but early medical therapy—in addition to alleviating pain—delays or possibly prevents joint deformities. There are two main categories of medications: NSAIDs and disease modifying antirheumatic drugs (DMARDs). NSAIDs relieve symptoms, but do not delay joint destruction. In the past, patients were initially treated with NSAIDs and DMARDs were started late in the disease. Now, the focus is on early treatment with DMARDs, to halt the underlying inflammation and delay or prevent joint destruction. No DMARD is universally effective in all patients, and they frequently have to be discontinued owing to side effects. These agents are tried in a stepwise manner, often in combinations, until inflammation is suppressed as indicated by ESR/CRP or symptoms.

Hydroxychloroquine is usually the first DMARD given, and in patients with mild disease may be effective alone. In patients with aggressive RA, methotrexate is the most often used DMARD and is usually given in combination with hydroxychloroquine. The treatment of RA has dramatically improved with the advent of new biologic agents: tumor necrosis factor alpha (TNFα) inhibitors and interleukin 1 receptor antagonist (IL-RA). The two TNFα inhibitors are etanercept and infliximab. Since these agents inhibit inflammatory cytokines that are used in normal inflammatory responses to infection, patients should be advised to seek medical attention if they develop serious fever and chills. Patients on TNFα inhibitors are at greater risk for TB. Other more toxic agents added or substituted when first line agents fail include gold salts, D-penicillamine, sulfasalazine, prednisone, cyclophosphamide, cyclosporin, chlorambucil, and azathioprine.

What surgical therapies are used for patients with RA?

Advances in orthopedic surgery have had a profound effect on the quality of life of patients with RA. Surgical synovectomy of a joint may temporarily improve symptoms, decrease joint destruction seen early in disease, remove debris interfering with normal function, and prevent tendon rupture. Total joint replacement of larger joints (hips, knees, shoulders) can markedly increase function and decrease pain. Other surgical options include repair of ruptured tendons, correction of valgus or varus deformities of the knee to realign weight-bearing bones, joint fusion to stabilize joints not easily replaced (e.g., ankle, wrist, thumb, cervical spine), correction of severe contractures, and metatarsal head excision to alleviate severe forefoot pain and improve gait.

K E Y P O I N T S

▶ RA causes symmetrical arthritis of peripheral joints, especially MCP and MTP joints.

▶ With RA, prolonged stiffness is most severe in the morning or after periods of inactivity.

▶ Extra-articular manifestations occur in 20% of patients with RA (usually in those with high rheumatoid factor).

▶ Early treatment with a DMARD, alone or in combination with other DMARDs, is essential to prevent destructive changes in patients with RA.

▶ Surgical therapy (such as joint replacement) is effective for severely damaged joints.

CASE 35–3. A 35-year-old woman reports gradual onset over the past two months of fatigue, pain involving the MCP, proximal interphalangeal (PIP) and wrist joints, and morning stiffness lasting one hour. On exam, MCP's, PIPs, and wrists are swollen bilaterally. The joints are tender and slightly warm.

   A. What is your differential diagnosis?
   B. What laboratory tests would you order?
   C. What do you recommend for treatment?

CASE 35–4. A 45-year-old woman is taking 7.5 mg of prednisone a day for sero-positive rheumatoid arthritis with multiple joint deformities. She reports that she cannot raise her left foot. On examination, she is slightly cushingoid. There is 2+ swelling of the MCP's, PIPs, wrist and ankles, and ulnar deviation, boutonnière and swan neck deformities. Flexion and extension of the wrist are markedly reduced. Her toes are cocked up. She cannot dorsiflex her left foot.

   A. What is the differential diagnosis of her left foot drop?
   B. What tests would you obtain?
   C. What do you recommend for treatment?

REFERENCES

Lee DM, Weinblatt ME: Rheumatoid arthritis. Lancet 358(9285):903–911, 2001.

Pisetsky DS, St. Clair EW: Progress in the treatment of rheumatoid arthritis. JAMA 286(22):2787–2790, 2001.

SYSTEMIC LUPUS ERYTHEMATOSUS

▶ ETIOLOGY

What is lupus?

Systemic lupus erythematosus (SLE) is a chronic immune disorder that involves many organ systems and causes a wide variety of symptoms. The severity ranges from nearly asymptomatic to life-threatening. Many patients have mild disease with a variety of skin lesions, alopecia, or arthritis, but some patients have serious complications such as renal failure, organic psychosis, or vasculitis. Survival rate in SLE is approximately 90% over the first ten years. Involvement of the kidneys or CNS is an unfavorable prognostic sign. Major causes of death are renal failure, infection often owing to the use of immunosuppressive drugs, and coronary artery disease.

Who gets lupus?

Lupus is most common among women of childbearing age, with a 9:1 female to male ratio. African-American women are affected three times more commonly than are whites, although blacks in Africa hardly ever get SLE. It usually develops between ages 13 and 40, but can occur at any age. Genetic factors are important as lupus is more common in relatives of affected patients.

What causes lupus?

Lupus is an autoimmune disease. For unidentified reasons, autoantibodies (Table 35–1) cause tissue injury when they are directed at a specific cell type, such as red blood cells, or if they form antigen-antibody (immune) complexes. Circulating immune complexes are deposited in blood vessels, initiating a cascade of complement-mediated injury. Certain drugs can cause a reversible drug-induced lupus. Common offenders include hydralazine, procainamide, and isoniazid.

TABLE 35–1

Important Antibodies in Lupus and Their Frequency

Antibody	Frequency (%)
Anti–double-stranded DNA • If positive, it is likely patient has lupus (high specificity) • Often increases with flares (doubling or increase of 30 in less than 10 weeks suggests disease flare)	70
Anti-Smith antibody • Nearly pathognomonic for SLE when it is present	30
Anti-RNP antibody • Can be present in other rheumatologic conditions	40
Anti-Ro antibody (SS-A) • Children of mother's with anti-Ro are at risk of neonatal lupus and congenital heart block	30
Anti-La antibody (SS-B) • Can be present in other rheumatologic conditions	10
Anti-histone antibody • Positive in 95% of patients with drug-induced SLE, 20% of patients with idiopathic SLE	70

Does pregnancy exacerbate lupus?

Active disease at conception is likely to worsen during pregnancy, but patients already in remission usually complete pregnancy without a clinical exacerbation. Nearly half of all lupus patients deliver prematurely, often by emergency C-section. Patients with a positive anti-Ro antibody are at risk of delivering a child with neonatal lupus or congenital heart block. Phospholipid antibody syndrome may occur in association with lupus and can cause fetal loss.

▶ EVALUATION

What are the most common manifestations of lupus?

The most common presenting symptom is symmetric arthritis, seen in about 65% of patients at presentation. Morning stiffness and distribution of joints involved is similar to RA. Other common manifestations are fatigue, skin rashes (some photosensitive), renal insufficiency, fevers, and hematologic cytopenias. Although fatigue is common in patients with lupus, fatigue also may be caused by other concurrent medical or psychiatric conditions and should not be ignored. Less common but interesting manifestations of the disease include pericarditis, pleuritis, oral ulcers, and psychiatric disturbances (Table 35–2). The disease characteristically has episodic

TABLE 35–2

Diagnosing Lupus (1982 American Rheumatism Association Criteria)*

Symptom, Sign, or Laboratory Abnormality	Frequency, %
Serositis–pleuritis, pericarditis	56
Oral or nasopharyngeal ulcers–painless	27
Arthritis—nonerosive, two or more peripheral joints	86
Photosensitivity–erythematous skin rash, raised or flat	43
Blood dyscrasias	
Hemolytic anemia (with reticulocytosis)	30
Leukopenia (WBC < 4000) on 2 or more occasions	40
Lymphopenia (<1500) on 2 or more occasions	
Thrombocytopenia (<100,000) in the absence of offending drugs	30
Renal–proteinuria, casts	50
Antinuclear antibody—in absence of drugs known to cause lupus	>95
Immunologic disorders	
Anti–double-stranded DNA	70
Anti-Smith: antibody to Smith nuclear antigen	30
False positive VDRL × 6 months, negative FTA-ABS	
Neurologic disorder–seizures, psychosis	50
Malar rash—flat or raised erythema, spares nasolabial folds	
Discoid rash—raised erythematous, scaling, follicular plugging, atrophic scarring	

*Classic lupus considered present when many criteria met; definite lupus when 4 criteria present; probable lupus when 3 criteria present; and possible lupus when only 2 criteria are present.

flares and remissions. Symptoms during flares can occur on a spectrum from catastrophic to low grade.

What questions should I ask if I think a patient may have lupus?

Do a thorough review of symptoms. Ask specifically about the many possible manifestations of lupus in various organs. If the patient has had three or more possible manifestations of lupus, further testing with an antinuclear antibody (ANA) is warranted.

What are features of drug-induced lupus?

Arthralgias, pleuritis, and pericarditis are common in drug-induced lupus (such as with hydralazine or procainamide), but renal and CNS manifestations are rare. Discontinuation of the drug typically resolves the syndrome. Nearly all patients with drug-induced lupus have a positive anti-histone antibody, but the anti–double-stranded DNA, found in 70% of patients with idiopathic lupus, is almost always absent.

How do I diagnosis lupus?

No one clinical abnormality or lab test establishes the diagnosis of lupus. In 1982, the American College of Rheumatism developed a classification system of 11 criteria (see Table 35–2). Lupus is diagnosed when patients meet at least four of these 11 criteria, either serially or at the same time. The ANA is positive in nearly all patients with lupus and is the best screening test, although it can also be positive with many other chronic inflammatory conditions.

What complications can occur?

Infection can be difficult to distinguish from a lupus flare. ESR, double-stranded DNA, and complement may be more abnormal with a flare than with infection. Osteonecrosis of the hips and knees, osteoporosis, and premature coronary artery disease all occur owing to long-term steroid use. Congenital heart block and neonatal lupus can occur when maternal anti-Ro antibodies are present.

▶ TREATMENT

What medications can be used for patients with lupus?

There is no cure for lupus. The goal of treatment is to relieve symptoms, suppress inflammation, and prevent future pathology (see Table 35–3). The risk-benefit ratio of potentially toxic drugs must be tailored to each individual. General measures involve rest and avoidance of stressful emotional experiences, sunlight, and drugs such as oral contraceptive pills that can trigger lupus flares. Patients with lupus should always wear sunscreen when they are exposed to sunlight.

TABLE 35–3

Drugs Commonly Used in Lupus Treatment

Drug	Use
NSAIDs	Mild arthritis or serositis
Steroids	
High dose	Potentially life-threatening severe neuropsychiatric conditions, pulmonary hemorrhage, rapidly progressing renal failure
Low dose	Hemolytic anemia, thrombocytopenia, NSAID-resistant arthritis, mild glomerulonephritis
Hydroxychloroquine	Mild disease, dermatitis, arthritis; steroid-sparing
Cyclophosphamide*	Severe organ involvement, glomerulonephritis, CNS disease
Azathioprine[†]	Potentially life-threatening disease, severe vasculitis, nephritis

*Cyclophosphamide can cause GI and bone marrow toxicity. Intravenous treatment can cause nausea and vomiting. Reversible alopecia occurs in 50% of patients. Infertility can also result.

[†]Azathioprine is less effective, but safer than cyclophosphamide and takes up to 3 months for the full effect. It can cause GI or bone marrow toxicity. Long-term use may result in a slightly higher rate of certain malignancies.

What features suggest a better or worse prognosis for patients with lupus?

The following are associated with a worse prognosis: renal disease, hypertension, male gender, young age or older age of onset, black race, poor socioeconomic status, antiphospholipid antibodies, and highly active disease.

K E Y   P O I N T S

▶ SLE is diagnosed clinically by satisfying at least 4 of 11 diagnostic criteria.

▶ The ANA is nearly always positive with lupus (greater than 95% sensitivity), but some patients with a positive ANA do not have lupus (not very specific).

▶ Anti–double-stranded DNA has low sensitivity and high specificity: Only 70% of patients with SLE have anti–double-stranded DNA, but when it is present, the patient usually has lupus.

▶ Double-stranded DNA levels predict flares when they are elevated, but ANAs do not.

▶ Photosensitivity is a very common problem in SLE.

CASE 35–5. A 30-year-old African-American woman reports six months of fatigue and painful swollen wrists, fingers, knees, and ankles that are worst for the first thirty minutes after she gets out of bed. In the past she has had intermittent episodes of rash after sun exposure, sharp chest pain, painless sores on the roof of her mouth, and a spontaneous abortion. Exam reveals normal vitals signs, an erythematous rash over her cheeks and nose that spares the nasolabial folds. Joint examination reveals tender but mild spongy swelling of the wrists, MCP joints, and ankles bilaterally.

     A. What is the most likely diagnosis, and what are some other possible diagnoses?
     B. Which of the 11 criteria of lupus does this patient meet?
     C. Which labs should you send next, and how will they affect your management of this patient?
     D. What initial therapy would you recommend for this patient?

VASCULITIS

▶ ETIOLOGY

What causes vasculitis?

Vasculitis results from inflammation of blood vessels, usually owing to immune complex deposition. This inflammation will affect the organ involved, e.g., renal failure in the kidney, purpuric rash in the skin, aortitis in large vessel disease, and foot drop in vasculitic neuropathy. Vasculitis can occur as a primary process or in association with various systemic diseases, such as rheumatoid arthritis or systemic lupus. When immune complexes play a role, size and charge may be important in determining which vessels and organ systems are involved. A good example of immune complex–mediated vasculitis is chronic hepatitis B and C infections causing renal failure and rash. Purpuric rash of cutaneous vasculitis can result from bacteremia with *Neisseria gonorrhoeae, Neisseria meningitidis,* or rickettsia. The cell type (lymphocytes, neutrophils, or eosinophils) also helps determine the pattern of vascular inflammation.

How are the various forms of vasculitis classified?

Classification is currently based on size of the vessels involved (large, medium, and small) with three major syndromes in each category (Table 35–4).

What illnesses can mimic vasculitis?

Patients with atrial myxoma or endocarditis can present with fever, weight loss, stroke-like symptoms, purpuric rash, Raynaud's phenomenon, and high ESR. Cholesterol emboli may cause livedo

TABLE 35–4

Examples of Vasculitis Categorized by Size of Vessel Typically Affected

Large Vessel	Medium Vessel	Small Vessel
Giant cell/temporal arteritis	Polyarteritis nodosa	Hypersensitivity: drugs, hepatitis C, HSP, SBE
Takayasu's arteritis	Churg-Strauss vasculitis	Wegener's granulomatosis
Systemic disease: RA, ankylosing spondylitis, syphilis	Connective tissue disease-associated: RA, lupus	Microscopic polyarteritis nodosa

reticularis (a diffuse, lacy, violaceous skin discoloration) and non-palpable purpura along with an elevated ESR, renal insufficiency, active urinary sediment, and eosinophilia. Cocaine use may also cause a vasculitis.

▶ **EVALUATION**

When should I consider vasculitis in the differential diagnosis?

Abnormalities of several organ systems at the same time, such as the kidneys (renal failure), skin (palpable purpura), and nerves (foot drop), are classic features of many forms of vasculitis. Systemic symptoms such as fever, anorexia, and weight loss are common. Diagnosis usually hinges on a biopsy showing vessel inflammation. Especially remember a foot drop or wrist drop as potential signs of vasculitis.

How does large-vessel vasculitis present?

Giant cell arteritis (temporal arteritis) is seen in people older than age 55 especially in those of Northern European extraction. Symptoms include headache, jaw claudication (pain in the chewing muscles with chewing), transient or permanent loss of vision, tenderness over the temporal scalp, fever, and weight loss. Polymyalgia rheumatica occurs in 50% of patients with giant cell arteritis and is characterized by proximal muscle pain without weakness, which distinguishes it from polymyositis. ESR is usually greater than 100. Diagnosis of giant cell arteritis is suggested by clinical picture and confirmed by temporal artery biopsy. Takayasu arteritis is most often reported in young women, especially Asian, and is one of the major causes of renovascular hypertension in Asian young adults. Inflammation and stenosis occurs in the aorta and vessels arising from the aortic arch. Renal and CNS arteries can also be affected. ESR is high.

Diagnosis is by arteriogram. Large artery involvement, especially of the proximal aorta, can be seen in miscellaneous systemic diseases such as ankylosing spondylitis, reactive arthritis, syphilis, relapsing polychondritis and, rarely, rheumatoid arthritis.

How does the patient with medium vessel vasculitis present?

Polyarteritis nodosa (PAN) affects small- and medium-sized muscular arteries. Target organs include the CNS, peripheral nerves, intestines, and kidneys. An isolated cutaneous form exists as well. PAN may be associated with chronic hepatitis B, hairy cell leukemia, HIV infection, or amphetamine abuse. ESR is often high and an active urinary sediment is frequently present. Diagnosis is based on arteriographic demonstration of vasculitis, with or without aneurysms especially in renal arteries. Biopsy of nerve, muscle, or testicular tissue is often useful. Churg-Strauss vasculitis affects similar vessels as PAN with less renal and much more pulmonary involvement. Distinctive features include a history of asthma in almost all patients, formation of granulomas, and eosinophilic infiltrates in the lungs and vessels. Diagnosis is similar to PAN. Connective tissue diseases such as rheumatoid arthritis or lupus may have an associated PAN-like vasculitis.

How does the patient with small vessel vasculitis present?

Wegener's granulomatosis classically involves a triad of upper respiratory tract, lung, and kidneys, but patients may present in a more limited fashion as well. Skin, eyes, and joints may also be involved. Antineutrophil cytoplasmic antibody is usually positive, with a cytoplasmic pattern of staining, called *c-ANCA*. This serology has not replaced the need for open lung biopsy to confirm diagnosis. Wegener's can be a culprit causing chronic sinusitis or saddle nose deformity. Microscopic polyarteritis nodosa (MPAN) is a small-vessel version of PAN with similar organ involvement. Both c-ANCA and p-ANCA (perinuclear antineutrophil cytoplasmic antibody) patterns are seen in these patients. Hypersensitivity vasculitis is a group of different diseases that typically causes a leukocytoclastic vasculitis of the skin, characterized by neutrophilic infiltrate with neutrophil fragmentation in and around the small capillaries and venules. Skin is most often involved, showing petechiae or purpura, especially on the lower extremities. Kidneys and bowel can also be involved depending on the cause. Etiologies include drugs (penicillin, sulfa) and other causes of serum sickness, subacute bacterial endocarditis (SBE), Henoch-Schönlein purpura (HSP), mixed essential cryoglobulinemia (now known to be caused primarily by hepatitis C), and other connective tissue diseases (Table 35–5).

What other vasculitis syndromes should I be aware of?

Primary CNS vasculitis is a small and medium vessel vasculitis limited to the CNS, which can cause stroke in young adults. It is seen in patients who abuse amphetamines, after recent herpes infection involving the eye, or with Hodgkin's lymphoma. Thromboangiitis obliterans (Buerger's disease) occurs most often in men who smoke and may represent a hypersensitivity to nicotine. It is characterized by panarteritis or panphlebitis with thrombosis and typically involves medium and small vessels of the lower extremities. Symptoms may include claudication (painful leg muscles with walking), Raynaud-like phenomena, and superficial thrombophlebitis.

TABLE 35-5

Common Clinical Manifestations of Vasculitic Syndromes

Syndrome	CNS	Lung	Kidney	Skin	Nerve
Large Vessel					
Temporal arteritis	Headache, blindness, rare stroke			Rare scalp infarct	
Takayasu's arteritis	Eye disease, strokes		Renovascular hypertension	Rare	
Medium Vessel					
Polyarteritis nodosa	Strokes	Infiltrates, hemoptysis	Hematuria to renal failure	Ulcers, ischemic digits, livedo reticularis	Mononeuritis multiplex, peripheral neuropathy
Churg–Strauss vasculitis	Strokes	Infiltrates very common, Hx of asthma	Rare	Similar to PAN	Similar to PAN
Small Vessel					
Hypersensitivity vasculitis	Rare	Rare infiltrates	Glomerulonephritis seen with several syndromes	Leukocytoclastic vasculitis typical	Peripheral neuropathy
Wegener's granulomatosis	Eye involvement, rare strokes	Infiltrates, nodules, cavitating lesions	Glomerulonephritis very common	Purpura, petechiae common	Peripheral neuropathy
Microscopic polyarteritis nodosa	Rare stroke	Infiltrates	Glomerulonephritis common	Purpura, petechiae common	Peripheral neuropathy

► **TREATMENT**

Treat giant cell arteritis with high-dose steroids to prevent blindness that can occur suddenly. Steroids and methotrexate are used for Takayasu's arteritis, with surgery if necessary to bypass stenotic vessels. Treat PAN, MPAN, and primary CNS vasculitis with steroids and cyclophosphamide. Cyclophosphamide is the drug of choice for Wegener's; methotrexate may be useful also. Some patients with mild, limited disease may also respond to TMP-SMX. For Buerger's disease, counsel patients to stop smoking. Surgery and immunosuppressive therapy may be of benefit to some of these patients.

K E Y   P O I N T S

► Headache or fever of unknown origin in the elderly could be from giant cell arteritis.

► Aortic regurgitation in a young man could be from ankylosing spondylitis or a reactive arthritis.

► Acute onset of foot drop or wrist drop could be polyarteritis nodosum.

► Polymyalgia rheumatica is an important cause of shoulder or neck pain and stiffness in elderly patients. About 10%–20% of these patients develop giant cell arteritis.

► Petechiae or purpura associated with vasculitis are raised and palpable; in contrast, noninflammatory disorders such as platelet abnormalities cause nonpalpable purpura.

► Think about primary CNS vasculitis in a young person with a stroke.

► Polyarteritis nodosum is often associated with chronic hepatitis B infection.

► Hepatitis C is an important cause of small vessel vasculitis by formation of cryoglobulins.

CASE 35–6. A 63-year-old white woman with a history of hypothyroidism and hypertension reports feeling unwell for one month. She has lost 5 lbs and has had frequent low-grade fevers as well as stiffness in the shoulders and low back when she awakes in the morning. She has a history of migraine headaches but over the last month she has had a more persistent right-sided headache. She attributes her weight loss to the fact that her jaw gets tired as she eats. She takes estrogen, progesterone, thyroxine, and acetaminophen with codeine. Exam reveals BP 140/85 in both arms, weight 154 lbs, T 38°C, mild tenderness of the right temporal scalp, and mildly reduced ROM in both shoulders.

A. What is the most likely diagnosis?
B. What are the appropriate diagnostic tests?
C. What would you recommend for treatment?

CASE 35–7. A 45-year-old white woman with a history of joint pain and positive rheumatoid factor presents with "red bumps" all over her legs. She reports using IV drugs as a teenager for six months. Current medication is ibuprofen 400 mg TID. On examination, there is no evidence of active swelling of joints of the hands, wrists, or feet. There are numerous palpable petechiae on the lower extremities below the knees.

A. What is the likely diagnosis?
B. What are the appropriate diagnostic tests?
C. What would you recommend for treatment?

36

Substance Abuse

ALCOHOL

▶ ETIOLOGY

How common are alcohol-related problems?

Up to half of all men have temporary alcohol-related problems, and 10%–20% of men and 5%–10% of women have persistent alcohol-related problems, defined as alcohol use causing legal, marital, physical, or interpersonal problems.

Why do patients who use alcohol have electrolyte problems?

Chronic use of alcohol causes renal magnesium wasting from tubular cells. Magnesium is important in maintaining a normal potassium level; low magnesium levels lead to potassium loss and hypokalemia. Adequate magnesium levels are also important in normal parathyroid hormone production and release. With hypomagnesemia, inadequate parathyroid hormone levels lead to low 1,25-dihydroxyvitamin D, calcium, and phosphate levels. Poor nutrition decreases phosphate intake, and phosphate loss in the urine occurs in the setting of hypomagnesemia.

Why do patients with alcoholism develop alcoholic ketoacidosis?

Alcoholic ketoacidosis occurs in the patient who habitually drinks heavily, but has stopped drinking one to two days before presentation. The patient often has not had anything to eat or drink over the preceding twelve to twenty-four hours due to nausea and abdominal pain. Blood gas findings show a moderate acidosis, chemistry shows a low HCO_3, and serum ketones are elevated with predominance of β-hydroxybutyrate. During the starvation state, counter regulatory hormones produce a marked increase in serum free fatty acids. Alcohol suppresses ketogenesis initially, but as the alcohol level falls, there is rapid conversion of fatty acids to ketones.

▶ EVALUATION

How can I recognize and diagnose alcohol-related problems?

Suspect alcohol abuse in patients with trauma, motor vehicle accidents, or unexplained abdominal pain. Consider alcohol use in patients with hypertension or osteoporosis because alcohol is an important secondary cause of osteoporosis, especially in men. Ask all patients if they consume alcohol. If the answer is no, ask if they have had problems with alcohol in the past. Patients who are currently using alcohol can be screened with CAGE questions (Box 36–1). CAGE questions have a sensitivity of 80% and a specificity of 85% if a cut-off of two or more positive responses is used. They are less sensitive in women and ethnic minorities.

What cardiovascular abnormalities are seen with alcohol abuse?

There is a firm link between chronic alcohol consumption and hypertension. This is seen in people who drink three or more drinks a day and is a common cause of secondary hypertension. "Holiday heart" is a syndrome of paroxysmal arrhythmias, the most common of which is atrial fibrillation, described in alcohol binge drinkers. Other arrhythmias include atrial flutter, paroxysmal atrial tachycardia, and ventricular tachycardia. Alcohol is an important cause in up to 50% of congestive cardiomyopathy cases. There is some reversibility of symptoms with cessation of alcohol use.

What are the acute and chronic effects of alcohol on the liver?

Alcoholic hepatitis from an acute alcohol binge presents variably from asymptomatic liver function test abnormalities to a florid, acute, life-threatening liver failure. Usually, it is insidious with

BOX 36–1

CAGE Questions Used to Screen for Alcohol Abuse

Have you ever felt you should Cut down on your drinking?
Have people Annoyed you by criticizing your drinking?
Have you ever felt Guilty about your drinking?"
Have you ever started the day by having a drink to get going or calm your nerves (Eye opener)?

anorexia, nausea, vomiting, abdominal pain, and low-grade fever. Physical exam usually reveals an enlarged, tender liver. Evidence of portal hypertension (severe hemorrhoids, ascites, and GI bleeding from esophageal varices) and hepatic encephalopathy may be present in severe cases. Liver enzymes are mildly or moderately elevated—AST more so than ALT (Table 36–1). Cirrhosis develops in 10%–20% of chronic alcoholics. It develops at a lower daily alcohol intake in women owing to 50% less alcohol dehydrogenase in their stomachs, resulting in decreased immediate metabolism of alcohol. In many patients, cirrhosis is unrecognized until a life-threatening complication such as esophageal variceal bleeding occurs. Check liver synthetic function with prothrombin time (PT) and albumin.

What are the different CNS complications seen with alcohol use?

Acute intoxication can cause ataxia, incoordination, and drowsiness. Large amounts of alcohol, especially in individuals without

TABLE 36–1

Lab Abnormalities Seen with Heavy Regular Alcohol Use

Abnormal Lab	Cause
Hematology	
Anemia	
Microcytic	Iron deficiency due to GI blood loss
Macrocytic with mildly increased MCV	Liver disease/direct effect on stem cells
Macrocytic with markedly increased MCV	Folate deficiency
Thrombocytopenia	Decreased platelet survival and/or hypersplenism due to cirrhosis
Leukopenia	Decreased marrow production of WBC
Abdominal	
Increased AST > increased ALT (AST rarely ever >300)	Alcoholic hepatitis
Increased GGT	"Alcohol use test", very sensitive to alcohol use
Decreased albumin	Alcoholic hepatitis or cirrhosis
Increased PT	
Increased amylase	Pancreatitis
Minerals/Electrolytes	
Decreased magnesium	Renal tubular magnesium wasting
Decreased potassium	Renal potassium loss worsened by magnesium deficiency
Decreased calcium	Hypomagnesemia decreases parathyroid hormone release, causing poor GI calcium absorption
Decreased phosphate	Poor nutrition, increased urinary loss

chronic use, can cause coma. Wernicke/Korsakoff syndrome is a nutritional neurologic disorder caused by thiamine deficiency. It commonly goes unrecognized. The clinical manifestations of Wernicke's encephalopathy are acute onset of oculo-motor abnormalities (bilateral abducens palsy, nystagmus, total ophthalmoplegia), ataxia, and global confusional state. Other symptoms that can occur include hypothermia, hypotension, and coma. All these symptoms may reverse with administra-tion of thiamine. Eighty percent of patients with Wernicke's encephalopathy who survive will develop Korsakoff's psychosis, which is characterized by retrograde and anterograde amnesia. Confabulation, the fabrication of stories, may be present. A sig-nificant proportion of patients with Korsakoff's psychosis do not recover and require long-term institutionalization. Chronic alco-hol use can cause peripheral neuropathy, which involves the feet first, then the hands in a "stocking and glove" distribution.

What are the symptoms of alcohol withdrawal?

Most patients with chronic alcohol use have mild withdrawal symptoms of tremor, sleep disturbance, and increased anxiety. In addition, tachycardia and increased temperature can occur. A small number (less than 5%) can have severe withdrawal with marked confusion and hallucinations (delirium tremens). Alcohol withdrawal seizures occur in a small percentage of patients, usu-ally in the first two days after cessation of alcohol. A history of withdrawal seizures increases the risk of recurrence with sub-sequent episodes of withdrawal.

▶ TREATMENT

How is alcohol withdrawal treated?

For mild withdrawal symptoms of tachycardia and jitteriness, a β-blocker can be helpful. Benzodiazepines are the mainstay of treat-ment of alcohol withdrawal. Longer-acting benzodiazepines, such as diazepam, are effective but are more likely to cause prolonged sedation owing to drug accumulation. Lorazepam has an inter-mediate half-life and thus better elimination in the elderly and in patients with renal insufficiency.

What other treatments should be given to hospitalized alcoholics?

Most patients have magnesium deficiency and should receive IV magnesium. All should receive thiamine 100 mg IV daily for three doses as well as a daily multiple vitamin with folate.

When should I hospitalize a patient with complications of alcohol use?

Hospitalize patients with the following:

■ Alcohol withdrawal with mental status changes or unstable vital signs
■ Metabolic disturbances that are severe (hypokalemia, alcoholic ketoacidosis)
■ Severe alcoholic hepatitis with recurrent emesis or signs of portal hypertension or encephalopathy
■ Patients desiring inpatient alcohol treatment, in order to facilitate transfer to a program

---

K E Y   P O I N T S

▶ Multiple mineral/electrolyte disorders occur with chronic alcohol use; hypomagnesemia is probably the most important and leads to hypokalemia and hypocalcemia.

▶ Alcoholic hepatitis can mimic acute cholecystitis with fever, leukocytosis, and RUQ pain.

▶ Transaminases are usually only modestly elevated with AST greater than ALT in alcoholic hepatitis.

▶ Alcohol use is an extremely common cause of secondary hypertension in the U.S.

CASE 36–1. A 39-year-old man with a history of alcohol abuse presents with nausea, vomiting, and abdominal pain. He has had low-grade fevers as well, and has been drinking 18–24 beers a day.

   A. What is your differential diagnosis for his abdominal pain?
   B. What lab tests would you order?
   C. His potassium is 2.9. What other electrolytes would you expect to be abnormal?

CASE 36–2. A 49-year-old man with a twenty-year history of alcohol abuse is admitted with confusion and weakness. His last drink was twenty-four hours ago. He usually drinks three to four bottles of wine daily. On exam he is tremulous with P of 128 and BP of 160/100. He is oriented only to person. Labs: Na–136, K–3.0, HCO_3–13, BUN–20, Creatinine–1.0, Glu–60, Cl–98, serum osmolality–280.

   A. What is the most likely cause for his metabolic acidosis? How would you treat it?

   B. What is appropriate therapy for his alcohol withdrawal?

REFERENCE

Chang PH, Steinberg MB: Alcohol withdrawal. Med Clin North Am 85(5):1191–1212, 2001.

COCAINE

► ETIOLOGY

How and why do people use cocaine?

Cocaine is derived from the leaves of the coca plant and has been chewed as a stimulant for thousands of years. The user gains a euphoric sense of boundless energy and self-confidence. Users can be hypersexual, angry, or violent. The drug is metabolized quickly, and the high is followed by a "crash," during which the user feels depressed and irritable. Drug craving sets in during this period. Powdered cocaine can be used intranasally (snorted), which gives a less intense high and is most expensive. Dissolved in water, cocaine can be injected intravenously, which gives an immediate and intense high. When no vein is available, cocaine can be injected subcutaneously ("skin-popping") or intramuscularly ("muscling").

"Crack" is a cheap smokable form of cocaine that gives a very brief but intense high. Its introduction in the 1980s was associated with a surge in drug-related crime, violence, and social problems across the country.

▶ EVALUATION

How do I know cocaine is causing a patient's problem?

Ask every patient about drug and alcohol use. People who do not offer information about their drug use at first will sometimes admit it if you tell them how important it is in order to treat their immediate problem. Urine drug screens detect cocaine for at least 48 hours after use.

What are the medical complications of cocaine use?

Cocaine causes centrally mediated sympathetic overdrive, with tachycardia, hypertension, and vasospasm of coronary and cerebral arteries. Seizures, hypertensive encephalopathy, and ischemic and hemorrhagic strokes are common neurologic sequelae. Chest pain and dysrhythmias, such as supraventricular tachycardia, ventricular tachycardia, and ventricular fibrillation, are the most common cardiac complications. Rhabdomyolysis, acidosis, fever, and coma are additional results that can be rapidly fatal. Less serious are nonhealing scabs and shallow skin ulcers that result from uncontrollable picking and the sensation of bugs on the skin (formication), which occurs even in noninjection users, and epistaxis and septal necrosis in intranasal users.

If cocaine is a stimulant, why do users present with decreased consciousness?

At very high doses, cocaine's local anesthetic effect predominates over its stimulant effect and causes life-threatening coma. People who have been on a cocaine binge become profoundly lethargic for hours or days after they stop, a condition called "post-cocaine depression" or "cocaine washed-out syndrome."

▶ TREATMENT

How do I treat cocaine-related medical problems?

Intravenous diazepam is the primary treatment for most types of cocaine toxicity. By decreasing centrally mediated sympathetic overdrive, diazepam reduces agitation, seizures, hypertension, tachycardia, and vasospasm-mediated chest pain. Even ventricular tachycardia and ventricular fibrillation, if cocaine-induced, should be treated with diazepam in addition to the usual defibrillation. If diazepam alone does not control blood pressure, labetalol and nitroprusside are good choices. Pure β-blocker drugs, such as esmolol and metoprolol, cause unopposed α-adrenergic stimulation and worsen the situation.

A patient with chest pain that resolves with diazepam and shows no ischemic ECG changes can be safely discharged, but ischemic changes on ECG and/or elevated cardiac enzymes require admission and standard therapy for acute MI. Rhabdomyolysis, confirmed by a high serum CPK and positive urine myoglobin, is frequently fatal and requires IV diazepam, IV bicarbonate, and aggressive hydration.

HEROIN

▶ ETIOLOGY

How and why are opioid drugs abused?

Opioids are naturally derived or synthetic drugs that mimic the effects of opium, producing pain relief, relaxation, sleep, and a powerful sense of well-being. These are also called narcotics. Oral narcotics, extensively used for medical pain relief, can be abused. A much more potent "high" comes from IV use. Heroin is the most commonly injected narcotic, but morphine, meperidine, and fentanyl are also available. Heroin may also be smoked or snorted. A "speedball" refers to injecting heroin and cocaine together.

▶ EVALUATION

What are the toxic effects of heroin?

A heroin overdose occurs when the user takes enough heroin to suppress the respiratory drive. He or she is found unconscious and apneic with pinpoint pupils. Prolonged apnea leads to hypoxic brain injury and may be complicated by aspiration, hypothermia, and/or rhabdomyolysis from prolonged immobility. With frequent use, tolerance develops to the respiratory depressant effect of opioids. A common situation for heroin overdose is a user who has been abstinent for a period of time, then uses the same amount to which he or she was previously accustomed. Noncardiogenic pulmonary edema can occur after IV narcotic use in both new and experienced users. Its etiology is unknown.

How can I identify heroin overdose?

Most overdose patients are treated by prehospital personnel with naloxone, an opioid antagonist, and are therefore alert when they reach the hospital. Naloxone can be safely used on any unconscious patient as a diagnostic maneuver. A response proves opioid intoxication.

How can I identify heroin withdrawal?

Narcotic withdrawal begins as soon as a chronic user misses an expected dose. The longest-acting opioids, such as methadone, produce the longest-lasting withdrawal syndrome. Along with dysphoria and drug craving, physical symptoms include some or all of the following: nausea, vomiting, diarrhea, abdominal cramping and pain, lacrimation, rhinorrhea, yawning, chills, diaphoresis, myalgias, piloerection (goose flesh, thus "quitting cold turkey"), and involuntary muscle jerks ("kicking the habit"). Fever is not part of narcotic withdrawal, and any heroin user with a fever needs an aggressive search for an infection.

▶ TREATMENT

When should I treat heroin overdose?

A patient who has hypoxia due to slow or ineffective respirations needs naloxone (IV or IM). If the patient does not immediately recover normal mental status, consider intubation to protect the airway and provide adequate air exchange. It is essential to consider other causes of depressed mental status in this case. Patients successfully treated with naloxone may become sleepy as the drug wears off, but if they are successfully oxygenating one hour after naloxone was given, are fully arousable, and have no infectious complications of their injection drug use, they may be safely discharged. Overdose of long-acting narcotics, usually methadone, requires frequent redosing of naloxone and, therefore, the patient should be admitted.

How can I treat heroin withdrawal in a hospitalized patient?

The symptoms of withdrawal are alleviated by substituting a longer acting narcotic such as methadone for heroin. Withdrawal from methadone also occurs, but a hospitalization can be a transition to a structured detoxification program or a long-term methadone maintenance program. Although heroin withdrawal is intensely uncomfortable, unlike alcohol or benzodiazepine withdrawal, the syndrome is not physically dangerous. Clonidine is an alternative to methadone as it lessens narcotic withdrawal symptoms.

INFECTIOUS COMPLICATIONS OF PARENTERAL DRUG ABUSE

▶ ETIOLOGY

What types of infections affect intravenous drug users?

Shared needles transmit viral infections from user to user, including hepatitis B, hepatitis C (present in about 80% of injection drug users), and HIV. Nonsterile injection also causes local bacterial infections, including open ulcers from "skin popping," deeper skin abscesses, and cellulitis from intravenous use, and large, deep intramuscular abscesses from "muscling." Injected cocaine causes local vasoconstriction and thus tissue necrosis, so cocaine-related abscesses are generally larger and more difficult to heal. Bacterial cultures reveal *staphylococci, streptococci, pseudomonads*, and oral flora including anaerobes (in users who lick their needles). Tetanus may be present. Every injection causes a transient bacteremia, with the potential for developing endocarditis, meningitis, septic pulmonary emboli, and lumbar osteomyelitis or epidural abscess. A depressed gag reflex during heroin use makes aspiration pneumonia common. Socioeconomic factors and poor immune function increase the risk of TB.

▶ EVALUATION

How do bacterial infections differ in drug users?

Because of impaired immunity, elevated WBC and fever are often absent in drug users with a serious infection. Cellulitis, abscesses, and osteomyelitis are best diagnosed by exam. CXR is essential to diagnosing pneumonia, although individuals with AIDS may have pneumonia but a normal film. If fever is present in an injection drug user, it strongly suggests infection.

What primary care might specifically benefit patients who use intravenous drugs?

Primary care for the injection drug user is an emerging concept currently lacking supporting data; these patients' high risk of acquiring and transmitting a variety of infections makes the following steps sound reasonable. Screen for HIV; hepatitis A, B, and C; and TB (by PPD). For patients who have not been exposed to hepatitis A or B, strongly consider vaccination. Hepatitis A vaccine is especially important in patients who have hepatitis C. Pneumococcal vaccine may also be warranted. Because up to

50% of women who are injection drug users participate in prostitution, regular screening for gonorrhea, *Chlamydia*, and cervical cancer is also wise.

▶ TREATMENT

Who needs hospitalization for a drug-associated bacterial infection?

Any injection drug user with a fever greater than 38.5°C should be hospitalized and treated presumptively for endocarditis with nafcillin and gentamicin. If another infection is present that could account for the fever, such as pneumonia or cellulitis, it is appropriate to tailor antibiotics to that illness while ruling out endocarditis with blood cultures. Cellulitis alone or a patient with an abscess that can be drained in the clinic can be treated on an outpatient basis with oral antibiotics, such as cephalexin or dicloxacillin. Abscesses should be packed once or twice a day.

K E Y   P O I N T S

▶ Cocaine has many potentially fatal toxic effects, most mediated by sympathetic overdrive.

▶ Heroin overdose causes respiratory depression and is reversible with naloxone.

▶ Heroin, cocaine, and methamphetamine do not have physically dangerous withdrawal syndromes, unlike alcohol or benzodiazepines.

CASE 36–3. A 19-year-old college student comes to you because of arm pain. Her left antecubital fossa has a 6 cm by 10 cm area of erythema, induration, warmth, and tenderness. You can easily see multiple tiny needle punctures along the vein. You suspect this is a complication of injection drug abuse.

   A. How would you approach asking her about drug use?
   B. What structures may be affected by this infection?
   C. What therapies are appropriate? How will her drug use change your management?

CASE 36–4. A 43-year-old man sees you in the office for chronic abdominal pain and constipation. He has seen multiple physicians for this problem but no diagnosis has been found. He is angry because his last doctor suggested that his main problem is addiction to pain pills. In fact, he has been taking large quantities of oral narcotics for many years, prescribed for multiple musculoskeletal pains.

A. If this assessment is correct, what do you think will happen if he stops taking all opiates?

B. How would you counsel this patient?

REFERENCE

Emergency Medicine Clinics of North America. 8(3):481–493, 495–511, 613–652, 665–681, 1990. The entire volume of this journal is devoted to diagnosis and treatment of complications of illicit drug use.

USEFUL WEBSITE

National Institute on Drug Abuse (NIDA) Website: Valuable information and resources for patients, families, health care providers, and researchers. http://165.112.78.61/NIDAHome.html

37

Women's Health

ABNORMAL PAP SMEARS

▶ ETIOLOGY

What causes abnormal Pap smears?

The Pap smear, or Papanicolaou test, is the most widely available screening test for cervical cancer. Risk factors for atypical Pap smears, also known as cervical dysplasia, include multiple sexual partners (more than two), early age of sexual intercourse (younger than age 17), history of sexually transmitted disease, HIV infection, oral contraceptive use, and tobacco use. Certain subtypes of human papillomavirus (HPV) appear to play a key role in most cases of cervical dysplasia. Other reasons for abnormal Pap smears include hormonal changes, inflammation related to vaginal infections, or artifacts related to Pap smear collection. Such changes are generally and easily identified by the cytopathologist.

▶ EVALUATION

How often should Pap smears be obtained?

Although prior practice has been annual Pap testing, some data suggest that a three-year period may be just as effective in women at low risk of acquiring HPV (those women with mutually monogamous partners, and with good records documenting multiple normal Pap smears). Women who have had a hysterectomy for reasons other than cervical cancer do not need pap smears.

How is the Pap smear result interpreted?

Most cytopathologists use the Bethesda classification system for reporting Pap smear findings. This system reports "squamous intraepithelial cell" lesions (cervical dysplastic changes) separately from "specimen adequacy" and "benign cellular changes."

Cervical dysplasia is a precancerous condition, requiring follow-up surveillance to detect progression to cancer. Cervical dysplasia is usually reported as ASCUS (atypical cells of undetermined significance), LGSIL (low-grade squamous intraepithelial lesion), or HGSIL (high-grade squamous intraepithelial lesion). Each finding should be triaged for appropriate follow-up (Figure 37–1), either repeated Pap smear or colposcopic examination. Colposcopy allows the clinician to view the cervix under low-power magnification and to biopsy cervical tissue to confirm cytologic findings of the Pap smear.

What role does HPV subtyping play in managing cervical dysplasia?

HPV strains have been differentiated into high, intermediate, and low risk types for causing cervical cancer. High risk types 16 and 18 are strongly correlated with carcinoma-in-situ or invasive carcinoma, and research is currently under way to identify vaccines against these strains. Use of HPV subtyping in triaging patients with ASCUS or LGSIL for colposcopy has been controversial. Most experts agree that, although HPV subtyping may be useful in managing women with ASCUS in the future, broader application requires further investigation.

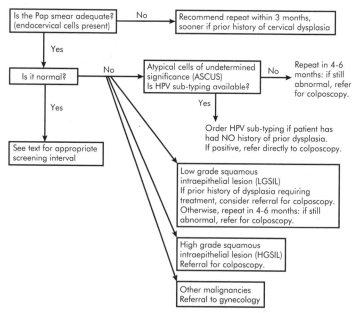

Figure 37–1. Algorithm for management of abnormal Pap smears.

▶ TREATMENT

How is cervical dysplasia treated?

Treatment options depend on the extent of disease and invasive potential. Conservative outpatient approaches include cryotherapy, laser vaporization, and the loop electrical excision procedure (LEEP). Surgical conization is indicated when patients have more severe dysplastic changes or when the transformation zone is not well visualized.

K E Y   P O I N T S

- ▶ Risk factors associated with cervical dysplasia include HPV infection, early first intercourse, multiple sexual partners, and tobacco use.

- ▶ Refer for colposcopy when HGSIL is identified.

- ▶ Refer for colposcopy when repeated ASCUS or LGSIL changes are found on follow-up surveillance.

CASE 37–1. A 39-year-old woman has a Pap smear result reading "atypical cells of undetermined significance (ASCUS), condylomatous changes present." Her history is negative for previous atypical Pap smears. When you call her to discuss the results, she seems very anxious. She has read that HPV causes cervical cancer. She insists on being referred to an oncologist.

   A. What will you recommend to her?
   B. What is the relationship between HPV and cervical dysplasia?

REFERENCE

Solomon D, Schiffman M, Tarone R: Comparison of three management strategies for patients with atypical squamous cells of undetermined significance: Baseline results from a randomized trial. J Natl Cancer Inst 93:293, 2001.

ABNORMAL UTERINE BLEEDING

▶ ETIOLOGY

How do we define abnormal bleeding?

Menstrual irregularity is one of the most frequent presenting symptoms in women. Normal menarche generally occurs before the age of 16 with a normal ovulatory cycle repeating approximately every 23 to 39 days and menstrual flow lasting from two to seven days. Abnormalities in menstrual cycle bleeding are characterized using specific terminology (Table 37–1), and any combination of these is possible.

What are common causes of abnormal uterine bleeding?

Differential diagnosis depends on age and bleeding pattern. Always consider pregnancy first with any abnormal bleeding pattern. Aside from pregnancy, other causes are structural, hormonal, infectious, or neoplastic (Table 37–2). Endometrial or cervical polyps, uterine fibroids, and coagulopathies can cause heavy bleeding, usually during menses without changing menstrual cycle timing. Irregular and infrequent bleeding that has persisted ever since onset of menarche is likely due to polycystic ovary syndrome (PCO). Intermenstrual spotting can occur with pelvic infection, normal ovulation (due to the physiologic abrupt fall in estrogen at mid-cycle), or ectopic pregnancy, especially if a period has been missed. Menstrual bleeding out of phase in postmenopausal women is suspicious for endome-

TABLE 37–1

Terminology Used to Describe Abnormal Patterns of Menstrual Bleeding

Terminology	Pattern
Amenorrhea	Lack of menses for 90 days or more
Menorrhagia (hypermenorrhea)	Heavy bleeding at regular intervals with menstrual cycle (bleeding lasts > 7 days and amount is > 80 mL/day or 6 pads/day)
Metrorrhagia	Irregular bleeding (can be too frequent, or too infrequent)
Oligomenorrhea	Infrequent bleeding
Intermenstrual bleeding	Bleeding between regular menstrual cycles
Polymenorrhea	Regular bleeding at intervals < 21 days
DUB (dysfunctional uterine bleeding)	Excessive uterine bleeding in the absence of identifiable organic pathology, not during a usual cyclic bleed

TABLE 37–2

Common Causes of Abnormal Vaginal Bleeding Based on Bleeding Pattern

| | Type of bleeding | | | |
	Menorrhagia	Metrorrhagia	Postcoital	Postmenopausal
Structural causes	Fibroid Polyp Coagulation disorder IUD	Polyp	Polyp	
Hormonal causes	Hypothyroidism DUB	Anovulation PCO syndrome anorexia OCPs		HRT
Neoplastic causes	Cervical cancer Endometrial cancer	Cervical cancer Endometrial cancer	Cervical cancer	Endometrial cancer
Infectious causes		Endometritis	Cervicitis Trichomonas	

trial cancer. Cyclic bleeding may be a normal occurrence with estrogen hormone replacement therapy, especially if hormones are cycled. Hyper- and hypothyroidism can cause abnormal bleeding patterns, usually amenorrhea and menorrhagia, respectively.

What causes anovulation and how does this affect menstrual periods?

Anovulation is common in adolescent girls and in women approaching menopause. Anovulation can occur suddenly and transiently with excessive weight changes, stress, illness, or endocrine disorders that disrupt function of the hypothalamic-pituitary axis. It can also be chronic, as in polycystic ovary syndrome. Patients with chronic anovulation have unpredictable, often infrequent, and heavy bleeding due to unopposed estrogen exposure (without ovulation, there is no progesterone produced). The unopposed estrogen causes buildup and unpredictable, periodic sloughing of the endometrial lining and increases risk of endometrial cancer.

Why do some patients have abnormal bleeding on oral contraceptives?

The low doses of estrogen in most modern oral contraceptives allow the endometrial lining to atrophy and become fragile, causing breakthrough bleeding between periods. Progesterone-only regimens cause unpredictable bleeding, especially early in their use.

▶ EVALUATION

How do I evaluate patients with abnormal uterine bleeding?

The pattern of abnormality helps guide diagnostic work-up. Patients presenting with changes over one to two cycles with an otherwise unremarkable history and exam should keep a menstrual log. Ask about duration of the problem, pattern of bleeding, amount of bleeding, use of birth control, and associated symptoms such as pain or fever. Quantifying vaginal bleeding can be a challenge. It may help to ask how many pads or tampons the patient has required over a twenty-four hour period of bleeding. History of medications is also key. For example, birth control pills or Depo-Provera shots frequently cause menstrual abnormalities. Include orthostatics if bleeding is brisk, and a pelvic exam to look for anatomic causes, such as fibroids or ectopic pregnancy. Verify normal secondary sexual characteristics and look for virilization or hirsutism.

What should be my approach for evaluating postmenopausal bleeding?

Bleeding occurring after menopause is concerning because of uterine malignancy. It is a common problem in women on estrogen/progesterone, especially when first starting the medication (see menopause section). Consider dose adjustments to hormonal regimen within the first six months of therapy. Obtain an endovaginal ultrasound and/or endometrial biopsy if bleeding persists or if the patient is not on hormonal replacement.

What lab tests or studies shall I order?

Order tests sequentially on the basis of H & P findings. Urine pregnancy test and TSH can almost always be justified, as pregnancy and thyroid abnormalities are among the most common causes for atypical menses. Order HCT to detect anemia, especially if excessive bleeding is reported. Platelets and coagulation studies may be indicated if underlying medical conditions or the clinical picture suggests a clotting problem. If ectopic pregnancy is suspected, send a β-HCG level. In addition, prolactin, LH, and

FSH can be helpful if an underlying endocrine problem is suspected.

Hyperprolactinemia can cause either amenorrhea or anovulatory bleeding. Hypothalamic hypopituitarism may be suggested on the basis of amenorrhea with low body weight. Polycystic ovarian syndrome may be a consideration in patients with hirsutism, obesity, glucose intolerance, and long-standing menstrual irregularity. Cervical cultures for chlamydia and gonorrhea may be taken during the pelvic exam if PID or endometritis is suspected. Ultrasound and/or endometrial biopsy may be required on occasion to evaluate for endometrial hyperplasia or tumor.

▶ TREATMENT

What is the treatment for abnormal uterine bleeding?

Management of abnormal uterine bleeding should be directed at resolving the underlying problem. Urgent cessation of bleeding with surgical intervention may rarely be indicated. Urgent medical treatment to stop prolonged bleeding is often desirable on the basis of low blood count or patient request. If contraindications to such therapy are excluded, short-term and rapid cessation of bleeding can often be achieved with a short course of progesterone (medroxyprogesterone 10 mg qd × 10 days).

Oral contraceptive pills are used commonly for treatment of chronic anovulatory states with abnormal bleeding, such as polycystic ovarian syndrome and hypothalamic dysfunction. Cervical polyps easily visualized can be removed by simple twisting with ringed forceps. Endometrial polyps require more invasive techniques for removal. Fibroids may be followed, although they should be removed if they are growing rapidly or causing significant anemia. Endometrial cancer usually requires hysterectomy.

Trichomonas or other STD diagnoses should be treated promptly with appropriate antibiotics and should prompt testing for syphilis and HIV. Patients with heavy, prolonged dysfunctional uterine bleeding should receive hormonal therapy with estrogen or progesterone to stop the bleeding, then remain on oral contraceptives.

When should I hospitalize or refer?

Indications for urgent referral and hospitalization include excessive vaginal bleeding causing hemodynamic changes, significant drop in blood count, or suspicion of ectopic pregnancy.

CASE 37–2. A nulliparous 22-year-old woman presents for routine annual exam. She reached menarche at the age of 11 and has always had irregular periods, which generally come two to four times a year. She is not interested in birth control and she assumes that since she has irregular periods, she cannot get pregnant. She uses topical isotretinoin for acne. On exam, height is 64 inches, weight is 180 pounds. She has mild hirsutism and acanthosis nigricans. Normal secondary sex characteristics are present, and there is no evidence of virilization.

A. How will you evaluate this patient for her irregular menses?
B. What other conditions would you wish to exclude?
C. How will you counsel her regarding treatment?

BREAST HEALTH

▶ ETIOLOGY

What normal and pathologic changes are seen in breast tissue?

Benign causes of lumps are simple cysts and fibroadenomas. Atypical hyperplasia, although benign, is a risk factor for subsequent development of cancer. Carcinoma in situ and invasive carcinoma of the ducts and/or lobules are malignant lesions.

What is mastalgia?

Mastalgia means breast pain. Prevalence studies show 20% of women experience moderate to severe breast pain. Bilateral tenderness is most commonly due to cyclic hormonal changes and does not require further evaluation. Although only 6% of cancers result in pain, persistent focal pain requires biopsy.

What are risk factors for breast cancer?

Breast cancer kills more than 40,000 annually in the U.S., but women may live many years with breast cancer. Age is an important risk factor: approximately 75% of breast cancer patients over age 50 have no risk factors aside from age. Other risk factors include early menarche, late menopause, nulliparity, and atypical cells on prior breast biopsy. A family history of premenopausal breast cancer in two or more first-degree relatives may suggest the presence of a genetic predisposition to breast cancer.

▶ EVALUATION

What screening is recommended for breast cancer?

Screening patients older than age 50 with annual examination and mammogram decreases mortality from breast cancer by 30%. Mammography for women ages 40 to 50 is reasonable, but benefits are smaller, and the risk of false positive findings is greater. Screen earlier with worrisome risk factors such as BrCA-1 or BrCA-2 gene mutation, first-degree relative, or atypia on breast biopsy.

How do I perform a good breast examination?

Inspect and palpate both breasts, compressing the tissue against the chest wall firmly but gently. Be certain to examine the entire breast systematically and thoroughly, including the axillae and sub-areolar areas. Document location, size, and quality of breast examination findings. Comparing one side to the other will reduce uncertainty about what is normal versus abnormal.

What clinical presentations are worrisome for underlying cancer?

Any palpable breast lump, asymmetric thickening, or focal pain should be regarded with suspicion. Breast cancer risk factors do not substantially alter pretest probabilities of cancer and so should not play a role in the decision to evaluate. Work-up is indicated for any focal finding or symptom. It is not possible to distinguish benign from malignant conditions on physical exam, but the presence of any of the following raises concern for malignancy (most breast cancers show none of these):

- A mass fixed to the chest wall
- Dimpling of the skin overlying the breast
- Recent onset, unilateral nipple inversion
- Spontaneous nipple discharge, especially if clear or bloody
- Scaly lesions of the nipple

■ Failure of breast inflammation to respond promptly to antibiotics
■ Persistent, focal breast pain

What are the first steps in the work-up of a breast lump, thickening, or focal pain?

Order a diagnostic mammogram in all patients age 25 years or older. This differs from a screening mammogram in that it requires more time, additional views, and direct supervision by a mammographer. Breast ultrasound, an important adjunct to the evaluation of breast masses, reliably identifies benign simple cysts, helps characterize solid lesions, and direct biopsy. Begin with ultrasound in women younger than age 25 because more dense tissue makes mammogram less accurate. When mammogram or ultrasound demonstrates a clearly benign finding, such as a simple cyst or calcified fibroadenoma, no further evaluation is needed.

When should a biopsy be obtained?

Refer the patient with highly suspect lesions such as those fixed to the chest or associated with dimpling for biopsy. Patients with lesions suggestive of cancer on imaging should also undergo core needle biopsy using ultrasound or stereotactic guidance. Other palpable masses or focal thickenings warrant close follow-up by repeat exam or fine needle aspiration (FNA), even if mammography findings are normal. FNA is not a true biopsy, but it is a useful procedure for sampling cells when clinical and radiographic suspicion for malignancy is low. An abnormal FNA mandates biopsy. A mass with negative "triple test" findings (negative FNA, combined with negative mammogram, and low-suspicion clinical breast exam) has less than a 3% chance of being a missed cancer and can be followed without biopsy.

What is the appropriate follow-up for focal breast problems with normal mammogram?

Since 10% of breast cancers are not detectable on mammography, plan close clinical follow-up. Have a low threshold for consultation with a breast specialist.

How does staging determine prognosis in breast cancer patients?

Many prognostic factors help you choose therapy. Your patient will do better if the tumor is small, if it has estrogen receptors, and if it has few "S" (synthesis) phase cells. The pathologist will determine this. The most important prognostic factor is the absolute number of positive axillary lymph nodes, and so node dissection is part of every lumpectomy or mastectomy.

▶ TREATMENT

How are simple cysts and fibroadenomas managed?

For ultrasound-demonstrated simple cysts, no further follow-up is necessary. If the cyst is bothersome or interferes with examination, it can be reduced through aspiration of fluid. Complex cysts may need to be biopsied. Fibroadenomas should be closely followed. Refer patients for resection when they have fibroadenomas that are more than 2 cm in size, or if they have grown rapidly or are painful.

What alleviates breast pain?

Well-fitting bra, low-fat diet, reduced caffeine, and cyclic hormonal supplements may be effective, but data are limited. Treat infection with antibiotics and abscess with drainage.

What is the best treatment for a breast cancer lump?

Treatment depends on the stage of the cancer. For stage I, lumpectomy with radiation is as good as modified radical mastectomy. Patient preference, diffuse cancer, or large tumors may call for mastectomy. Most women are cured surgically. Patients with negative nodes, tumors smaller than 1 cm, and favorable histology have excellent prognosis and usually do not require adjuvant chemotherapy. Hormonal therapy with tamoxifen is used for estrogen receptor (ER)-positive tumors of low risk. Chemotherapy is substituted or added for ER-negative tumors, high-risk histology, or older age.

How is metastatic breast cancer treated?

Most metastases are to bone, brain, or liver. Chemotherapy is the only option for ER-negative disease. Hormonal manipulation is helpful in ER-positive patients: oophorectomy for premenopausal women and tamoxifen for postmenopausal women. If the disease progresses, progestins and androgens may be tried. Radiation can be used to control disease locally for palliation.

How effective is therapy?

Ten-year disease-free survival is nearly 75% for node-negative cancer, and 30% for invasive tumors or many positive nodes. Many people live with cancer that needs to be managed, if not cured.

K E Y   P O I N T S

▶ Most breast cancer occurs in the absence of risk factors aside from age.

▶ Physical examination cannot reliably distinguish benign from malignant conditions.

▶ Begin with diagnostic mammography for evaluation of most breast symptoms in women older than age 25.

▶ Palpable masses must be followed up with repeat exams or FNA even if mammogram findings are normal.

CASE 37–3. A 48-year-old woman reports a month-long history of a sensation of fullness in the upper outer quadrant of her left breast. You detect a 2 cm lump with indistinct margins that is mobile and without overlying skin dimpling.

    A. What is the first step in the evaluation?
    B. If the diagnostic evaluation is negative, what follow-up should be planned?
    C. What should prompt a referral to a breast surgeon?

CASE 37–4. A 28-year-old woman presents with a 2.5 cm mobile, slightly tender mass in the inferior left breast. Mammogram is negative although breast tissue is very dense.

    A. What other tests are indicated?
    B. What is appropriate follow-up if studies suggest a fibroadenoma?
    C. What is appropriate follow-up if studies suggest a simple cyst?

MENOPAUSE

▶ ETIOLOGY

What is menopause?

Natural menopause is the permanent cessation of menses and it marks a woman's entry into the postreproductive phase of life. The final menstrual period (FMP) is defined retrospectively after twelve consecutive months of amenorrhea. The menopause transition includes the years before the FMP when variability of the menstrual cycles increases. This transition period and the twelve months following the FMP are defined as the perimenopause. The perimenopause is a period of physiologic disruption due to fluctuating levels of hormones and symptoms. Following menopause, the incidence of both coronary artery disease and osteoporosis increases significantly.

What is a hot flash?

A hot flash (HF) is a symptom complex caused by the sudden downward resetting of the central core temperature set point. This results in a sensation of heat and the initiation of heat-dissipating mechanisms such as vasodilatation, sweating, and reflex tachycardia. Hot flashes are more frequent and can be quite severe in the perimenopause and decline in following years. They are a common reason women seek care at perimenopause.

Can menopause cause depression?

Major depression and anxiety disorders are not associated with menopause and are in fact less prevalent than earlier in life. Mood swings may be associated with sleep problems leading to daytime irritability, forgetfulness, and fatigue. Perimenopause is also a time of profound social and psychologic change for women: children leave home, elderly parents need assistance, work roles and relationships with spouses may change. The stresses and health effects of these life events may be falsely attributed to coincidental biologic changes associated with menopause. Major depression, if present, requires treatment and will not respond to hormone therapy alone.

Why is osteoporosis particularly prevalent in postmenopausal women?

Whereas both men and women show age-related decline in bone mineral density after age 40, most women have an accelerated phase of bone loss associated with the cessation of ovarian estrogen production in the five years following menopause. Men are protected against osteoporosis because they achieve higher peak bone mass, and they do not have an abrupt fall in sex hormones.

▶ EVALUATION

How does one determine if a woman is perimenopausal?

Perimenopause can be identified clinically by a combination of age and characteristic symptoms. The median age of onset of the menopausal transition occurs at 47.5 years, and the FMP at 51 years. The characteristic symptoms of hot flashes, sleep disturbance, and mood swings peak in perimenopause and diminish in the years following. Vaginal dryness and urinary frequency manifest later in the transition and in the postmenopausal years. Classic symptoms do not occur in every woman, may precede the transition by years, and may be caused by other conditions.

Are blood tests helpful in defining perimenopause?

Blood tests such as follicle stimulating hormone (FSH) have no place in defining this phase of life in nonhysterectomized women. FSH levels fluctuate markedly during this time and do not reliably correlate with stage of perimenopause or predict transition events. By contrast, women who have undergone hysterectomy will not manifest menstrual changes, so an elevated FSH is helpful in deciding when to begin hormone replacement. Unusual patterns, such as cycle irregularity at an early age, warrant further testing for unexpected pregnancy, thyroid disease, and hyperprolactinemia with β-HCG, TSH, and prolactin levels, respectively.

What are the expected bleeding patterns in the transition phase?

Most commonly, menstrual cycles become further apart and the volume of menstrual blood flow is reduced, reflecting the waning production of estrogen by the ovaries and the increasing frequency of anovulatory cycles. In 10% of women, menses cease abruptly.

What bleeding patterns should prompt further evaluation?

Heavy menstrual bleeding, prolonged menses (longer than seven days), and more than two cycles in a one-month period should prompt investigation for endocrine (hypothyroidism) or structural abnormalities. Endovaginal ultrasound detects uterine fibroids and uterine polyps, which may cause heavy bleeding. In addition, ultrasound is useful for ruling out endometrial carcinoma: an endometrial stripe of less than 5 mm makes endometrial cancer very unlikely. Endometrial sampling using a pipette catheter can also detect endometrial hyperplasia or carcinoma.

▶ TREATMENT

What are the options for treatment of perimenopausal symptoms?

Hot flashes, mood swings, and sleep disturbances are most effectively treated with estrogen replacement therapy. The relatively new selective estrogen receptor modulators (SERMs) such as raloxifene do not prevent hot flashes. Other treatment modalities are less effective but may be useful in women who cannot or do not wish to take ERT. These include clonidine, soy products, paroxetine, venlafaxine, and environmental control such as maintenance of cool ambient temperature and cotton clothing. A number of alternative medicines are available but to date none has demonstrated effectiveness. Combination HRT (estrogen and progesterone) increases the risk of thromboembolic and cardiovascular disease and breast cancer. Use should be limited to the patient with symptomatic perimenopausal period with occasional attempts to taper off.

What are the currently available replacement hormones?

For women with an intact uterus, HRT should consist of an estrogen and a progestin, the latter to protect against endometrial proliferation and uterine cancer. The most commonly used estrogens in the U.S. are conjugated equine estrogen (oral), micronized estradiol (oral), $17\text{-}\beta$ estradiol (transdermal patches and vaginal creams), and piperazine estrone sulfate (oral). The available progestins are medroxyprogesterone acetate (MPA) and micronized progesterone (MP).

What replacement therapy regimens are currently used?

One of the estrogens described above is usually taken daily. Progestins may be given cyclically (e.g., medroxyprogesterone acetate 5 mg on days one to fourteen) or continuously (e.g., 2.5 mg daily). The cyclic regimens should result in regular bleeding starting on day nine or later and are particularly useful in the early perimenopausal patient to regulate cycles. The daily continuous regimen should, after the first six to twelve months of therapy, lead to amenorrhea. Out-of-phase bleeding should result in adjustment of the regimen and/or evaluation of the endometrium by ultrasound or endometrial biopsy to rule-out hyperplasia or cancer. Adjustment in the estrogen/progesterone regimen is an appropriate approach if bleeding occurs within the first six months of replacement therapy. If bleeding continues beyond six months, work-up with endovaginal ultrasound or endometrial biopsy is appropriate. For isolated symptoms, the estrogen ring is an appropriate alternative; it is placed vaginally by the patient, and releases hormone locally. The ring is changed every three months.

What are the risks of hormone replacement therapy?

The results of a large, randomized, controlled trial showed that combination HRT (estrogen/progesterone) produced a higher number of adverse events (stroke, coronary artery event, thromboembolic disease, and breast cancer). Its use is no longer recommended for primary prevention of disease. An arm of the trial is continuing with estrogen alone.

K E Y　P O I N T S

▶ The symptoms of perimenopause are hot flashes, sleep disturbances, mood swings, and irregular menses, although not all women require or desire treatment.

▶ Evaluate heavy or frequent bleeding out of phase in the perimenopause for uterine pathology by endovaginal ultrasound or endometrial biopsy.

CASE 37–5. A 48-year-old woman seeks care for a six month history of bothersome hot flashes and infrequent menses. She is otherwise in good health and has a normal physical exam.

    A. What tests are required to assure she is in the menopause transition?

    B. What type of HRT would you prescribe?

    C. Three months later she reports prolonged menses lasting fourteen days. What should you do next?

    D. What other regimen might you prescribe?

OSTEOPOROSIS

▶ ETIOLOGY

What is osteoporosis?

Osteoporosis is a state of low bone mass and skeletal fragility due to microarchitectural deterioration of bone tissue. Osteopenia is a precursor to osteoporosis.

Why is osteoporosis a problem?

Long-term sequelae of osteoporosis include fractures of the hip, spine, and other bones, chronic fracture pain and kyphosis with compression of internal organs from repeated vertebral compression fractures. The most severe and common result of osteoporosis is hip fractures, occurring in 15% of elderly women. Only one third of hip-fracture patients return to prefracture independence. As our population ages, the number of hip fractures is expected to triple by the year 2040.

Who gets osteoporosis?

Osteoporosis affects an estimated 30% of postmenopausal white and Asian women in the U.S. Rates are lower, although not inconsequential, among other groups: approximately 10% of African American women and 13% to 16% of Hispanic women age 50 and older have osteoporosis. Women are four times as likely to get osteoporosis as men, although men have more disability after hip fracture. In men, hypogonadism accelerates bone loss. Alcoholism is also a major risk factor.

What are other secondary causes of osteoporosis?

Early menopause, such as with oophorectomy, corticosteroid therapy, hyperthyroidism, and hyperparathyroidism, can cause bone loss.

What are risk factors for osteoporosis?

Key, easily identifiable risk factors include

- Age
- Family history of fracture in first-degree relative, particularly prior to age 80
- Personal history of fracture after age 40
- Current cigarette smoking
- Low body weight, less than 127 lbs

Additional risk factors include white or Asian ethnic descent. Lifestyle issues also play an important role including inadequate vitamin D and calcium intake, tobacco, alcohol and caffeine use, and sedentary habits. Osteoporosis is also associated with hyperthyroidism, hyperparathyroidism, and chronic inflammatory conditions such as collagen vascular diseases. Medications such as corticosteroids, heparin, anticonvulsants, and methotrexate also predispose the individual to the development of osteoporosis.

▶ EVALUATION

Who should be screened for osteoporosis?

Recommendations vary, but screening for premenopausal women is not indicated. The National Osteoporosis Foundation recommends screening for

- All women over age 65
- Postmenopausal women older than age 50 with one or more risk factors

Validated prediction rules like SCORE (simple calculated osteoporosis risk estimation) perform better than more broad-based screening guidelines.

How is osteoporosis diagnosed?

Diagnosis is made by T-score on DXA of less than −2.5 *or* by fragility fracture regardless of T-score (Box 37–1). A fragility fracture is a fracture that occurs with minimal or no trauma, for example, a vertebral compression fracture.

What are T-scores and Z-scores?

The T-score represents the patient's bone density in standard deviations compared with the average 25-year-old woman. The Z-score is the age-matched result. The T-score has been chosen as the marker for osteoporosis.

What site is best to view with DEXA, and how often should the DXA be repeated?

Site of DXA measurement, hip/spine/wrist, best predicts fracture at that site. Since degenerative arthritis can falsely raise spine DXA values, hip DXA measurement is the best overall fracture risk predictor. DXA should not be repeated more frequently than every 2 to 5 years unless you expect rapid loss, such as with steroid use.

BOX 37-1

Interpretation of DXA Results

T-score greater than −1.0 = normal
T-score between −1.0 and −2.5 = osteopenia
T-score less than −2.5 = osteoporosis

BOX 37-2

When to Start Osteoporosis Treatment

T-score less than −2.0
or
T-score less than −1.5 plus one or more risk factors
or
Fragility fracture regardless of T-score result

▶ TREATMENT

When should treatment be started?

Although common sense dictates that treatment should start before full osteoporosis develops, a large scale national study found benefit only in patients with T-scores less than −2.5, that is, patients with osteoporosis. Nonetheless, the current National Osteoporosis Foundation (NOF) recommendations are listed (Box 37–2). These guidelines may be revised, so visit the NOF website for the most recent information.

What are options for treatment?

Calcium, vitamin D, and weight-bearing exercise are baseline treatments in any patient with osteoporosis and for prevention in all women. Pharmacologic treatment recommendations vary. Choices include bisphosphonates, SERMs, calcitonin, and estrogen. Prospective data show roughly equivalent fracture reduction rates of approximately 50%, although slightly less for calcitonin.

Bisphosphonates are available in several formulations (alendronate and risedronate). Optimal duration of therapy is unknown. Alendronate comes in a once-weekly formulation. Bishosphonates may cause erosive esophagitis, and patients must take precautions to remain upright for 30 minutes after intake. Whether bone loss resumes after therapy is stopped is controversial. The currently available SERM, raloxifene, is contraindicated in a woman with a history of thromboembolic disease, as it increases the risk of venous thromboembolic disease.

Estrogen improves bone mass and helps treat menopausal symptoms of vaginal atrophy and hot flashes. It increases rates of breast cancer, cardiovascular disease, and thromboembolic disease with long-term therapy, however. Uterine cancer is increased with postmenopausal estrogen, but it can be offset by simultaneous progesterone. Bone density loss resumes when the hormone therapy is stopped. For men with hypogonadism, testosterone is the first line of therapy.

Can osteoporosis be prevented?

It is becoming increasingly clear that prevention of osteoporosis is a far more effective intervention in reducing morbidity and mortality than treatment of established disease. It is critical that conditions, which may predispose the individual to inadequate bone mass development, be identified in adolescence and early adulthood because peak bone mass is reached in the late twenties for women and mid-thirties for men. Conditions that predispose individuals to inadequate bone mass include eating disorders, hypothalamic conditions leading to amenorrhea, tobacco and alcohol use, sedentary lifestyle, and intolerance of dairy products. Smoking cessation is vital. In addition, it is important to recognize that low bone mass alone is not predictive of fracture. Fall risk is a major contributing factor to the development of fractures, particularly in the elderly. Providers should be aware that gait instability, poor vision, unsafe home environment, and medications that alter consciousness are potentially avoidable causes for falls in this population.

Prevention should start in the teenage years or earlier with vitamin D and calcium (Box 37–3). Further benefit is gained from weight-bearing exercises on sites susceptible to fracture (walking for hip and spine density, weights for wrists).

BOX 37–3

Recommended Total Daily Intake for Calcium and Vitamin D

Calcium

800 mg for children 4–8 years old
1300 mg for children and young adults 9–18 years old
1000 mg for adults 19 to 50 years old
1200 mg for adults over age 50

Vitamin D*

200 IU daily for children and adults to age 50
400 IU daily for adults age 50 to 70
600 IU daily for adults over age 70
800 IU daily for adults who are homebound or institutionalized

---

*Less vitamin D may be required if sunlight is abundant and no sunscreen is used.

KEY POINTS

▶ Main risk factors for osteoporosis are age, female sex, low weight, family or personal history of fracture, and cigarette smoking.

▶ Screen for osteoporosis with DXA in women over age 65 and women over age 50 with risk factors.

▶ Diagnosis of osteoporosis is made by DXA T-score less than −2.5, or by fragility fracture regardless of T-score.

▶ Prevent osteoporosis with adequate vitamin D, calcium intake, and reasonable weight-bearing exercise starting in the teenage years.

▶ Bisphosphonates and estrogen are the main therapies for osteoporosis.

CASE 37–6. A 62-year-old Asian woman with eczema, reflux, and tobacco use is in the office for her annual health maintenance examination. She is lactose intolerant and does not exercise. On exam, she weighs 120 lbs, has normal vital signs, and somewhat stooped posture, which she reports is similar to her mother's posture.

A. What are her risk factors for osteoporosis?
B. Should she be screened?
C. What test would you use for screening?
D. Prior to her test results, what treatment would you recommend?

CASE 37–7. A 57-year-old woman has a screening DXA because she has a family history of osteoporosis. Her T-score is −2.3. She is not having menopausal symptoms currently. She has a history of spontaneous deep venous thrombosis.

A. Does she have osteoporosis or osteopenia?
B. Does she require treatment?
C. What treatment would you recommend?

REFERENCE

Kado DM: Vertebral fractures and mortality in older women: A prospective study. Study of Osteoporotic Fractures Research Group. Arch Intern Med 159(11):1215–1220, 1999.

USEFUL WEBSITES

www.osteoed.org
www.nof.org

Case Answers

5–1, A–B. Learning Objective: *Recognize what actions the duty of confidentiality requires.* The duty to maintain confidentiality remains strong in this case because information about the patient does not directly concern others' health, welfare, or safety. There is no imminent danger to others here. The wife is certainly affected by her husband's health and prognosis, however. Every effort should be made to encourage sharing of information, although it remains his right to do so or not.

5–2, A–B. Learning Objective: *Recognize effective ways to address patient participation and respect for persons in decision making.* The patient seems to understand what is at stake with his treatment refusal. Because he is competent, you have a duty to respect his decision. You should be sure to explore his reasons for refusing treatment and consider alternative treatments or ways of reducing his risk. You can be clear that his treatment refusal will be honored, but that it is not necessarily the end of the discussion.

▶ Practical Skills for the Medical Student Answers

6–1, A. Learning objective: *Use sensitivity, specificity, and pretest probability to generate a 2 × 2 table and to calculate positive predictive value.* Assume 1000 patients. Using pretest probability of 25%, 250 will have disease and 750 will have no disease. Then, working backwards, use the sensitivity and specificity of 98% to calculate the number of true positives (A = 98% of 250 = 245) and true negatives (D = 98% of 750 = 735). Quadrant B is total disease absent – true negatives (750 – 735 = 15). Quadrant C is total disease present – true positives (250 – 245 = 5). With all quadrants filled in, you can calculate PPV and NPV. With a calculated PPV of 94%, we can say that with a positive test, this high-risk patient is 94% certain to have HIV infection (see table).

Predictive Value Calculations for HIV Test in a High-Risk Patient

Pretest probability = 25%
Assume N = 1000

		DISEASE			
		Present in 250		Absent in 750	
TEST	Positive	A	245	B	15
	Negative	C	5	D	735

$$PPV = \frac{245}{(245 + 15)} = \textbf{94\%}$$

$$NPV = \frac{735}{(735 + 5)} = \textbf{99\%}$$

6–1, B. Learning objective: *Recognize that a low pretest probability markedly decreases positive predictive value.* When applied to high-risk patients, the HIV test has excellent PPV and NPV. The results are quite different when applied to low-risk populations (see table). What is striking is that although this test is highly sensitive and specific, a positive test result in a low-risk patient has only a 5% likelihood of reflecting true disease.

Predictive Value Calculations for HIV Test in Low-Risk Patient

Pretest probability = 1/1000
Assume N = 1000

		DISEASE			
		Present in 1		Absent in 999	
TEST	Positive	A	0.98	B	20
	Negative	C	0.02	D	979

$$PPV = \frac{0.98}{(20 + 0.98)} = \textbf{5\%}$$

$$NPV = \frac{979}{(979 + 0.02)} = \textbf{99.9\%}$$

6–2. Learning objective: *Understand that the pretest probability affects the predictive value of a test and use this concept to carefully select patients for testing.* The predictive value of the test can be increased by carefully selecting whom you use it in. By choosing to test a population of patients who have an increased risk of having the condition you suspect, you increase the pretest probability and thus the predictive value of the test.

▶ **Abdominal Pain Answers**

7–1, A. Learning Objective: *Recognize a very ill patient and generate an appropriate differential diagnosis for a young woman with sudden onset, right lower quadrant pain and signs of shock.* Differential diagnosis includes ectopic pregnancy, most concerning because of its potential to cause rapid hypovolemic shock. With such an acute onset, also consider a ruptured ovarian cyst or ovarian torsion. Less likely (because symptoms should build more gradually or precede an acute onset) are ruptured duodenal ulcer, pancreatitis, appendicitis, pyelonephritis, right renal stone, PID, and tubo-ovarian abscess.

7–1, B. Learning Objective: *When patients are acutely ill with abnormal vital signs and abdominal pain, call for help and perform rapid work-up to exclude or confirm potentially life-threatening causes.* Inform your senior resident immediately of your concerns, even before finishing a full evaluation in a patient with severe abdominal pain and abnormal vital signs suggesting shock. Call a surgical consult and ask your patient not to eat, in case surgery will be required. Order a pregnancy test and rapid pelvic imaging, preferably with a bedside pelvic ultrasound or CT scan. Order urgent labs: CBC with platelets, protime, and prothrombin time to rule out blood loss, DIC, and to prepare for probable surgery, as well as electrolytes, renal function, amylase, sedimentation rate, and urinalysis. Re-evaluate your patient frequently to assess for worsening status.

7–2, A. Learning Objective: *Generate an appropriate differential diagnosis for an elderly man with diffuse abdominal pain.* Differential diagnosis includes ischemic bowel until proved otherwise, especially in light of his age, recent weight loss, risk factor of hypertension, relatively benign abdominal exam in the presence of severe diffuse pain, and guaiac-positive stool. Peptic ulcer disease is possible in light of aspirin and alcohol use and guaiac positive stool. A GI malignancy, such as gastric or colon cancer, is possible with a history of weight loss and guaiac-positive stool. Constipation, obstipation, and diverticulitis should always be considered in elderly patients. As guaiac testing in patients who have not undergone diet preparation can be a false positive finding, don't use this finding to limit your differential diagnosis. Pancreatitis from gallstones, alcohol, or hydrochlorothiazide should be considered. He could have bladder outlet obstruction from BPH with or without associated cystitis or pyelonephritis. (Fever can be absent in elderly patients.) Although pain is diffuse, don't forget the possibility of cardiac or pulmonary disease, occurring atypically in an elderly patient.

7–2, B. Learning Objective: *Recognize a very ill patient and design a work-up to investigate diffuse abdominal pain in an elderly man.* Inform your team of your patient's abnormal vital signs, discuss your concerns for ischemic bowel, and consider a surgical consult. A blood pressure of 100/60 should be concerning in a patient with a history of hypertension, especially with concurrent tachycardia. Order electrolytes and ABG to look for acidosis, renal function, liver function tests, CBC, amylase, urinalysis with postvoid residual, ECG, and chest and abdominal films. Order abdominal CT. Re-evaluate your patient frequently.

▶ Anemia Answers

8–1, A. Learning Objective: *Recognize jaundice as a presenting sign of hemolytic anemia.* At first glance, this patient appears excessively anticoagulated from the coumadin and may be bleeding as a consequence. An elevated reticulocyte count and a resultant elevated MCV are consistent with a GI bleed. She could also have anemia from poor production due to renal insufficiency, although you would not expect an elevated reticulocyte index. More likely, this patient has a destructive process, or hemolytic anemia, in light of her jaundice. Furthermore, the clinical features suggest thrombotic thrombocytopenic purpura (TTP), an uncommon syndrome that occurs with microangiopathic hemolytic anemia, thrombocytopenia (low platelets), neurologic disorders (usually confusion), renal insufficiency, and noninfectious fever.

8–1, B. Learning Objective: *Design appropriate evaluation of a patient with hemolytic anemia, including hospitalization for a patient with TTP.* This patient needs hospitalization owing to her symptoms that suggest end-organ hypoxia (tachycardia, tachypnea), new acute renal failure, and life-threatening TTP. To confirm the diagnosis of hemolytic anemia, look for prominent schistocytes on peripheral smear and order an indirect bilirubin, haptoglobin, and LDH.

8–2, A. Learning Objective: *Always pursue work-up for anemia, even in the elderly.* Anemia is not normal, even in the elderly, and the cause of anemia should always be investigated. This man has mild anemia with a reduced MCV and most likely has iron deficiency. The cause must be investigated upon presentation. He cannot merely be treated with iron.

8–2, B. Learning Objective: *Pursue work-up to confirm diagnosis in a patient suspected of having iron deficiency.* Review of the peripheral smear should show a population of small cells with central pallor (hypochromia). Iron deficiency can be confirmed by a low serum iron, elevated TIBC, and low transferrin saturation. Sigmoidoscopy is an inadequate study to assess for colon cancer in an older patient with iron deficiency anemia. He should have a colonoscopy and, if negative, an EGD to look for a source of bleeding.

▶ Chest Pain Answers

9–1, A. Learning objective: *List causes of pleuritic pain.* The most likely causes of pleuritic pain in this patient include pericarditis, pulmonary embolus, costochondritis, rib fracture, pneumonia, or pleurodynia (pleuritis). Other less likely causes to consider include angina, pneumothorax, and esophageal spasm.

9–1, B. Learning Objective: *Identify clinical features that support a diagnosis of either pericarditis or pulmonary emboli.* The patient's recent viral illness, her absence of dyspnea or calf pain, and increase in her pain when lying down favor pericarditis. Her smoking history and oral contraceptive use increase her risk for a pulmonary embolus. Pleuritic pain can occur with either pericarditis or pulmonary embolus.

9–1, C. Learning objective: *Recognize clinical features and ECG findings of pericarditis.* This patient's pleuritic pain (worsened by lying down), her recent viral illness, and ECG findings of diffuse ST elevations, along with PR depression, all suggest a diagnosis of pericarditis.

9–1, D. Learning objective: *Recognize the pertinent exam findings of pericarditis.* The most helpful exam finding to support a diagnosis of pericarditis is the presence of a pericardial friction rub. This is a high-pitched, scratching sound heard best with the patient sitting up and exhaling. If a patient has a large pericardial effusion associated with pericarditis, exam may reveal distant heart sounds, distended neck veins, and pulsus paradoxus (see Table 9–1).

9–1, E. Learning objective: *List the causes of pericarditis.* The patient's recent viral illness would make a viral etiology the most likely cause for her pericarditis. Viral causes for pericarditis include coxsackievirus, echovirus, adenovirus, and influenza. Other causes of pericarditis include renal failure, autoimmune disorders, metastatic cancer, drugs, trauma, myxedema, radiation, and bacterial, fungal, or tuberculous infections.

9–2, A. Learning objective: *Identify cardiac risk factors.* This patient's risk factors include being a man older than age 44, tobacco use, hypertension, family history of premature coronary artery disease (present in a first-degree male relative younger than age 55 or a first-degree female relative (younger than age 65), and hypercholesterolemia. He does not have diabetes.

9–2, B. Learning objective: *Create a differential diagnosis for chest pain appropriate for the patient's history and exam.* Given his description of his symptoms and his multiple cardiac risk factors, angina or myocardial infarction is the most likely diagnosis. Esophageal spasm, reflux, aortic dissection, pulmonary embolus, pericarditis, chest wall pain, pneumothorax, pneumonia, and biliary colic should be considered, but are less likely causes in this patient.

9–2, C. Learning objective: *Recognize the ECG findings of ischemia.* This patient's ECG shows evidence for anterolateral ischemia, with ST depression and T wave inversions in leads I and V3–V6 and isolated T wave inversions in lead II. This patient has either unstable angina or myocardial infarction. Serial cardiac enzymes and ECGs are required to determine if he has had an infarction. This patient should be admitted to the CCU; given aspirin, nitroglycerin, and heparin; and would benefit from a β-blocker.

▶ Cough Answers

10–1, A. Learning objective: *List the likely causes of acute or subacute cough in a young person.* Most likely in this young man is postinfectious bronchospasm or postnasal drip. Because he has a history of allergies, cough-variant asthma should also be considered. Although up to 40% of people have cough for several weeks following upper respiratory infection, 25% of adults with acute cough greater than or equal to 3 weeks have pertussis.

10–1, B. Learning objective: *Identify helpful historical or examination clues in making a diagnosis in acute cough.* A history of "barking cough" is unlikely to be asthma. Severe "whooping" after coughing spells or post-tussive vomiting suggests pertussis. Clues that might suggest cough-variant asthma include personal or family history of asthma or eczema, or sensitivity to NSAIDs or aspirin. Sputum production only in the morning is a clue to PND. Ask about ill contacts, pets, and occupational and hobby exposures. Helpful examination findings include posterior pharyngeal cobblestoning or nasal exudates suggesting PND and wheezing with or without rapid forced expiration and eczema suggesting asthma.

10–1, C. Learning objective: *Recognize features suggestive of pertussis and consider testing to treat contacts.* No testing is usually needed for acute/subacute cough since most cases of acute tracheobronchitis are viral and self-limited. Office spirometry may confirm bronchospasm by an FEV_1/FVC ratio less than 75%, but a therapeutic trial of bronchodilators may be as effective at confirming the diagnosis. Physicians should be on the lookout for cases of pertussis. Nasopharyngeal swab for pertussis PCR should be considered because contacts should be treated.

10–1, D. Learning objective: *Treat postinfectious cough with inhaled albuterol.* Empiric albuterol is more effective for postviral cough than cough syrups. Sedating (drying) antihistamines may be helpful for PND and cough at night. Narcotic cough syrups should be considered only when cough seriously interferes with eating or sleeping and other measures have failed. Importantly, antibiotics are not helpful in this setting because pneumonia is highly unlikely with normal vital signs.

10–2, A. Learning objective: *List the likely causes of chronic cough in older patients.* GERD, PND, and asthma are common causes of chronic cough and many patients do not have other specific reflux, nasal congestion, or asthma symptoms. A "loose" productive cough in a smoker suggests chronic bronchitis. Many patients have multiple causes. Cancer and TB should be considered in patients older than age 50. ACE inhibitors cause dry cough in up to 30% of patients.

10–2, B. Learning objective: *Elicit pertinent history and physical findings in patients with chronic cough.* Ask about fever, weight loss, night sweats, hemoptysis, PPD testing, TB exposure, history of asthma, allergies, eczema, and PND; ask about cough after meals or at night (GERD/PND); timing related to URIs and ACE inhibitor use; CHF symptoms; and occupational exposure. Physical findings helpful in making the diagnosis include pharyngeal cobblestoning (PND), increased AP chest diameter (COPD), lung wheezes (asthma/COPD) or crackles (apical-TB, basal-CHF, bronchiectasis, scarring), lymphadenopathy (TB or cancer), clubbing (COPD), and cyanosis (hypoxia—usually COPD).

10–2, C. Learning objective: *Order appropriate tests and interventions for patients with chronic cough.* In this case, a CXR and office spirometry might be helpful. Stop his ACE inhibitor for one week then restart and assess cough. If cough resolves, use an ace-receptor-blocker (ARB) instead. Give albuterol and inhaled ipratropium, if COPD, for two to four weeks. Cigarette cessation is key. Empiric medications for PND include sedating antihistamines and nasal steroids. If cough persists, consider pH probe testing and/or a three-to six-month trial of proton pump inhibitors to diagnose and treat GERD.

10–2, D. Learning objective: *Recognize cough as a symptom of CHF in the appropriate clinical setting.* An S_3 and crackles are signs of heart failure, as are cough made worse with exercise and when recumbent, and these should prompt work-up for CHF. If the S_3 is right-sided, consider interstitial lung disease (i.e., Velcro crackles on exam).

▶ DIARRHEA ANSWERS

11–1, A. Learning objective: *List most likely cause of diarrhea in this patient with recent antibiotic use and new medications.* Mrs. J has two main risk factors for diarrhea: medications and prior antibiotic therapy. Both medication-induced diarrhea and *Clostridium difficile* colitis can occur as a mild, indolent, chronic process.

11–1, B. Learning objective: *Outline how to evaluate for C. difficile colitis and medication-associated diarrhea.* In deciding whether to work-up or treat her symptoms, you must first think about the natural history of these two processes. Most patients with mild (less than 6 stools per day, T less than 38.5°C, WBC less than 12K) *C. difficile*–induced diarrhea improve 48–72 hours after stopping antibiotics and do not need specific therapy. Patients with more severe disease or persistent symptoms or those who are elderly or debilitated should always be treated. *C. difficile* toxin should be sent. Other lab work at this time is unnecessary.

11–1, C. Learning objective: *Outline treatment options for C. difficile and medication-associated diarrhea.* You could start her empirically on metronidazole (250 mg PO qid × 10 days) now or wait until the test results are available. If the toxin assay is negative, then changing medications would be the next step. Diarrhea due to the β-blocker should resolve once she stops the medication. Atenolol is working well for her angina, and her symptoms are relatively mild so you can investigate other causes first.

11–2, A. Learning objective: *Identify appropriate initial evaluation and treatment for a patient with ongoing bloody diarrhea.* Mr. D. has chronic inflammatory diarrhea. Given his age and the absence of other risk factors, this most likely represents inflammatory bowel disease. Your job in clinic is to make sure that the effects of diarrhea (volume and electrolyte loss, anemia) are under control until definitive diagnosis and treatment can be made. Mr. D. was given 1 L of normal saline and was no longer orthostatic. A stat hematocrit was 35 and his electrolytes were normal.

11–2, B. Learning objective: *Outline initial outpatient management for a patient with chronic bloody diarrhea.* A flexible sigmoidoscopy should be performed within the next week or so. Instruct the patient to drink 2 L of fluid a day and return to the ED or clinic if dizziness, bleeding, or fatigue increases.

11–3, A. Learning objective: *Identify likely causes of acute diarrhea in a traveler.* This patient most likely has travelers' diarrhea. Another possibility would be viral gastroenteritis. Travelers' diarrhea is caused by bacteria in 90% of patients and is almost always benign and self-limited.

11–3, B. Learning objective: *List appropriate testing in mild travelers' diarrhea.* In the absence of bloody stool or high fever, no further diagnostic testing is needed.

11–3, C. Learning objective: *Outline treatment of travelers' diarrhea.* Travelers' diarrhea is usually self-limited and typically lasts one to five days. At this point antibiotic therapy will not change the course of disease, but she should be given education about replacement fluids and medications, such as Imodium to reduce stool frequency.

► DIZZINESS AND SYNCOPE ANSWERS

12–1, A. Learning objective: *Recognize a cardiac cause of syncope, hypertrophic cardiomyopathy.* Syncope with exertion in a young adult suggests cardiac outflow obstruction or arrhythmia. When the patient goes from squatting to standing, the ventricular chamber size gets smaller. The relative obstruction due to hypertrophy gets more severe, and the murmur of hypertrophy gets louder. Virtually all other systolic murmurs, except some mitral valve prolapses, become softer. This is a potentially serious cause of dizziness. He should be told not to participate in strenuous exercise until further evaluation is obtained. Many athletes have died owing to this abnormality.

12–1, B. Learning objective: *Identify echocardiogram as the appropriate test for evaluation of patient with syncope and significant murmur on exam.* This abnormality is best confirmed with a cardiac echo. CXR and ECG are nonspecific. If the echocardiogram is normal, Holter monitoring is the next step to evaluate for a significant arrhythmia.

12–2, A. Learning objective: *Diagnose benign positional vertigo.* The type of dizziness he is describing is vertigo, and the most common cause is benign positional vertigo (BPV). This is a classic presentation for BPV: a) occurs in older people, b) is worse with head movement, c) symptoms and nystagmus show latency and are fatigable with repeated confrontation, and d) cerebellum is not involved. (Important to rule-out a rare cerebellar hemorrhage.)

12–2, B. Learning objective: *Recognize that the diagnosis of BPV is confirmed by history and exam only.* We don't always need another test! This presentation, with positive Dix-Hallpike maneuver (see figure 12–1) is very specific for this disease. He can be treated with fatiguing exercises (repeatedly doing head movements that bring on symptoms in order to hasten recovery), mild anti-dizziness medication (e.g., meclizine), and reassurance. He should be told the expected course of the illness (slowly better over three to ten days) and to report back if he is not better or gets worse.

▶ DYSPEPSIA ANSWERS

13–1, A. Learning objective: *List a differential diagnosis for epigastric pain.* The differential diagnosis includes PUD, functional dyspepsia, and gastric and pancreatic cancer. It is difficult to distinguish these diseases based on history alone, but in older patients, recent onset of symptoms should raise concern over serious organic pathology.

13–1, B. Learning objective: *Design appropriate evaluation for epigastric pain in a patient with red flags (age greater than 45).* Given his age is greater than 45 years he should undergo prompt endoscopy to rule-out complicated PUD or gastric malignancy. Remember, any patients with such red flags (dysphagia, bleeding, weight loss, and new onset of symptoms later than age 45) should have endoscopy. The "test-and-treat" for *Helicobacter pylori* strategy is reserved for patients younger than age 45 without alarm symptoms.

13–2, A. Learning objective: *List lifestyle modifications for treatment of patients with GERD.* The patient should avoid smoking and alcohol and late meals because these can exacerbate reflux. Sleeping on pillows increases intra-abdominal pressure and worsens GERD. Some physicians instruct the patient to raise the head of the bed by tilting up the whole frame (about six inches), but the benefit of this is uncertain. Weight loss is helpful, as well as looser waistbands, to decrease intra-abdominal pressure. If the patient is refractory to lifestyle modifications, prescribe H_2RAs or PPIs.

13–2, B. Learning objective: *Refer patients with long-standing GERD for EGD to look for Barrett's esophagus.* Because long-standing GERD may be associated with a premalignant lesion, Barrett's esophagus, she should undergo endoscopy.

▶ DYSPNEA ANSWERS

14–1, A. Learning objective: *Recognize PE and silent ischemia as potential serious causes of acute dyspnea in an older patient without chest pain or cough.* Dyspnea at rest in a patient with diabetes and unrevealing chest exam is concerning for either cardiac ischemia or pulmonary embolus, particularly with tachycardia on exam. Silent ischemia (myocardial ischemia without chest pain) is more common in patients with diabetes. Pneumonia is possible, but much less likely in the absence of cough or fever.

14–1, B. Learning objective: *Select appropriate diagnostic tests for a patient with dyspnea of uncertain etiology.* Initial diagnostic tests for this patient should include CBC, ECG, CXR, and pulse oximetry. If these are not revealing, an ABG is warranted. If historical details (vein trauma, stasis, hypercoagulable state) and ABG suggest pulmonary embolus, consider ordering a sequence of tests to include one or more of the following: D-dimer, lower extremity venous duplex, pulmonary ventilation-perfusion scan, and chest CT scan.

14–2, A. Learning objective: *List causes of acute dyspnea associated with pleuritic chest pain.* Diagnoses to consider with acute dyspnea associated with pleuritic chest pain include pulmonary embolus, pneumonia, pericarditis, and pneumothorax. Although she is a smoker, at her age COPD is unlikely.

14–2, B. Learning objective: *Distinguish pulmonary embolus, pericarditis, pneumonia, and pneumothorax by their associated clinical features.* Her tobacco and oral contraceptive use increase her risk of having a PE. Pleuritic pain, tachycardia, and hypoxia are also consistent with this diagnosis. Although she has no leg symptoms or signs of deep venous thrombosis (DVT), up to 70% of patients with PE have no symptoms to suggest a DVT. Her recent URI increases her risk for both pericarditis and pneumonia. Some patients with pericarditis complain of dyspnea because of the pain associated with taking a breath. The absence of a rub on her cardiac exam makes pericarditis less likely. Pneumonia is possible, but is unlikely in the absence of fever or productive cough and a normal chest exam. Although pneumothorax may be associated with dyspnea and pleuritic pain, this is a relatively uncommon condition. She has no history of risk factors for pneumothorax (trauma, tall body habitus, or pneumocystis pneumonia). Her breath sounds are symmetric, but this does not exclude pneumothorax. A CXR may identify a small pneumothorax not detectable on exam.

14–2, C. Learning objective: *Order appropriate diagnostic tests in a patient with dyspnea, pleuritic chest pain, and risk factors for PE.* The initial evaluation of this patient should include CBC, CXR, ECG, and ABG. Because of her multiple risk factors for PE, workup should be obtained with testing as noted in 14–1, B.

▶ **FATIGUE ANSWERS**

15–1, A. Learning objective: *Recognize features of fatigue suggesting an underlying medical diagnosis.* The relatively short duration of her fatigue, association with exertional dyspnea, and history of unprotected sex are all concerning for physical disorders.

15–1, B. Learning objective: *Obtain a focused history to assist in finding a medical cause of fatigue.* Ask about menstrual history; weight loss or gain; symptoms of thyroid disease, such as temperature intolerance and changes in bowel habits; dryness of hair or skin; orthopnea; cough; allergy symptoms; or symptoms of sexually transmitted diseases, such as rashes or vaginal discharge; and history of exposure to TB.

15–1, C. Learning objective: *Order appropriate tests for a patient with fatigue and a history suggesting an underlying medical condition and risks for sexually transmitted disease.* Order TSH, CBC, electrolytes, renal function, glucose, bilirubin, hepatic transaminases, pregnancy test, cervical swabs for gonorrhea and chlamydia, RPR or VDRL, HIV, and viral hepatitis serology. Consider a CXR and PPD testing.

15–2, A. Learning objective: *Recognize possible chronic fatigue syndrome and use your history to rule-out other causes of fatigue, to establish rapport, and to set reasonable expectations for work-up and recovery.* Take a more thorough sleep history, focusing on symptoms of sleep apnea, such as snoring, cessation of breathing noted by a bed partner, and daytime somnolence. Ask also about symptoms of depression and social stressors. Ask the patient what he is most concerned that his symptoms might represent, how it has affected his life, and what further evaluation he might like. Acknowledge that these symptoms are worrisome and frustrating. Tell him that his symptoms are real, and that even though the tests so far show no evidence of physical disease, there are things that can be done to help him cope with how he's feeling, although this may take time.

15–2, B. Learning objective: *Perform a thorough physical exam in patients suspected of chronic fatigue syndrome to validate and address patient concerns and rule-out serious medical illness.* A thorough physical exam will indicate to the patient that you take his concerns seriously. Because he has mentioned headaches and joint pain, do a thorough neurologic and joint exam, and tell the patient what you are checking as you do it.

15–2, C. Learning objective: *Recognize that no further testing is required if history and exam are negative in a patient with long-standing fatigue.* Tell the patient that you would like to consult with your attending before deciding on any tests. Do not offer the diagnosis of chronic fatigue syndrome until you have discussed the case with your preceptor and reviewed the criteria carefully with the patient.

▶ GASTROINTESTINAL BLEEDING ANSWERS

16–1, A. Learning objective: *Recognize clues to distinguish upper from lower GI bleeding.* Bright red blood from the GI tract can be from either a lower or a brisk upper GI bleed. The clue here is the elevated BUN. The BUN-to-creatinine ratio is often greater than 25 in upper GI bleeding due to the absorbed nitrogen load of blood in the small intestine. She has an upper GI bleed from an NSAID-induced (rofecoxib and aspirin) ulcer. Though COX-2 inhibitors are less likely to cause GI bleeding than other NSAIDs, they still can induce GI bleeding, especially in the setting of other risk factors, such as aspirin use, advanced age, smoking, alcohol use, and *Helicobacter pylori* infection.

16–1, B. Learning objective: *List common causes of GI bleeding in older patients.* Common causes of GI bleeding in older patients include diverticuli, angiodysplasia, PUD, and hemorrhoids. Less common but important causes to consider include GI malignancy and ischemic bowel.

16–1, C. Learning objective: *State the treatment options to reduce the occurrence of NSAID-induced ulcers.* Overall, chronic NSAID use over a year carries a 2%–4% risk of serious GI bleeding. NSAIDs with the least risk of GI bleeding include the COX-2 inhibitors (rofecoxib, celecoxib) and salsalate. Ibuprofen carries moderate risk, and piroxicam and ketorolac carry the greatest risk. Proton pump inhibitors offer some protection against NSAID-induced ulcers, as does misoprostol, a stomach protective prostaglandin E_1 analogue, whose use is limited by diarrhea.

16–2A. Learning objective: *Recognize signs of liver disease and suspect esophageal variceal bleeding or peptic ulcer as the source of GI bleeding.* Spider telangiectasias, bulging flanks suggestive of ascites, palmar erythema, and Terry's nails are signs of chronic liver disease. The most common causes of GI bleeding in this setting are esophageal varices, peptic ulcer, and gastritis. Other findings to look for that suggest liver disease include gynecomastia, jaundice, caput medusa, shifting dullness to abdominal percussion, and abdominal fluid wave. It is important to recognize liver disease-associated esophageal bleeding because it carries a 30%–50% mortality and requires rapid resuscitation and intervention. This patient has a variceal bleed. When he is more stable it will be useful to find out the cause of liver disease.

16–2B. Learning objective: *Appropriately resuscitate patients with large-volume GI bleeding.* Admit this patient to the ICU for frequent monitoring and aggressive resuscitation. Call GI and surgical consults early. Assess vital signs and orthostatic changes in pulse and pressure for volume depletion. Obtain IV access with two large-bore catheters or a central venous catheter. Give IV normal saline for volume repletion. Type and cross to keep multiple units of blood in the hospital; follow serial hematocrits every two to four hours; and check platelets, PT, and PTT for signs of coagulopathy. Give packed red cells to keep hematocrit above 25 in young patients and above 30 in frail, older patients. Give fresh frozen plasma if protime INR is greater than 1.5. Give platelets if platelet count is less than 50,000. Follow calcium levels and replace if multiple transfusions lower them. Intubation may be required to prevent aspiration in patients with confusion and large volume upper GI bleeding. Reassess your patient frequently for signs of continued or worsened blood loss.

16–2C. Learning objective: *Use octreotide to slow variceal and other causes of GI bleeding.* Octreotide, a synthetic analogue of somatostatin, is the drug of choice to reduce splanchnic and hepatic blood flow, thereby reducing the rate of bleeding in patients with rapid GI bleed of any source. Beta-blockers must not be used during an acute variceal bleed, but they do prevent first variceal bleed and rebleeding in stable patients with portal hypertension.

16–2D. Learning objective: *State the appropriate use of endoscopy, balloon tamponade, and TIPS for treatment of bleeding esophageal varices.* Endoscopic variceal ligation of bleeding varices is the procedure of choice to stop variceal bleeding, with an 86% success rate. Sclerotherapy is less effective and has higher complication, rebleeding, and mortality rates than does variceal ligation. Balloon tamponade with a Sengstaken-Blakemore or Minnesota tube is an older and less-effective technique that can be applied only for a short time period. Transjugular intrahepatic portosystemic shunt (TIPS) is effective at controlling bleeding and reducing rebleeding, but it also carries a higher complication rate than ligation. The shunt is placed angiographically in the liver between a hepatic artery and portal vein.

▶ HEADACHE ANSWERS

17–1, A. Learning objective: *Diagnose migraine headaches based on history.* This young woman's unilateral, throbbing headache, accompanied by nausea and phonophobia, is classic for migraine. No red flags are present for ominous cause.

17–1, B. Learning objective: *Imaging is not required for headache with benign history and exam.* Studies have shown that with a normal neurologic exam, and no red flags for an ominous cause, imaging is not necessary.

17–1, C. Learning objective: *Identify abortive treatment for migraine.* Given her infrequent symptoms, a nonsteroidal, such as Naprosyn, is a reasonable choice at the first sign of headache. There may be gastroparesis, so consider adding a promotility agent, such as metoclopramide. Warn the patient of overuse of analgesics and the propensity to cause withdrawal headaches. If she develops more severe symptoms that do not respond to the Naprosyn (e.g., unable to work for more than a day, vomiting,) consider sumatriptan. Before you prescribe sumatriptan, review risk for cardiovascular disease. In a young person, CV disease is unlikely.

17–1, D. Learning objective: *Recognize the importance of prophylactic treatment for frequent headaches.* With the increased frequency of her headaches, consider prophylactic treatment. The first choice would be riboflavin or Naprosyn taken daily. If this doesn't work, β-blockers are a reasonable choice.

17–2, A. Learning objective: *Identify warning signs for headache from a worrisome cause.* Age older than 50 and new headache is a concerning combination in this woman. Her fatigue and diffuse muscle aches raise further questions about overall health.

17–2, B. Learning objective: *Know appropriate work-up for concerning headache history.* This woman gives a history consistent with polymyalgia rheumatica and associated temporal arteritis. On exam, she likely has tenderness with palpation over the temporal artery and diffuse muscle pain with normal strength. In one study, temporal arteritis was as common as migraine in this age group. The most targeted test for PMR is the sedimentation rate and, if elevated in this setting, is diagnostic. If TA is a concern, obtain a temporal artery biopsy, because steroid dose is higher in this condition than in PMR alone. If the diagnosis is not clear, screen with basic labs of CBC, electrolytes, and liver function. Consider contrast CT scan, looking for structural disease, such as tumors, in this age group.

17–3, A. Learning objective: *Recognize presentation of SAH.* This man has a subarachnoid hemorrhage until completely proved otherwise. The sudden onset, association with weight-lifting, and severity all point to this diagnosis.

17–3, B. Learning objective: *Outline the appropriate testing for SAH.* Although his CT scan is negative, there is still a 5% chance of a missed bleed. You must perform an LP for xanthochromia.

▶ HEALTHY PATIENTS ANSWERS

18–1, A. Learning objective: *Know what preventive health counseling is appropriate for young healthy males.* The leading cause of death in this age group is motor vehicle accidents and other unintentional injuries, homicide, suicide, malignant neoplasms, and heart disease. General screening considerations are height, weight, activity level, blood pressure, and assessment for substance abuse. Counseling is directed at injury protection, such as seat belt use, motorcycle helmets, safe use of firearms; avoidance of the use of tobacco, excessive alcohol intake, and illicit drug use; safe sex practices; healthy diet and adequate physical activity; use of sunscreen protection; and good dental health.

18–1, B. Learning objective: *Identify key immunizations for this age group.* Immunizations include tetanus, hepatitis B, and measles-mumps-rubella (MMR) if not previously immunized. Other interventions may be indicated if, by history, he is in a high-risk population.

18–1, C. Learning objective: *Recognize that prostate screening has no role in young men.* There is no indication for prostate cancer screening in this age group.

18–2, A. Learning objective: *Apply the model for change to patient's own process.* This young man is in stage 2, contemplation. Although he is discouraged, he is still contemplating trying again.

18–2, B. Learning objective: *Design an approach to help patient move through stages of change.* Focus questions on what barriers interfered with success on his last attempts. Work to increase motivation by helping him identify personal benefits of weight loss.

18–2, C. Learning objective: *Recognize and support the determination stage.* Now that he has determined to lose weight again, work on specific plans of action. Explore what medical and social supports are available to him. Re-address barriers and motivations. Make explicit plans for date to start and next follow-up appointments.

▶ JOINT AND MUSCULAR PAIN ANSWERS

19–1, A. Learning objective: *Recognize osteoarthritis (OA).* Her obesity is a risk factor for OA. The slow onset of symptoms and essentially benign exam also suggest OA. Effusion is common but is not inflammatory if tapped. Sense of fullness is due to the effusion and may progress to a Baker's cyst.

19–1, B. Learning objective: *Design appropriate work-up for low-grade, pauciarticular joint pain.* Exam should include tender points to rule-out fibromyalgia. X-ray will confirm the diagnosis of OA. Gout is unlikely in this case because it is uncommon in the knee, is usually not bilateral, and is exquisitely painful. Arthrocentesis would rule-out gout and infection, but is not needed when OA can be confirmed by x-ray. A normal uric acid level is not helpful in ruling out gout. No history suggests polyarticular, inflammatory disease. Bursitis, although common in this population, is not supported by exam.

19–1, C. Learning objective: *Appropriately treat OA.* Give Tylenol at adequate doses for pain relief. Suggest weight loss and non-weight-bearing exercise such as swimming or simple knee extension exercises. Glucosamine, an over-the-counter food supplement, may also decrease pain and increase function in patients with OA.

19–2, A. Learning objective: *Identify causes of systemic arthritis in a young person.* By history of acute onset, prolonged stiffness, and exam findings of skin rash and synovitis, autoimmune arthritis-like SLE or RA is high on the list. Although fever can be consistent with autoimmune processes, fever makes infection more likely, so disseminated gonococcal infection (DGI) should be a concern. Other causes of septic arthritis, usually *Staphylococcus,* are rarely polyarticular.

19–2, B. Learning objective: *Recognize importance of sexual history and symptoms of other organ involvement in systemic arthritis.* Ask about unprotected sex to gauge the risk of gonorrhea infection. Obtain a good review of symptoms including constitutional symptoms (fever, weight loss, fatigue), skin rash, and pulmonary symptoms. See SLE and RA chapters for specifics of history regarding autoimmune processes.

19–2, C. Learning objective: *Recognize importance of arthrocentesis in this setting.* Fever, multiple joint involvement, and unprotected sex indicate DGI until proved otherwise by arthrocentesis, blood culture, and swabs of the throat, cervix, penile urethra, and rectum. Facial rash may indicate SLE. This and RA are most likely if DGI is ruled out. Further examination for systemic signs is needed, with appropriate serum tests (see Chapter 35).

19–3, A. Learning objective: *Recognize common causes of muscle pain.* This is a classic presentation for fibromyalgia with sleep disruption and multiple tender points. It is important to rule-out thyroid disease, which can cause myalgias and depression. PMR is unlikely in a woman her age.

19–3, B. Learning objective: *Identify appropriate tests for workup of diffuse muscular pain.* Nothing in this patient's history or exam indicates an autoimmune process. Her exam and history are consistent with fibromyalgia. It is reasonable to obtain a TSH, and if she demonstrates muscle weakness, a CPK. An ANA is a very nonspecific test and would not be helpful in this clinical setting.

19–3, C. Learning objective: *Appropriately treat fibromyalgia.* Provided her thyroid disease is adequately treated, prescribe exercise and low-dose tricyclic antidepressants for sleep.

19–4, A. Learning objective: *Identify main causes of shoulder pain*. Most likely this represents rotator cuff tendinitis with accompanying bursitis. Other causes to consider are thyroid disease, nerve impingement in the neck, PMR, and malignancy given weight loss and age.

19–4, B. Learning objective: *Recognize warning sign of weight loss in shoulder pain.* Given her age and weight loss, obtain an x-ray to look for lytic lesions, an ESR to screen for atypical presentation of PMR, and a TSH.

19–4, C. Learning objective: *Recognize the signs and symptoms of rotator cuff tear.* This patient's decreased active range of motion could indicate a tear. Pain may limit her, so an injection of lidocaine for acute pain control with subsequent repeat strength testing is indicated. With the limitation of both active and passive range of motion, frozen shoulder is a possibility, as well.

▶ LOW BACK PAIN ANSWERS

20–1, A. Learning objective: *Identify that acute low back pain does not require further testing if red flags are not present.* In this healthy woman without significant trauma, risk for infection, or cancer, there is no reason to investigate her back pain further.

20–1, B. Learning objective: *Outline appropriate initial treatment in acute low back pain.* NSAIDs, brief bed rest, and physical therapy are the appropriate initial management for acute low back pain in the absence of warning signs or symptoms.

20–1, C. Learning objective: *State the limitations for returning to work with acute low back pain.* She should return to work as soon as possible; however, she will need light duty. By the guidelines in the chapter, she should not lift anything heavier than 20 pounds until this episode resolves.

20–1, D. Learning objective: *Outline the expected time course for acute low back pain.* She should be significantly improved in four weeks. If she is not, consider further evaluation.

20–2, A. Learning objective: *Identify red flags for pathologic causes of low back pain.* Her red flags are age, time course, and pattern of pain (worse at night, prolonged duration, worsening rather than improving).

20–2, B. Learning objective: *State the appropriate initial testing in patients with low back pain and red flags for pathologic cause of pain.* Lumbosacral x-ray and sedimentation rate are warranted. In addition, with her history of anemia and mild renal failure, a complete blood count and chemistry panel are important to assess her current status. In this particular case, you should also obtain a serum and urine protein electrophoresis to screen for multiple myeloma, which can result in back pain, renal dysfunction, and anemia.

▶ LOWER EXTREMITY PAIN, SWELLING, AND ULCERS ANSWERS

21–1, A. Learning objective: *Recognize when to evaluate for systemic causes of peripheral edema.* She has new onset bilateral extremity edema and possibly generalized edema by history. The

most common cause of bilateral peripheral edema is venous insufficiency, but this would not explain more generalized edema. The
differential diagnosis includes hypothyroidism, low albumin states,
medication, renal insufficiency, and CHF. Because she has no
known chronic diseases and has a normal exam except for ankle
edema, the two most likely causes are either medication or
hypothyroidism.

**21-1, B. Learning objective: *Know the appropriate tests to screen
for systemic causes of edema.*** Obtain a TSH, albumin, BUN, and
creatinine to screen for hypothyroidism, low-albumin states, and
renal insufficiency. CHF is unlikely given her normal cardiopulmonary exam and lack of symptoms. Because estrogen, medroxyprogesterone, and ibuprofen all can cause generalized edema,
find out if there have been any dose changes or if one was started
recently. If so, undergo a trial of witholding the appropriate medication to see if fluid retention resolves.

**21-2, A. Learning objective: *List and differentiate the presenta-
tion of common causes of chronic unilateral lower extremity pain
not associated with edema or erythema.*** Peripheral vascular disease (PVD), radiculopathy, and spinal stenosis all can cause lower
extremity pain extending from the hip to the foot. The diagnosis
of PVD is supported by his diminished left posterior tibialis pulse
and pain always occurring with a set amount of exercise. Although
PVD is more common in elderly people, he has multiple risk factors including diabetes and hypertension. Radiculopathy and
spinal stenosis are usually associated with back pain.
Radiculopathy worsens with sitting or forward flexion and is associated with paresthesias. Spinal stenosis, more common in the elderly, is usually bilateral and does not resolve with rest while
standing, but requires sitting or forward flexion.

**21-2, B. Learning objective: *Order appropriate evaluation when
you suspect peripheral vascular disease.*** Ankle/brachial indices
(ABIs) may be artificially high due to noncompressible calcified
arteries in patients with diabetes and, therefore, misleading.
Further testing with a lower extremity arterial duplex and/or angiography may be necessary. His ABIs were 1.0 on the right and 0.82
on the left. After exercise treadmill testing, his ABIs decreased
significantly to 0.63 (right) and 0.41 (left). An arterial duplex
showed a 50% narrowing of the bilateral common iliac arteries,
50% narrowing of mid-distal superficial femoral artery, and focal
occlusion of the left anterior tibial artery. He subsequently under-
went arteriography, bilateral iliac transluminal angioplasty, and
stent placement.

21-2, C. Learning objective: *List modifiable risk factors for PVD.*
Patients with PVD have the same relative risk of death from cardiovascular causes as do patients with a history of coronary or
cerebrovascular disease. It is imperative to address modifiable risk

factors, which include hypertension, hyperlipidemia, diabetes, and smoking cessation.

▶ LYMPHADENOPATHY ANSWERS

22–1, A. Learning objective: *List the causes of axillary lymphadenopathy.* The most likely diagnoses are breast cancer metastatic to the axilla, lymphoma, cat scratch disease, or staphylococcal or streptococcal infection of the arm or hand.

22–1, B. Learning objective: *Order the appropriate tests for axillary adenopathy in an older woman.* If there has been no exposure to cats and there is no evidence for a superficial infection of the arm, then a CXR, CBC, and diagnostic mammogram are indicated. Early referral to a surgeon for a biopsy is necessary.

22–2, A. Learning objective: *List causes of generalized lymphadenopathy with splenomegaly.* There are several common causes of generalized lymphadenopathy with splenomegaly: infectious mononucleosis, chronic lymphocytic leukemia, Hodgkin's disease, non-Hodgkin's lymphoma, and other leukemias. Mononucleosis is unlikely at his age. The indolent presentation points to CLL or lymphoma.

22–2, B. Learning objective: *Order and interpret the appropriate tests for patients with generalized lymphadenopathy and associated splenomegaly.* The CBC will immediately suggest CLL if the absolute lymphocyte count is elevated. Often it is greater than 25,000 and constitutes greater than 90% of the white cell differential. The WBC differential also discloses an acute leukemia. In addition, a CXR showing hilar lymphadenopathy suggests either Hodgkin's or non-Hodgkin's lymphoma. If the CBC does not support CLL, immediate referral for biopsy is appropriate.

22–3, A. Learning objective: *Recognize a mono-like syndrome and know the differential diagnosis.* Influenza is very difficult to diagnosis with certainty on the basis of history, exam, and routine labs. All of the symptoms mentioned are seen with influenza although coryza, sore throat, and cough are expected. Classic flu usually has an abrupt onset (patients can recall the exact onset of illness) and resolves in two to five days. His significant adenopathy, especially outside the neck area, with fever, fatigue, and pharyngitis describes a mono-like syndrome. Lymphadenopathy would not be seen in influenza.

Differential diagnosis: infectious mononucleosis, acute HIV infection, acute CMV infection, acute toxoplasmosis, rubella, secondary syphilis, sarcoidosis, meningitis, and Hodgkin's disease. Rarer infections (e.g., typhoid fever, leptospirosis, brucellosis) may occur similarly but generally have some distinguishing feature.

22–3, B. Learning objective: *Gather a complete sexual history to assess risk of HIV infection.* A detailed sexual history may raise the concern for HIV: any male-to-male contacts, visits to prostitutes, lack of condom use, visits to an STD clinic, and history of genital sores. Note that in spite of the recent drop in mortality from AIDS, the incidence of new HIV infections has not declined. Review the risk for toxoplasmosis: new pet cat or eating undercooked meat, especially lamb or pork. Presence of photophobia or neck stiffness raises the probability of meningitis.

22–3, C. Learning objective: *Order appropriate test for the mono-like syndrome.* Order CBC with white cell differential, Monospot, electrolytes, BUN, creatinine, ALT/AST, LDH, and CXR. If you suspect primary HIV infection, order an HIV RNA and HIV ELISA/Western blot. The HIV tests require the patient's consent. In primary HIV infection, the ELISA is negative and HIV RNA is positive. An indeterminate Western blot can be seen. The CD_4 count is useless because many infections can transiently suppress this. Any suspicion of meningitis necessitates a lumbar puncture to rule-out bacterial meningitis. If the patient is not dehydrated and initial laboratory testing does not disclose any significant abnormalities, outpatient management is legitimate. Use your clinical judgment. If you are not completely comfortable sending the patient home, admit for observation.

22–4, A. Learning objective: *Identify the importance of examining for generalized adenopathy.* In this young woman with relatively recent symptoms, viral or bacterial pharyngitis is the most likely explanation. Your examination is incomplete without screening for other adenopathy and splenomegaly. These, if present, indicate another differential diagnosis list.

22–4, B. Learning objective: *Recognize the limited role for laboratory testing under these circumstances.* This patient requires a strep throat culture or rapid strep detection. If negative, no other testing is warranted. Her symptoms are of short duration.

22–4, C. Learning objective: *Design a follow-up plan for significant lymphadenopathy.* Although clinical improvement is reassuring, her cervical lymph nodes are quite large (greater than 1.5 cm) and should be re-examined in several weeks to be certain they have resolved or significantly decreased in size.

▶ SLEEPING ABNORMALITIES ANSWERS

23–1, A. Learning objective: *Recognize sleep problems as a cause of daytime fatigue.* Fatigue has many potential causes, including iron deficiency and hypothyroidism. This patient reports falling asleep inappropriately during the day, suggesting that her sleep at night is insufficient for some reason.

542

Case Answers

23–1, B. Learning objective: *Pursue a screening sleep history when a patient reports fatigue or excessive daytime sleepiness.* On specific questioning, this patient reports obtaining only four to five hours of sleep each night because of troublesome leg "cramps." On further description, the "cramps" are actually an uncomfortable crawling sensation in both legs that begins each night at bedtime. She gets up and shakes her legs or walks to obtain relief. When she lies back down, the sensation recurs. This happened occasionally during her pregnancies several years ago, but now the problem is more debilitating and more persistent. She thinks her father may have the same problem.

23–1, C. Learning objective: *Identify restless legs syndrome (RLS) by history.* Her description is classic for RLS. Patients may also describe their limb sensation as itching, painful, burning, or aching, or may find it difficult to describe. The key features are restlessness, overwhelming urge to move the limbs, and symptoms that occur or are worse in the evening or night and with rest. Other family members may also be affected.

23–1, D. Learning objective: *Seek and treat the underlying cause of RLS, if one is present.* This patient has iron deficiency as a likely explanation for active symptoms of RLS. Replacement of iron, and folate or B_{12} deficiency if identified, is the appropriate next step.

23–2, A. Learning objective: *List conditions that reversibly impair the alertness or response time of a driver, including sleep disorders.* Alcohol and other substance use, hypoglycemia, seizures, and malignant arrhythmias are all causes of potential driver impairment, for which the privilege of driving may be suspended in most if not all jurisdictions. Sleep deprivation and sleep disorders also increase the chance of moving vehicle accidents (MVAs), especially in a driver who reports sometimes dozing off at the wheel and in one who has had prior MVAs.

23–2, B. Learning objective: *Inquire further into the sleep history in patients with motor vehicle accidents.* This patient probably fell asleep at the wheel, and he has findings on H & P exam suggestive of OSA. In this case, his wife was interviewed and reported that he snores, loudly and often, and sometimes stops breathing in his sleep. The patient denied daytime sleepiness but did admit to nodding off at times, including while driving.

23–2, C. Learning objective: *Identify key pieces of advice for a patient with OSA.* This patient should be advised of the likelihood that he has OSA. Because of his history, he should be advised not to drive until this question can be evaluated further and appropriate treatment is begun. Weight loss, methods to encourage side-sleeping, and avoidance of alcohol and sedatives before bedtime may lessen the frequency and severity of obstructive apneas and allow him more restorative sleep.

23–2, D. Learning objective: *Refer a patient with probable sleep disorder to a sleep medicine specialist.* This patient almost certainly has a sleep disorder, most likely OSA. He needs further evaluation with a nocturnal sleep study. If OSA is confirmed, he needs treatment with CPAP and attempt at weight loss.

► CARDIAC ARRHYTHMIAS ANSWERS

24–1, A–B. Learning objective: *Recognize atrial fibrillation as a cause of exercise intolerance and choose appropriate therapy.* The rhythm strip shows atrial fibrillation. This is a common arrhythmia, especially in the setting of CHF. Because of the rapid rate and absence of atrial contraction, the left ventricle does not fill well during diastole. This results in a decreased cardiac output, which may cause fatigue and shortness of breath with activity. Atrial fibrillation accompanied by a rapid ventricular rate should be treated with an agent to slow the rate of conduction through the AV node (usually a β-blocker or calcium channel blocker). Patients without contraindications to anticoagulation should also be placed on coumadin.

24–2, A–B. Learning objective: *Recognize ventricular tachycardia and treat appropriately with emergent cardioversion and antiarrhythmic therapy.* The ECG tracing shows ventricular tachycardia. The rhythm is fast and the QRS is wide. This potentially lethal condition occurs most often as a complication of myocardial ischemia or infarction. Treatment consists of immediate cardioversion and administration of antiarrhythmic drugs such as lidocaine or amiodarone. Quick treatment is the key to patient survival.

► CONGESTIVE HEART FAILURE ANSWERS

24–3, A. Learning objective: *State common symptoms and signs of CHF.* Her presentation is explained by her previous MI with ensuing CHF. Ask about orthopnea (how many pillows does she need and has this changed recently?), PND, and prior vs. current edema. Quantify exercise capacity and ask about other reasons for shortness of breath. Ask about weight, diet (salt intake), and medication compliance. Check vital signs; weight; JVP; PMI; heaves; heart sounds; lung exam for rales; wheezes or dullness (effusions); abdominal bruits or abdominojugular reflux; and extremities for cyanosis, clubbing, edema, and perfusion.

24–3, B. Learning objective: *Design appropriate work-up for new-onset CHF.* CBC, chemistry panel, ECG, oxygen saturation, CXR, and echocardiogram should be ordered. ECG may reveal evidence of further ischemia or an arrhythmia, such as atrial fibrillation, which can contribute to CHF. Consider a TSH if signs or symptoms are consistent. Cardiac enzymes may be helpful if you suspect she has had more ischemia recently. She may need repeat catheterization to reassess the angioplasty results.

24–3, C. Learning objective: _Adjust therapy for moderate CHF._ This patient has moderate CHF with new edema and DOE indicating volume overload. Hospitalization should be considered. Start furosemide, e.g., 20-40 mg PO qam, and increase ACEI to maximum dose, e.g., enalapril 20 mg PO bid, over one to two weeks. Check creatinine and potassium every two to three days and, if outpatient, see her at least weekly until asymptomatic. Once she is no longer volume overloaded, start a β-blocker for ischemic heart disease and CHF. Patients with diabetes on β-blocker should be warned that β-blockers decrease adrenergic symptoms of hypoglycemia (palpitations and shakiness). She should rely on sweating as the main symptom.

24–4, A. Learning objective: _Recognize diastolic dysfunction in CHF._ Diastolic dysfunction is highly likely given this patient's hypertension with clinical volume overload and CHF and the presence of S_4, and LVH on ECG.

24–4, B. Learning objective: _Design appropriate work-up for suspected diastolic dysfunction._ This patient has a long history of hypertension making resultant diastolic dysfunction the most likely cause for his CHF symptoms. Obtain a CXR to evaluate heart size and an echocardiogram. Both heart size and ejection fraction may be normal. Other causes of diastolic dysfunction include hemochromatosis, amyloidosis, and sarcoidosis. Of these, the most likely in this elderly man would be amyloidosis from multiple myeloma. Thus, serum calcium, SPEP, and UPEP might be revealing. Hemochromatosis would probably have occurred earlier, but a screening ferritin and iron saturation would rule-out this possibility.

24–4, C. Learning objective: _Prescribe appropriate initial treatment for diastolic dysfunction._ Treatment to slow the heart rate and increase diastolic filling time is indicated. A β-blocker would be the medication of choice. Because he is volume overloaded, diuretics (e.g., furosemide 20 mg PO qam) should be initiated.

▶ ISCHEMIC HEART DISEASE ANSWERS

24–5, A. Learning objective: _Recognize atypical symptoms of myocardial ischemia._ This patient's age and risk factor profile place her at high risk for CAD. While she does not have frank chest pain, her symptoms are otherwise typical in that they are brought on with exercise and relieved with rest. Her ECG shows T-wave inversions in the inferior leads, consistent with the diagnosis of myocardial ischemia. Based on history and ECG, she has a high likelihood of CAD as the cause of her symptoms. Because these symptoms are new, she meets criteria for the diagnosis of unstable angina.

24–5, B. Learning objective: *Order appropriate lab testing in patients with possible active coronary ischemia.* Goals of testing are to 1) assess risk for progression to acute MI or sudden cardiac death, 2) detect conditions that could be provoking or exacerbating ischemia, and 3) identify modifiable CAD risk factors. CK (with MB fraction, which is more specific for myocardial tissue) and troponin I should be ordered to detect myocardial injury and to evaluate risk. Elevated cardiac enzyme levels place this patient in a higher risk category and support a more aggressive approach to management. CBC, thyroid testing, toxicology screen, and oxygen level determination will help identify conditions that may be increasing myocardial oxygen demand or decreasing oxygen delivery. A lipid panel will identify patients who will benefit from long-term lipid reduction therapy.

24–5, C. Learning objective: *Appropriately triage and treat patients with unstable angina.* Recognize and hospitalize patients with unstable angina. While this patient is not having ischemic symptoms in your office, she has a low-to intermediate risk, based on new onset angina of moderate severity with an abnormal resting ECG, for progressing to acute MI in the near future. Treat her with medications that will 1) relieve symptoms and 2) reduce risk for MI. Initial management should include aspirin and a β-blocker. If the patient is intolerant or hypersensitive to aspirin, clopidogrel or ticlopidine should be used. If ischemic symptoms develop or if cardiac enzymes are elevated, start heparin and nitrates. For ongoing ischemia despite these measures, or for planned angiography with stent/plasty, the American College of Cardiology recommends adding a platelet GP IIb/IIIa receptor antagonist agent (eftifibatide or tirofiban). A similar medication, abciximab, is not recommended because of its high cost.

24–5, D. Learning objective: *Use features of the clinical course to guide further testing in patients with new onset angina.* If the patient remains symptom-free in the hospital and has a stable ECG and normal cardiac enzymes, she should undergo further testing to evaluate risk with either an ETT or a nuclear medicine perfusion study. If she has recurrent symptoms, evolving ECG changes, elevated cardiac enzymes, or significant ischemia by ETT or nuclear medicine perfusion study, she should be referred for coronary catheterization.

24–6, A. Learning objective: *Recognize acute MI.* Chest pain radiating to the shoulders and associated with diaphoresis increases the likelihood of acute MI. You should have obtained the ECG tracing within five minutes of his presentation and immediately diagnosed acute MI based on the presence of ST segment elevation in the anterior leads.

24–6, B. Learning objective: *Initiate reperfusion therapy within 30 minutes of presentation for patients with MI.* Admit him to an ICU and treat with aspirin (chewed, not swallowed whole), a β-blocker, and nitrates if necessary to relieve pain. The anterior location of his MI places him at significant risk for hemodynamic instability and, indeed, he is already tachycardic and hypotensive. He needs close monitoring. As soon as is feasible, reperfusion therapy should be initiated with either thrombolytics (assuming the patient has no contraindications to the use of these medicines) or coronary catheterization if readily available.

24–6, C. Learning objective: *Recognize complications of acute MI.* Arrhythmias are the most common complication of acute MI and generally occur near the time of presentation. Delayed complications include papillary muscle rupture, ventricular rupture, and LV clot. This patient's holosystolic murmur could be produced by either mitral valve regurgitation or rupture of the intraventricular septum. Order urgent echocardiogram to distinguish between these two possibilities.

▶ VALVULAR HEART DISEASE ANSWERS

24–7, A. Learning objective: *Recognize aortic regurgitation with an associated Austin-Flint murmur.* Only aortic regurgitation is present. The murmur at the apex is an Austin-Flint murmur that is caused by obstruction of mitral flow produced by partial closure of the otherwise normal mitral valve by the regurgitant jet.

24–7, B. Learning objective: *Recognize ankylosing spondylitis as a cause of AR.* The presentation of chronic back pain, morning stiffness, and reduced spine flexibility in a young man suggests ankylosing spondylitis, which can be associated with aortic regurgitation and AV conduction abnormalities, especially in patients with long-standing, severe disease.

24–7, C. Learning objective: *Design an appropriate initial work-up for an asymptomatic pathologic murmur.* Obtain an ECG to look for LVH, a CXR to look for left ventricular prominence, and an echo to visualize the valves, grade the severity of the regurgitation, and measure LV function. Image the spine and sacroiliac joints. Obtain a sedimentation rate and consider checking HLA-B27 status.

24–7, D. Learning objective: *Appropriately manage a pathologic murmur.* Afterload reduction with an agent such as an ACEI or a vasodilating calcium channel blocker is appropriate. Indications for referral for correction of aortic insufficiency include moderate to severe symptoms, ejection fraction below 55%, and LV end-systolic dimension greater than 55 mm.

24–7, E. Learning objective: *Remember to offer antibiotic prophylaxis for dental procedures.* He should receive 2g of amoxicillin PO one hour prior to the extraction.

24–8, A. Learning objective: *List clinical features of severe aortic stenosis.*

1. The murmur peaks later in systole.
2. The aortic component of the second heart sound diminishes. There is reversed splitting of the second sound.
3. The carotid upstrokes become diminished and delayed.
4. There is a palpable left ventricular heave or thrill.
5. There is a lag between PMI and carotid artery upstroke.
6. A previously loud murmur becomes softer as cardiac output decreases.

24–8, B. Learning objective: *Avoid exercise testing in patients with symptomatic aortic stenosis.* Patients with symptomatic aortic stenosis should not undergo exercise testing because this may precipitate syncope or myocardial ischemia. Patients with aortic stenosis can have chest pain due to the stenosis alone, and anginal symptoms do not always indicate underlying atherosclerotic disease. The aortic stenosis should be evaluated first by echocardiogram. If you wish to rule-out atherosclerosis, an angiogram is probably a better idea.

▶ DERMATOLOGY ANSWERS

25–1, A. Learning objective: *Recognize conditions associated with eczema and its typical distribution pattern.* This is a typical presentation of eczema. Some clues: young age, history of another "atopic" condition, and distribution of the rash on the flexor surfaces of her arms.

25–1, B. Learning objective: *Recognize the potential for secondary bacterial infection of an excoriated rash.* The yellow crusting is concerning for secondary bacterial infection. The appearance is similar to the "honey-crusting" seen with impetigo. Impetigo is usually caused by common skin flora, such as staphylococcal or streptococcal species.

25–1, C. Learning objective: *Design treatment for eczema with secondary bacterial infection.* The patient should first receive an antibiotic with activity against skin flora, such as cephalexin. Antihistamines may be added, especially at night, to minimize scratching. Keep fingernails short. Once the infection has cleared, treat with a medium-potency topical steroid with liberal application of a lanolin-free moisturizer.

25–2, A. Learning objective: *Recognize the typical presentation of herpes zoster.* This is a very typical presentation of herpes zoster. Clues are the patient's older age, the painful prodrome of the rash and the characteristic dermatomal distribution of the rash.

25–2, B. Learning objective: *Recognize the efficacy of antiviral therapy in the acute treatment of zoster.* Start immediate antiviral therapy with either oral acyclovir or valacyclovir in order to speed healing of the rash and to shorten the course of postherpetic neuralgia, should it occur. Antivirals are more effective the sooner they are given. Efficacy is unclear if given more than 72 hours after the onset of symptoms.

25–2, C. Learning objective: *Recognize the risk of corneal involvement in facial zoster and the seriousness of this condition.* Because the patient has lesions on his forehead, he should be evaluated urgently by an ophthalmologist to rule-out corneal involvement. If there are early signs of corneal lesions on careful exam, the patient should be given immediate high-dose intravenous acyclovir to prevent corneal scarring and possible blindness. Topical steroid drops and cycloplegics may be required if there is an associated uveitis.

25–3, A. Learning objective: *State the features of a suspicious mole.* In addition to noting the lesion's asymmetry, flatness, and size, ask whether the lesion has been itching or bleeding and note whether it has any color variation. A complete exam should also include examination of the rest of the skin and whether regional lymph nodes are enlarged.

25–3, B. Learning objective: *Recognize a mole that is highly suspect for melanoma.* The primary concern is for malignant melanoma. When a patient notes that a pigmented lesion has been growing, especially if the borders are asymmetric, the suspicion for melanoma should be high.

25–3, C. Learning objective: *Design appropriate diagnostic evaluation of a highly suspect mole.* Given the high clinical suspicion for melanoma, the most appropriate initial procedure should be definitive excision.

▶ ADRENAL DISORDERS ANSWERS

26–1, A. Learning objective: *Recognize acute adrenal crisis.* This patient is in adrenal crisis. Differential diagnosis includes adrenal crisis, hypoxia, bleeding, myocardial infarction, and sepsis. History of COPD suggests steroid dependence with resulting adrenal suppression. He may not have received stress-dose steroids prior to surgery. Hypotension unresponsive to saline challenge is a common finding in adrenal crisis.

26–1, B. Learning objective: *Design a work-up that includes screening for adrenal insufficiency (prior to administering steroids) in hypotensive patients with risk factors for adrenal insufficiency.* Obtain serum cortisol immediately (prior to treatment) and do not wait for results to begin treatment. There is no indication that a single dose of steroids will worsen outcome if the patient has sepsis instead. A cortisol less than 20 µg/dL is diagnostic. Obtain

ABG, blood cultures, CBC, serial hematocrits, urinalysis, basic chemistry, CXR, and ECG to rule-out hypoxia, infection, and bleeding.

26–1, C. Learning objective: *Appropriately treat adrenal crisis with high-dose hydrocortisone.* Treat emergently with hydrocortisone (100 mg IV Q8 hours), volume repletion with glucose and IV saline, and other supportive measures as needed. Empiric antibiotics may be warranted while culture results and cortisol level are pending.

26–2, A. Learning objective: *Recognize common findings that may mimic Cushing's.* Cushing's syndrome is rare. The estimated annual incidence of pituitary-dependent Cushing's disease is 0.1–1 new cases per 100,000. Cushing's syndrome is 0.5–5 per 100,000. Obesity and depression (affects approximately 25% of adults), however, are much more common. Obesity remains the most frequent reason for Cushing's syndrome evaluation. Other explanations for this woman's symptoms might be sleep apnea with resultant hypertension and increasing obesity, polycystic ovaries, and hypothyroidism.

26–2, B. Learning objective: *Design appropriate testing to detect Cushing's syndrome.* If initial testing for thyroid disease, PCO, and sleep apnea are normal, you may want to screen for Cushing's. Initial evaluation can be a 24-hour urine cortisol level. If these results are equivocal, perform a 48-hour, low-dose dexamethasone suppression test followed by CRH stimulation. This maneuver suppresses plasma cortisol levels in normal people but not in Cushing's syndrome. Dexamethasone (0.5 mg every 6 hours) is taken orally eight times starting at 1200 hours, then CRH (1 μg/kg IV) is given at 0800 hours (2 hours following the last dexamethasone dose). In normal individuals, the cortisol concentration is less than 39 nmol/L following CRH and greater than 40 in those with Cushing's syndrome.

▶ DIABETES ANSWERS

26–3, A. Learning objective: *Distinguish between type 1 and type 2 diabetes.* Glucose results confirm diabetes. Based on age, symptoms (polyuria, polydipsia, weight loss) and in the setting of obesity, she has type 2 diabetes. Type 2 diabetes more commonly occurs in patients older than age 40, but insulin resistance can precipitate type 2 diabetes earlier, especially in ethnic groups at risk. If she were thinner, islet cell antibodies or GAD antibodies would be helpful (positive in approximately 80% of patients with type 1 diabetes). Although ketones in the urine should always lead to consideration of type 1 diabetes, in her case, ketones in the urine are likely due to starvation (anorexia).

26–3, B. Learning objective: *Design appropriate initial insulin therapy.* Dose based on weight at 0.5–1 U/kg/d (higher end of dosing range used for obese patients with insulin resistance). In her case, she required approximately 100 U/kg (220lb = 100kg) over the first 24 hours; it is reasonable to dose her at the high end. For basal bolus regimen, start 50% of insulin as basal insulin, e.g., 50 U of glargine at bedtime. Have her check Chemstrips four times daily (qac and qhs, meaning before meals and before sleep). Goals are a fasting glucose of less than 110 mg/dL and glycated hemoglobin of 6.5%. The remaining 50 U should be distributed as lispro insulin with meals, e.g., 15 U at breakfast, 15 U at lunch, and 20 U with dinner, depending on actual planned caloric intake at those times. Patients on this regimen need to learn carbohydrate counting, typically using 1 U lispro/15 gm carbohydrate.

26–3, C. Learning objective: *Order appropriate screening tests in a patient newly diagnosed with type 2 diabetes.* Order urine for microalbuminuria, fasting lipid panel, and TSH because hypothyroidism is common and complicates diabetes and lipid management. Only type 1 patients have an increased incidence of autoimmune thyroid disease. Initial protein on Chemstrip may be due to renal disease, but may be a false positive because the diabetes is out of control. Repeat it when the diabetes has stabilized. She needs an eye examination now.

26–4, A. Learning objective: *Perform appropriate initial evaluation for a patient with new type 2 diabetes.* She probably has type 2 diabetes based on her random glucose and nocturia. Check fasting glucose twice to confirm the diagnosis. Obtain further history on diet and exercise as well as risk factors for and symptoms of CVD. Initial exam should include eye exam for retinopathy, foot exam for peripheral neuropathy and deformities that increase the risk for foot ulcers. Skin exam can search for acanthosis nigricans (indicates insulin resistance), necrobiosis lipoidica diabeticorum, and signs of peripheral vascular disease with decreased pulses or ulcers on the feet. Order A1C, fasting lipids, urine protein/creatinine ratio for microalbuminuria, BUN and creatinine, and obtain a baseline ECG.

26–4, B. Learning objective: *Convert A1C to average blood glucose levels.* Start with 120 mg/dL (normal) and add 30 mg/dL for every 1% of A1C over 6%. If 6% = 120 mg/dL, then 9% = 120 mg/dL + (3 × 30) = 210 mg/dL. Her A1C is just below this at 8.8% or about 200 mg/dL. Check A1C every three months while changing therapy or working toward the goal of less than 6.5% (this may not be appropriate for all patients) and every six months when stable at or near goal.

26–4, C. Learning objective: *Start appropriate therapy for patients with newly diagnosed type 2 diabetes.* Initial treatment is with diet, referral to a nutritionist, and exercise. Consider an exercise treadmill if multiple cardiac disease risk factors or symptoms exist. She should return with serial blood pressure and glucose measurements after a four to six week trial. Given an A1C of 8.8%, an oral agent will probably be needed. Because of her obesity, metformin is the drug of choice if creatinine is less than 1.4 mg/dL and if she does not have CHF or liver problems. Start slow to avoid GI side effects with 250 mg a day; double the dose every three to five days until you reach 500 mg bid. Titrate up as needed for good control or maximum dose of 850 mg PO tid over several weeks. Warn about GI side-effects that affect compliance.

26–4, D. Learning objective: *Choose appropriate initial therapy for hypertension and hyperlipidemia in type 2 diabetes.* For hypertension, start an ACEI (e.g., benazepril 5 mg PO qd). Patients with diabetes should be started on therapy for LDL greater than 130 with a goal LDL less than 100. Dietary counseling is appropriate in all patients. Statins, e.g., pravastatin and simvastatin, are the drugs of choice because niacin increases insulin resistance.

▶ HYPERLIPIDEMIA ANSWERS

26–5, A–E. Learning objective: *Know whom to screen, and how to screen for hyperlipidemia.* For A, order a complete lipid panel. For B, no screening is necessary because the patient is young and her father had a heart attack older than age 55. For C, order a TG level only as you are looking for a cause of her pancreatitis. For D, order a TC and HDL because this is a young person with no risk factors for CAD. For E, order a complete lipid panel because you want to know the LDL in this patient with elevated TC.

26–6, A. Learning objective: *Be able to calculate LDL, or use an estimate of LDL when TG levels are high.* Use the formula in the chapter to calculate LDL. Substitute the number 400 in this formula for TG levels to estimate LDL when TG levels are greater than 400. This approach actually overestimates LDL, but allows treatment decisions to be made based on estimated LDL.

26–6, B. Learning objective: *Appropriately treat hypertriglyceridemia in the absence of known CAD or high LDL levels.* Recommend diet, exercise, and weight loss. Be sure to diagnose and treat other causes of hypertriglyceridemia (alcohol excess, hyperglycemia, hypothyroidism, and nephrotic syndrome).

26–7, A. Learning objective: *Use the NCEP guidelines to determine LDL treatment goals.* The goal LDL is less than 130; she has two risk factors, age and hypertension.

26–7, B. Learning objective: *Recognize and treat causes of secondary hyperlipidemia before starting medications for hyperlipidemia.* She has evidence of hypothyroidism (elevated TSH), which can cause hyperlipidemia. Treat the hypothyroidism first with thyroid replacement therapy. If the LDL is still too high, despite diet and exercise therapy and thyroid replacement, consider a statin.

▶ MALE HYPOGONADISM ANSWERS

26–8, A. Learning objective: *Distinguish between primary and secondary hypogonadism.* Elevated gonadotropins indicate primary hypogonadism (testicular failure).

26–8, B. Learning objective: *Identify the most common causes of primary hypogonadism.* Klinefelter's syndrome (XXY karyotype) is the most common cause of primary hypogonadism. Klinefelter's syndrome is associated with small testes. Other common causes of primary hypogonadism include trauma, bilateral orchidectomy, and postpubertal mumps orchitis.

26–8, C. Learning objective: *Understand the goals of therapy in primary and secondary hypogonadism.* Androgen replacement therapy is considered for all men with hypogonadism. Men with primary hypogonadism are generally infertile, although an occasional man with primary hypogonadism might conceive with assisted reproductive techniques. Men with secondary hypogonadism may be fertile with appropriate hormonal therapy (gonadotropin-releasing hormone or gonadotropin therapy). Androgen replacement therapy is much cheaper than hormone therapy for fertility.

26–9, A. Learning objective: *Recognize the presentation of male hypogonadism.* The differential diagnosis of these vague symptoms includes depression, congestive heart failure, adverse drug effect (β-blocker), and hypogonadism.

26–9, B. Learning objective: *Understand the evaluation of secondary hypogonadism.* Order a pituitary MRI to exclude a macroadenoma and iron studies to exclude hemochromatosis. Perform a careful H & P to look for Cushing's syndrome.

▶ THYROID DISEASE ANSWERS

26–10, A. Learning objective: *Recognize apathetic hyperthyroidism in an elderly patient.* His weight loss with anorexia, proximal muscle weakness, as evidenced by his difficulty with stairs, and atrial arrhythmia are classic signs of apathetic hyperthyroidism in an older person. If thyroid function tests are normal, rule-out depression or occult malignancy. He also needs treatment for atrial fibrillation.

26–10, B. Learning objective: *Interpret thyroid function tests and identify the most likely cause of hyperthyroidism based an features of the clinical setting.* This patient has a suppressed TSH and an elevated free T_4, consistent with clinical hyperthyroidism. Toxic multinodular goiter is suggested by his lumpy thyroid exam findings and is common in the elderly. Acute thyroiditis is unlikely because the thyroid is not tender. Graves' disease usually occurs in younger women, so is less likely here.

26–10, C. Learning objective: *Describe treatment of toxic multinodular goiter.* Initially, start methimazole or PTU. Once he is euthyroid, radioactive iodine ablation can be performed. Propranolol may control his heart rate while antithyroid medication takes effect. Propranolol should be used during radioactive iodine ablation to avoid thyrotoxicosis from gland destruction.

26–11, A. Learning objective: *Recognize myxedema coma and list other common problems in the differential when an elderly patient presents with altered mental status.* Differential includes MI, infection, hypothyroid myxedema coma, stroke, metabolic derangement (hypo- or hypernatremia and hypercalcemia), drug overdose, and alcohol ingestion.

26–11, B. Learning objective: *Recognize and name seven features of myxedema coma.* Elevated TSH, low free T_4, depressed mental status, hypothermia, bradycardia, hypoventilation, macroglossia, cool dry doughy skin, constipation, congestive heart failure, and probable pericardial effusion are all classic signs and symptoms for myxedema coma, a potentially fatal condition.

26–11, C. Learning objective: *Describe medications and supportive therapies for myxedema coma.* Give IV levothyroxine and high-dose glucocorticoids for her life-threatening myxedema coma. She needs intensive supportive care. Her respiratory status is in jeopardy: hypoventilation and aspiration risk due to somnolence warrants ABG and probable intubation. Even with clinical response to medical therapy, some patients require prolonged ventilatory support, presumably due to accompanying, slow-to-resolve respiratory muscle weakness. Cardiac status is also worrisome (bradycardia, CHF, and probable pericardial effusion). Pericardial effusion in hypothyroidism usually develops slowly, does not lead to tamponade, and often responds to medical therapy without requiring urgent pericardiocentesis. For hypothermia, gentle rewarming is usually sufficient. Myxedema coma is often precipitated by infection, so look for this with exam, blood, urine, sputum cultures and CXR and begin antibiotics if indicated.

26–11, D. Learning objective: *Describe lab abnormalities associated with hypothyroidism.* CPK, SGOT, LDH, and cholesterol can all be elevated and usually normalize with levothyroxine. Hematocrit and sodium may be low.

26–11, E. Learning objective: *List the likely causes of hypothyroidism.* Radioiodine ablation for Graves' disease is the most common cause of hypothyroidism. In this case, she also may not have been taking prescribed thyroxine. Hashimoto's thyroiditis is also common. If this is the case, her symptoms could have developed insidiously or perhaps were attributed to old age. Because she lives in the U.S. where salt is supplemented with iodine, and there was no mention of a goiter on her exam, iodine insufficiency is unlikely.

▶ BILIARY TRACT DISEASE ANSWERS

27–1, A. Learning objective: *Identify key history, exam, and labs that help narrow your differential diagnosis in a woman with right upper quadrant pain.* Has she had this before (gallstones or peptic ulcer)? How much alcohol does she use (pancreatitis)? Is she having unprotected sex, traveling, or using injection drugs (hepatitis)? Has she had recent dysuria, hematuria, frequency, flank or back pain (pyelonephritis)? Has she had any changes in her bowel habits (gastroenteritis or bowel obstruction)? Has the stool been abnormally colored (melena suggests peptic ulcer; pale stools suggest common bile duct obstruction)? Examine for signs of sepsis with orthostatic vital signs, for signs of retroperitoneal hemorrhage suggesting pancreatitis, for jaundice suggesting hepatitis or cholangitis, and for peritoneal signs suggesting perforated viscus. CBC looks for signs of infection. Electrolytes may show an acidosis from sepsis or bowel perforation. Bilirubin and alkaline phosphatase identify biliary obstruction; SGOT and SGPT identify hepatocyte inflammation. Amylase and lipase help evaluate for pancreatitis. Abdominal films find free air or bowel obstruction. Urgent abdominal ultrasound or CT scan provides evidence of biliary tree obstruction, cholecystitis, or gallstones. In her case, CBC, alkaline phosphatase, and bilirubin are high.

27–1, B. Learning objective: *Identify three potentially life-threatening conditions that cause right upper quadrant pain.* You don't want to miss perforated ulcer, ascending cholangitis, or pancreatitis because these can rapidly worsen and are potentially fatal. With her clinical picture and elevated CBC, bilirubin, and alkaline phosphatase, cholangitis is very likely.

27–1, C. Learning objective: *Appropriately triage a patient with possible ascending cholangitis and sepsis to intensive care.* This patient is very ill. High pulse and low blood pressure (especially low relative to her usual hypertension) are worrisome indicators of sepsis. Respiratory rate is high, increasing concern for sepsis, acidosis, and a compensatory respiratory alkalosis. She needs inpatient intensive care for resuscitation, rapid diagnosis, and treatment.

27–1, D. Learning objective: *Recognize potentially lethal cholangitis and appropriately treat with urgent ERCP and empiric antibiotics.* RUQ pain and signs of early sepsis make cholangitis possible. She needs urgent GI consult for ERCP. Start empiric IV antibiotics. Ampicillin/sulbactam or other β-lactam/β-lactamase is more cost-effective than any three-drug therapy. Give IV fluids and monitor closely because her condition may quickly deteriorate.

▶ LIVER DISEASE ANSWERS

27–2, A. Learning objective: *State the differential diagnosis for jaundice.* The differential diagnosis includes viral, alcoholic, autoimmune, and drug-induced hepatitis. Biliary obstruction due to gallstone or neoplasm is also possible. Hereditary causes of liver disease are not likely in this patient due to the acute onset and older age, although hemochromatosis occasionally occurs later in women because of the phlebotomy-like effect of menses.

27–2, B. Learning objective: *Order appropriate laboratory studies in a jaundiced patient.* Given jaundice, order a broad panel including ALT, AST, bilirubin, albumin, PTT, PT INR, and alkaline phosphatase. If transaminases are elevated to a greater degree than bilirubin and alkaline phosphatase, order hepatitis A, B, and C serologies. If bilirubin and alkaline phosphatase are more elevated, order a right upper quadrant ultrasound to rule-out biliary obstruction.

27–2, C. Learning objective: *Do a thorough history to look for potential exposures as the cause of an acute hepatitis.* Quantitate alcohol intake. Ask about potential toxic exposures and medications, especially in the elderly or in the setting of ongoing heavy alcohol use. Be sure to include over-the-counter remedies, particularly acetaminophen. This patient had elevated aminotransferases in the 1000 range and a bilirubin of 10.2. Hepatitis serology studies were normal except for a positive HAV IgG antibody indicating old infection. A careful review of his medical history revealed that he had been recently hospitalized with an MI and had been discharged on trazodone to help with sleep, a possible cause of drug-induced hepatitis. Withdrawal of trazodone resulted in resolution of his symptoms and normalization of bilirubin and aminotransferases.

27–3, A. Learning objective: *Identify appropriate diagnostic studies in the evaluation of hepatitis C.* HCV RNA tests, viral load, and liver biopsy are useful diagnostic studies for determining the extent of disease. The alanine aminotransferase level is an inexpensive and useful test that is best for monitoring HCV infection and the efficacy of therapy in the intervals between molecular testing. HCV genotype is useful for planning the duration of potential treatment because it is advisable to treat those infected with genotype 1 for 48 weeks and those infected with genotypes 2 and 3 for 24 weeks.

27–3, B. Learning objective: *Identify factors that would influence treatment of hepatitis C.* Hepatitis C treatment is appropriate for patients who are at the highest risk for progression of their disease. This includes patients with detectable levels of HCV RNA who have persistently elevated alanine aminotransferase levels and liver biopsy results demonstrating moderate necrosis and inflammation.

27–3, C. Learning objective: *Recognize the main factor that accelerates progression to cirrhosis.* Advise patients with any form of chronic hepatitis to abstain from alcohol ingestion in order to prevent acceleration and progression to cirrhosis of the liver.

▶ PANCREATITIS ANSWERS

27–4, A. Learning objective: *List three disorders in which abdominal pain can radiate to the back.* Pancreatitis, abdominal aortic aneurysm, pyelonephritis, osteomyelitis, perforated peptic ulcer, and epidural abscess all can cause back pain in association with abdominal pain.

27–4, B. Learning objective: *Identify key features of the clinical presentation that help differentiate causes of abdominal pain radiating to the back.* Pancreatitis is likely with long-standing use of alcohol. Young age makes abdominal aortic aneurysm (AAA) unlikely even though he smokes. Check for other risk factors of AAA including hypercholesterolemia, hypertension, family history of AAA, or signs of other vascular disease, such as carotid bruits or diminished pulses. He does not have a chronic bladder catheter, prostatic enlargement with bladder obstruction, or history of urinary tract stones or symptoms to put him at risk for pyelonephritis. He lacks TB exposure or intravenous drug use to place him at risk for vertebral or epidural infection.

27–4, C. Learning objective: *Order appropriate labs to diagnose pancreatitis and assess prognosis.* Amylase and lipase are sensitive and specific for pancreatitis. Assess prognosis using Ranson criteria. This patient has two criteria thus far: WBC greater than 16, SGOT greater than 250. Follow hematocrit, fluid requirement, calcium, BUN, and PaO_2 in the first 48 hours to assess all criteria. If no further criteria are met, his mortality risk is 2%.

27–4, D. Learning objective: *Design appropriate therapy for acute pancreatitis.* Order bowel rest, pain control, and NG tube suction to decrease emesis. Common clinical practice is to give IV meperidine rather than morphine for pain control because there is a theoretic risk of sphincter of Oddi spasm and worsening pancreatitis with morphine, although no evidence suggests a difference in outcome. If orthostatic, give normal saline boluses and recheck. Add dextrose to IV fluids for basal energy needs because he is not eating. If his illness persists, requiring prolonged bowel rest, start parenteral nutrition. He needs close monitoring for complications.

► GERIATRICS ANSWERS

28–1, A. Learning objective: *Understand clinical diagnostic criteria necessary to establish a diagnosis of dementia.* Memory deficits alone are not sufficient to make a diagnosis of dementia. Impairments must also be present in other areas of cognition and must be severe enough to impair usual function. Although this patient is having difficulty completing her tasks at work, there is no history of other cognitive impairments besides memory complaints. Although many patients with isolated short-term memory impairment do later develop other deficits sufficient to make a diagnosis of dementia (about 10% per year), the diagnosis of dementia is not made until all diagnostic criteria are met.

28–1, B. Learning objective: *Recognize that depression is a common cause of "reversible dementia" and that this patient has many features suggestive of depression.* Drugs and depression are the most common causes of reversible cognitive impairment and should be considered for all patients who present with memory or other cognitive complaints. Patients who are depressed often emphasize their disabilities, e.g., difficulty with recall and concentration, whereas patients with Alzheimer's disease often deny, or are untroubled by, their impairments. This patient relates a fairly defined period of onset ("a few months ago") with steady worsening over a relatively short period, both features that are atypical of the usual insidious onset and slow decline of Alzheimer's and most other dementing illnesses. Her symptoms of decreased energy, sleep disturbance, and poor concentration are classic features of depression and, although she denies depressed mood, this is common, particularly in older adults. Her poor effort with serial calculations on MMSE testing is another hallmark of depression in that such patients often won't or can't concentrate to perform requested tasks and give up easily, compared with Alzheimer's patients who commonly cheerfully respond, albeit often with incorrect answers.

28–1, C. Learning objective: *Recognize that medications and medical conditions also need to be thoroughly reviewed and considered as potential causes in patients presenting with cognitive impairment.* This patient has been taking Tylenol PM, which contains diphenhydramine, a common over-the-counter antihistamine with anticholinergic effects that can impair memory. She also has significant risk factors for vascular disease (diabetes and hypertension) and, although her nonfocal neurologic examination argues against a stroke, this remains a possibility. Consider hypoglycemia in this patient who recently started on glipizide.

28–1, D. Learning objective: *Plan appropriate work-up for patients presenting with cognitive impairment.* Although this patient does not meet criteria for dementia, she does have cognitive complaints and memory deficits. Medical conditions that can cause both depressed mood and cognitive impairments (e.g., hypothyroidism and vitamin B_{12} deficiency) should be tested for with TSH and B_{12} levels, along with usual metabolic studies of electrolytes, renal and liver function, and CBC. Given the lack of focal neurologic signs or symptoms and history suggestive of other possible diagnoses (depression and drugs), a head CT scan isn't necessary now, but might be considered in follow-up if other tests are unrevealing.

28–1, E. Learning objective: *Stop medications that might worsen cognitive function, and consider a trial of an antidepressant in patients with cognitive impairment.* Before starting new medications, old drugs that might be having adverse effects should be discontinued. This patient's Tylenol PM should be discontinued and her glucose levels should be closely monitored to rule-out hypoglycemia. Unless she improves markedly with these changes, a trial of an antidepressant (usually an SSRI) should be initiated.

28–2, A. Learning objective: *Recognize overflow incontinence and diagnose by testing postvoid residual.* His history of markedly worsened hesitancy and force of stream, along with small volume incontinence is most consistent with overflow incontinence. He does not relate symptoms of urgency and, although urine loss with bending is consistent with stress incontinence, this can also occur in patients who incompletely empty their bladders. Stress incontinence tends to be a problem that mostly affects women. The key diagnostic test to detect overflow incontinence is a postvoid residual, which was 265 mL after a 300 mL void, confirming incomplete emptying and overflow incontinence.

28–2, B. Learning objective: *Recognize new, acute incontinence and consider causes in the DRIP mnemonic.* This patient has a history of several years of mild BPH symptoms (hesitancy, decreased force of stream, and nocturia), but when incontinence is new or suddenly worse, as in this case, DRIP causes should be considered. He is on two drugs that can impair bladder emptying: amlodipine, a calcium channel blocker, can decrease smooth muscle contractility (bladder); and Dimetapp contains brompheniramine (an antihistamine) that can impair bladder contractility due to anticholinergic effects; and pseudoephedrine (an α-agonist) that can impair emptying by increasing internal urethral sphincter tone. Over-the-counter allergy remedies frequently contain similar ingredients that can cause urinary retention in men with BPH. Other components of the DRIP mnemonic do not appear likely by history but a urinalysis should be obtained to rule-out infection.

28–2, C. Learning objective: *Review treatment options for BPH and recognize that referral to urology is appropriate in light of PVR more than 100 mL.* This patient does have potentially reversible causes of his overflow incontinence and it is reasonable to adjust his medications and re-evaluate before referring to urology. Discontinue Dimetapp and change amlodipine to an alternate antihypertensive, such as the α-blocker doxazosin, which treats both hypertension and BPH. If PVR remains above 100 mL after these medication changes, the patient should be referred to urology for possible surgery (TURP).

▶ BLEEDING DISORDERS

29–1, A. Learning objective: *Suspect ITP when petechiae appear in the setting of autoimmune disease.* The most likely diagnosis is ITP. Her autoimmune history puts her at a slightly higher risk of acquiring additional autoimmune complications such as ITP. The combination of ITP and autoimmune hemolytic anemia is known as Evans' syndrome and is seen in patients with underlying autoimmune disorders, such as lupus and rheumatoid arthritis.

29–1, B. Learning objective: *Order appropriate labs for the work-up of low platelets.* CBC will yield the most pertinent information for acute management. Typical platelet counts with an initial diagnosis of ITP are less than 50,000, and they can be as low as 1–5000. Evaluating for the presence of antiplatelet antibodies is not helpful, because they do not correlate with the presence of ITP or with disease activity in patients with chronic ITP.

29–1, C. Learning objective: *Treat ITP appropriately with steroids; add IVIG only if acute bleeding is present.* The highest risk for life-threatening bleeding associated with ITP is in the first month with a platelet count of less than 20,000. She has evidence of a primary hemostasis problem (petechiae or purpura), but no acute bleeding at present. She can therefore be treated with prednisone (1 mg/kg/day) for two to seven days, followed by a very slow taper over a month or more. If she had evidence of acute bleeding (and she does not), then IVIG (1 gm/kg/day × two days) is indicated, because the onset of action of IVIG is within hours rather than days.

▶ CLOTTING DISORDERS

29–2, A. Learning objective: *Develop a differential diagnosis for DVT in young patients.* Statistically, the two most likely diagnoses are an inherited factor V Leiden mutation (activated protein C resistance; genetic frequency of approximately 5%) and a prothrombin G20210A mutation (genetic frequency of approximately 3%).

29–2, B. Learning objective: *List appropriate diagnostic tests in the work-up of hypercoagulable state.* The most important studies to perform, in terms of probability, are DNA/PCR screening for factor V Leiden and the prothrombin mutation. These are not affected by anticoagulation therapy. Blood should be drawn to test for other autosomal dominant hypercoagulable disorders, such as protein C, protein S, and antithrombin III deficiencies, with careful consideration of how heparin (antithrombin III) or warfarin (proteins C and S) will affect the results. Note that in the setting of acute thrombosis, the measured levels of protein C, protein S, and antithrombin III may be falsely lowered.

29–2, C. Learning objective: _Order appropriate anticoagulant therapy._ Anticoagulation therapy should be initiated with heparin, followed by warfarin for six months. Prophylaxis in future situations with risk of thrombosis (surgery, trauma, immobilization) is recommended. It is not recommended during pregnancy.

29–2, D. Learning objective: _Recognize the heritable nature of many coagulation disorders and know the appropriate approach to family members._ The family history strongly suggests a heritable disorder. Screening of family members with a history of thrombophilia is indicated if it has not already been done. First-degree relatives of patients with one or more abnormal test results should be examined to determine whether they should receive primary prophylaxis (e.g., anticoagulation during elective surgery). Whether to screen all potential carriers who have not been affected is somewhat more controversial. In all of medicine, the issue of genetic susceptibility on the basis of specific testing is becoming a management issue. In general, any genetic testing in an otherwise healthy individual should be performed in conjunction with the help of a genetic counselor who is able to clearly describe the relative risks and benefits of obtaining such information. There are real concerns about discrimination involving e.g., third-party insurance carriers and potential employers, which must be considered. If a family history indicates that the genetic vulnerability poses a risk only as an adult, testing is usually deferred until the family member reaches the age of 18.

► ONCOLOGY ANSWERS

29–3, A. Learning objective: _Design appropriate work-up for a solitary pulmonary nodule._ Perform complete history and exam to identify other causes of this nodule besides lung cancer (perhaps an aspergilloma or a metastatic gastric cancer). Review old CXR to establish the history of the lesion. Characterize the lesion by chest CT and look for enlarged chest nodes. Bone scan may reveal bony metastases causing back pain. Chance of cancer is high. An early stage NSCLC that might be cured by excision is the best possible tumor you could find.

29–3, B. Learning objective: _List CXR features of pulmonary nodules that suggest malignancy._ Malignant nodules are more likely to double in volume (not diameter) between 7 and 465 days.

Nodules unchanged for two years are unlikely to be cancer. Eccentric or stippled calcifications, irregular shape, and poorly defined borders all suggest malignancy. The "pretest probability" is also important, (e.g., a nodule in a 25-year-old nonsmoker is unlikely to be lung cancer).

29–3, C. Learning objective: *List potential causes of hypercalcemia in a man with a pulmonary nodule.* A squamous cell lung cancer might produce parathyroid-like hormones, or less likely, bony metastases (remember his sore back) causing elevated calcium. Other potential causes unrelated to lung cancer include hyperparathyroidism, immobility, and multiple myeloma. CXR showed an eccentrically calcified nodule, work-up for nodes and metastases was negative, FEV_1 was high enough to allow lobectomy that showed adenocarcinoma with negative regional nodes. High calcium persisted, and eventually a parathyroid adenoma was removed. The patient knew it was a close call, and this helped him to quit smoking!

29–4, A. Learning objective: *Think of leukemia when someone has dyspnea, fatigue, and bleeding.* Common causes of "low energy" such as depression and CHF don't cause bleeding. The nosebleed may be coincidental; consider other diagnoses such as pneumonia, TB, anemia, or lung cancer. History of other bleeding really helps distinguish incidental from worrisome cause. She reports bleeding from her gums too.

29–4, B. Learning objective: *Learn how to diagnose acute leukemia.* Look for gum infiltration, adenopathy, petechiae, lung consolidation, meningitis, and focal neurologic deficits. Peripheral smear with blasts is a strong hint, but a bone marrow biopsy showing greater than 30% blasts defines leukemia. Auer rods—those red cigars in the cytoplasm—clinch the diagnosis of AML. Next, you need the hematopathologist to subtype the AML by identifying characteristic membrane antigens using flow cytometry.

29–4, C. Learning objective: *Anticipate the common complications of AML.* Look for sepsis (fever, tachycardia, hypotension) and check coagulation studies to rule-out DIC. If the white count is greater than 150,000, worry about sludging and tumor lysis with renal failure. CNS involvement is not common in adults, but if she develops a seventh nerve palsy, she needs head CT and LP.

29–5, A. Learning objective: *List cancers that can cause nodes in the supraclavicular fossa.* Virchow's node is a left supraclavicular node from metastatic intestinal cancers (stomach, colon). He is at risk for colon cancer because of his brother's colon cancer. Testicular cancers can appear in the neck—but he is a bit old. Perform a testicular exam to be sure. His 50 pack-years of smoking increases lung cancer risk. Fever could be due to postobstructive pneumonia, a "B" symptom of lymphoma, sarcoidosis, or tuberculosis.

29–5, B. Learning objective: *Describe the work-up for chest lymphadenopathy.* Although node biopsy is tempting, further imaging first helps you decide between a needle biopsy (for lung cancer or intestinal cancer) or excisional biopsy (for lymphomas). Chest and abdominal CT show no lung mass, but there is diffuse adenopathy and splenomegaly that you and your attending missed on exam. The biopsy shows an intermediate grade lymphoma, that is stage III-B.

29–5, C. Learning objective: *Learn the long-term effects of some cancer treatments.* He undergoes intensive chemotherapy with CHOP (cyclophosphamide, doxorubicin, vincristine, and prednisone). He is alive at five years, but is sterile and has an increased risk for a second primary cancer at any site.

29–6, A. Learning objective: *Understand the principles and methods of screening for colon cancer.* Almost all colon cancers could be prevented if their antecedent polyps were discovered and removed. Current recommendations are for screening to start at age 50 or earlier, if there is a family history or other risk factors. Colonoscopy is the most effective method, but compared with flexible sigmoidoscopy plus fecal occult blood testing, it has greater immediate costs, inconvenience, and modestly increased chance of complications.

29–6, B. Learning objective: *Understand Dukes' classification and the necessary work-up*. Refer to Table 29–5. The normal CT, CXR, and liver tests suggest that there are no metastases. Regardless of the depth of invasion of the original cancer, the involvement of regional lymph nodes defines Dukes' stage C. Before surgery, you would have ordered a carcinoembryonic antigen level to help you prognosticate.

29–6, C. Learning objective: *Understand the role of adjuvant chemotherapy in the treatment of colon cancer.* For her stage C tumor, you would recommend fluorouracil (5-FU) and leucovorin for six months. Less advanced tumors are simply excised. Treatment for metastatic disease varies but may include resection of isolated metastases, chemotherapy, or comfort care.

29–7, A. Learning objective: *Understand the evaluation of a prostate nodule.* Most palpable prostate nodules are benign and caused by calcification, scarring, or other processes. Suspicious ones may be evaluated by measuring the prostate-specific antigen (PSA), transrectal ultrasound, and often biopsy. In this case, the PSA was "high-normal" and a biopsy showed a tiny focus of intermediate grade. (The exam findings were coincidental.) The grade, or Gleason score, is based on histologic appearance and may predict the aggressiveness of the tumor.

29–7, B. Learning objective: *Counsel patients about difficult treatment decisions.* Your patient faces a potentially difficult decision because he is 70 years old, his tumor is very small, the benefits of treatment are not certain, but the morbidity of treatment is substantial. Help your patient make a list of questions that he should have answered in order to decide about treatment. For example, what might happen if he does nothing? What are the common complications of treatment? Then guide your patient through a discussion that defines his particular values, fears, and goals. Does he value most the chance to live a long time, or is he particularly fearful of the incontinence and impotence that may occur after therapy?

29–7, C. Learning objective: *Understand how screening decisions for prostate cancer are influenced by individual patient characteristics.* Screening is not appropriate for the son or the uncle, even with their family history and elevated risk for prostate cancer. Because prostate cancer is so rare at age 35, the grandson's PSA will be either normal or perhaps falsely elevated. The chances for a true positive are very small. The 92-year-old man has a high chance of having prostate cancer, but no treatment would be indicated unless he had symptoms; therefore, there is no reason to screen.

▶ GENITAL INFECTIONS ANSWERS

30–1, A. Learning objective: *State the differential diagnosis for vaginal itching in a 47-year-old woman.* Vaginal itching is a very nonspecific symptom and does not confirm the diagnosis of candidal vaginitis, although that is on the differential. Other possibilities include irritation from either the increased physiologic or pathologic discharge, atrophic vaginitis (if peri- or postmenopausal), BV, gonorrhea, chlamydia, trichomoniasis, or herpes simplex. Vulvar dermatitis is also in the differential, whether a variant of eczema or a contact dermatitis from her ongoing use of topical antifungal agents. With persistent scratching, lichen sclerosus may ensue. Urinary tract infections can also cause pruritus in some women.

30–1, B. Learning objective: *Outline an appropriate exam for a woman with vaginal itching.* Start with an external perineal exam and proceed to vaginal/cervical exam, with microscopic review of vaginal discharge for hyphae, white cells, clue cells, and trichomonads. Consider microbiologic testing for gonorrhea, chlamydia, fungal culture, and sensitivity. If her exam is consistent with candidal vaginitis, check her glucose level to screen for diabetes and review HIV risk factors.

▶ HIV INFECTION PRIMARY CARE ANSWERS

30–2, A. Learning objective: *Understand when to start antiretroviral therapy and what agents to use.* Current guidelines recommend starting antiretroviral therapy in patients with CD_4 counts less than 350 and/or in patients with viral load greater than 55,000. Although this patient has a CD_4 count of 405, his viral load of 75,000 is high, warranting treatment with a potent antiretroviral regimen. He has been on AZT + ddI so may be resistant to these. Patient adherence is another important factor to evaluate before starting therapy. These regimens are very complex and require a high level of patient commitment. Poor compliance can result in only intermittent antiretroviral therapy; this quickly leads to resistance. Noncompliance may be reason to defer therapy. Combination therapy is the rule with at least three drugs. The goal is to use at least two drugs the patient has not been given before. Given this patient's high viral load of 75,000, a protease inhibitor is a cornerstone for combination treatment. One option is a protease inhibitor (indinavir or nelfinavir) + AZT + 3TC, giving the patient two new drugs (a protease inhibitor plus 3TC) and a combination of AZT + 3TC, because 3TC often restores AZT sensitivity. Another option is to include a non-nucleoside drug: d4T + 3TC + efavirenz. Efavirenz is a non-nucleoside analogue that works well with nucleoside analogues. Never use single-drug therapy. It is not wise to use another two-drug nucleoside combination.

30–2, B. Learning objective: *Order appropriate routine testing for HIV-infected individuals.* This patient needs a PPD, VDRL, toxoplasmosis titer, LFTs, hepatitis serologies, cholesterol panel, CBC, and platelet count. VDRL is important because of the increased incidence of syphilis (especially in those with a history of male to male sexual contact or injection drug use). Toxoplasmosis titer assesses risk for developing future infection: patients with positive IgG titers are at greater risk of toxoplasmosis infection. LFTs and hepatitis serologies provide a baseline and assist in determining if hepatitis B vaccine is needed. Cholesterol panel provides a baseline for evaluating the effect of protease inhibitors. CBC provides an important baseline, particularly if zidovudine is restarted but causes anemia and neutropenia. Platelet count is important because of a fairly high incidence of immune-mediated thrombocytopenia (ITP) in patients with HIV. Vaccines against *pneumococcus* and hepatitis B (if nonimmune) are warranted. If a patient has hepatitis C, they should receive hepatitis A vaccine, otherwise it is optional.

▶ HIV INFECTION COMPLICATIONS ANSWERS

30–3, A. Learning objective: *Recognize that the severity of seborrheic dermatitis correlates with immune function and CNS disease.* Seborrheic dermatitis is extremely common in patients with HIV. Some 80% have it at some point. Severity worsens with declining immune function or CNS disease. Interestingly, this holds true even for non–HIV-infected patients in whom seborrheic dermatitis is commonly seen with Parkinson's disease.

30–3, B. Learning objective: *Recognize that molluscum suggests declining immunity; HL suggests more rapid disease progression.* Molluscum contagiosum is seen usually when CD_4 is less than 100 and is a sign of declining immunity, especially with giant molluscum. Oral hairy leukoplakia is specific for HIV disease and may be a marker for increased risk of disease progression.

30–3, C. Learning objective: *Discuss the differential diagnosis for headache in an AIDS patient.* This patient presents with headache, encephalopathy, and fever. On physical exam he has focal findings on the left side. The most likely diagnosis is cerebral toxoplasmosis. This is made even more likely because the patient was not on toxoplasmosis prophylaxis (TMP/SMX is the best prophylactic drug). Other possibilities include CNS lymphoma and progressive multifocal leukoencephalopathy (PML)—both cause focal motor findings and can cause encephalopathy but usually not fever.

30–3, D. Learning objective: *Order CNS imaging for AIDS patients with headache and fever.* Because of the focal neurologic exam, CNS imaging is key. Options are contrast CT scan or MRI. MRI is more sensitive, but about two and a half times as expensive. PML usually does not show up on CT scans but does on MRI. Serum IgG for toxoplasma is an important part of the work-up. If the MRI scan is negative, which is very unlikely, then LP is appropriate.

▶ MENINGITIS ANSWERS

30–4, A. Learning objective: *Plan appropriate work-up for mental status change in an elderly patient.* This patient needs a glucose level, urinalysis and culture, blood cultures, oxygen saturation, ECG, and a CXR. Based on results of these tests you will decide if he needs more invasive testing (LP).

30–4, B. Learning objective: *List the most common causes for delirium in the elderly.* This patient has had a sudden change in mental status in the setting of fever and an elevated WBC. Mental status change may be the only symptom of infection in the elderly. The most common causes of acute delirium in the elderly are urinary tract infection and pneumonia. Meningitis is a rare cause. Another very important cause of delirium is medication side effects. This patient probably has a UTI. If urinalysis and x-ray are normal, then an LP would be appropriate. Fever makes MI less likely, although always consider this possibility in confused elderly patients.

30–5, A. Learning objective: *Order appropriate tests to evaluate for meningitis.* This patient presents with high fever, seizures, evidence of pneumonia and alcoholism—important risk factors for pneumococcal disease. Order blood cultures, ABG, and head CT scan. A CT scan is obtained here prior to LP because the patient is obtunded, can't give a history, and has seized. This increases the likelihood of a mass lesion. The risk of herniation is low (6%) even in the setting of increased intracranial pressure but is a complication worth avoiding. If contrast CT does not show shift, perform an LP. Order CSF protein, glucose, WBCs, Gram's stain, and culture. A CIE can also be ordered. Give antibiotics before the patient goes to the CT scanner.

30–5, B. Learning objective: *Recognize pneumococcal meningitis.* Most pneumococcal meningitis is seeded from a pneumonia, as in this case. *Listeria* and meningococcus are less likely to have concurrent pulmonary infection. This patient could have a brain abscess causing the seizure, seeded from the lung. This usually occurs in the setting of a pulmonary shunt or right-to-left cardiac shunt.

30–5, C. Learning objective: *Design appropriate empiric therapy for patients with probable pneumococcal meningitis.* This patient should have empiric therapy to cover meningococcus, pneumococcus (because of his pulmonary infiltrate), and *Listeria* (because of his alcohol use). Vancomycin + ceftriaxone + ampicillin is appropriate. Vancomycin is given because of increasing penicillin-resistant pneumococcus. Vancomycin controls bacteremia but does not penetrate the CNS well. Ceftriaxone penetrates the CNS well and is effective against intermediate PCN-resistant pneumococcus. Ampicillin is added to cover for *Listeria*. As soon as CSF Gram's stain or culture are positive, simplify therapy.

▶ PNEUMONIA ANSWERS

30–6, A. Learning objective: *List likely organisms causing pneumonia in an older smoker.* Abrupt onset cough with rusty sputum and shaking chill suggest community-acquired pneumonia. Pneumococcus is most likely. *Haemophilus, Moraxella,* and, much less likely, *Legionella* are also possible because of her smoking history. Because she does not live in an institution, TB, *Staphylococcus*, and *Pseudomonas* are unlikely. There is no history of alcohol, sedating medications, or neurologic disease to suggest aspiration. Her pulse is unexpectedly low for the degree of fever, a finding called *pulse-temperature dissociation* and sometimes associated with *Legionella*, although this can occur with any pneumonia.

30–6, B. Learning objective: *Design appropriate work-up for a patient who likely has pneumonia.* Check vital signs, pulse oximetry, and orthostatic changes in pulse or pressure to determine IV fluid requirements and detect early sepsis. Perform lung exam looking for signs of consolidation or effusion (dullness, fremitus, egophony, bronchial breath sounds). Send CBC, electrolytes, creatinine, BUN, blood culture, blood gas, sputum Gram's stain, and culture. Order CXR.

30–6, C. Learning objective: *Choose appropriate empiric antibiotic coverage based on details of the clinical setting.* A second or third generation cephalosporin (cefuroxime, cefotetan, ceftriaxone) is adequate to cover potentially β-lactam resistant pneumococcus, *Haemophilus*, or *Moraxella*. Although *Legionella* is not as likely, it is potentially life-threatening. Adding high-dose erythromycin to cover *Legionella* is quite reasonable in light of her smoking and pulse-temperature dissociation.

30–6, D. Learning objective: *Recognize the usual course of response to therapy in patients with pneumonia.* Patients may spike fevers two to four days into therapy, although in general the peak temperature gradually drops over that time. Leukocytosis may not resolve until up to four days of therapy. Continue current therapy and monitor for any signs of deterioration. Generally, empiric antibiotics are broad and left unaltered over the first 72 hours of therapy unless an organism is found or the patient gets rapidly worse.

30–6, E. Learning objective: *Recognize deviation from the usual course of response to therapy and design appropriate work-up to detect complications.* Fever should be abating at this point. Look for a resistant organism, an empyema or other complication, a drug fever or a noninfectious cause of fever. Order repeat CXR, blood and sputum cultures. If CXR shows fluid, obtain bilateral decubitus films to see if the fluid is free-flowing (amenable to pleural tap) and tap the fluid immediately.

30–7, A. Learning objective: *Recognize altered mental status as a presentation of pneumonia in an elderly patient and generate a broad differential diagnosis.* Differential includes pneumonia, PE, MI, electrolyte disturbance (hyponatremia or hypercalcemia), sepsis (from a UTI, ischemic bowel, meningitis or cholecystitis), or pancreatitis.

30–7, B. Learning objective: *Design work-up in an older patient with altered mental status.* Aside from careful history and exam, obtain electrolytes, calcium, amylase, liver function tests, CXR, oxygen saturation, ABG, ECG, and urinalysis to start with, looking for the entities in answer 30–7, A. Consider lumbar puncture if fever or elevated WBC is found with no apparent source of infection. Stiff neck or other meningeal signs mandate head CT and LP.

30–7, C. Learning objective: *List most likely organisms causing pneumonia in an elderly patient who resides in a nursing home.* *Pneumococcus, Staphylococcus aureus, Pseudomonas aeruginosa,* other gram-negative rods, TB, and anaerobes are all possible causes of infection in this nursing home resident with altered mental status. Alcohol use, poor dentition, or impaired swallowing due to underlying neurologic disease make aspiration even more likely.

30–7, D. Learning objective: *Describe factors making atypical presentations of pneumonia more likely.* Elderly patients may not have the vigorous immune response necessary to produce sputum, cough, or fever. Pain localization can be inaccurate and lower lobe pneumonia can present as abdominal pain.

▶ TUBERCULOSIS ANSWERS

30–8, A. Learning objective: *Know the appropriate differential diagnosis for patients with subacute pulmonary symptoms and weight loss.* An appropriate differential diagnosis for this patient would include TB, lung cancer, lung abscess, and HIV-related pulmonary disease. His risk factors for TB are homelessness (including spending time in shelters), history of spending time in jail, and to a lesser extent, alcoholism, and his symptoms are compatible with TB (weight loss, cough, and hemoptysis). Lung cancer is also an important diagnostic concern given the combination of hemoptysis, weight loss, and smoking history. His alcoholism puts him at risk for aspiration pneumonia and subsequent development of lung abscess. Typical features of lung abscess include weight loss, cough, and low-grade fevers. This patient should have further questioning about HIV risk factors. HIV disease is more common in individuals who have been in prison. HIV-related pulmonary diseases to consider include PCP as well as an increased risk for lung cancer.

30–8, B. Learning objective: *Know the typical CXR findings of pulmonary TB.* Upper lobe infiltrates are the hallmark of reactivation tuberculosis. Pleural thickening and cavity formation can occur. Elderly patients and patients with advanced HIV disease may have lower lobe infiltrates.

30–8, C. Learning objective: *Understand how to treat active TB.* This patient would be best treated with directly observed therapy. Nonadherence to therapy increases the risk of development of drug resistant TB. It may be most appropriate to admit him to the hospital to start his treatment and set up monitoring. In most cases patients with TB do not need to be hospitalized to start therapy. His homeless status and alcoholism make hospitalization a good option. An appropriate medication regimen would be four drugs (isoniazid, rifampin, pyrazinamide, and ethambutol) given three times a week with direct observation. Length of therapy would be six months with testing at three months to make sure the culture is negative. Most patients with TB take daily medications. In patients where nonadherence is likely, using three times a week directly observed therapy is preferable because it is usually easier in the public health system to administer drugs three times a week than daily.

▶ URINARY TRACT INFECTION ANSWERS

30–9, A. Learning objective: *Recognize complicated cystitis and risk factors for other conditions.* This woman has complicated cystitis based on her age alone. She is likely off hormone replacement therapy because of her breast cancer, so she may have atrophic vaginitis causing her symptoms. Although patients with STDs such as HSV might also present in this way, this is unlikely in this monogamous woman. If she had atypical symptoms or other risk factors, you could consider a gynecologic evaluation. Most important is to ascertain if she has had frequent UTIs and, if so, whether cultures have been done recently. For this scenario, assume that she has not had recent UTIs.

30–9, B. Learning objective: *Outline a treatment regimen for complicated cystitis.* This woman has not been exposed to many antibiotics, so TMP/SMX is a reasonable choice for her. The duration is key: seven to 14 days should be adequate. If her symptoms recur or persist, obtain urine culture and sensitivities and perform a gynecologic exam if these have not been done recently, to evaluate for STDs and atrophic vaginitis. If the latter is present, you could consult with her oncologist and consider topical estrogen therapy.

▶ ACID-BASE DISTURBANCES ANSWERS

31–1, A. Learning objective: *Identify the primary acid-base derangement.* Alkalemia with a pH of 7.5 is a primary respiratory alkalosis because pCO_2 is low.

31–1, B. Learning objective: *Recognize that a compensatory metabolic acidosis should be a nongap acidosis.* Low HCO_3^- suggests a metabolic acidosis. One might be tempted to call this compensatory, but a compensatory metabolic acidosis should be a nongap acidosis because it is generated by renal bicarbonate loss. His anion gap acidosis is, instead, a coexisting primary process.

31–1, C. Learning objective: *Identify all coexisting primary acid-base derangements by calculating anion gap, osmolar gap, and delta-delta.*

Anion gap is elevated at 22 (140 – (103 + 15)), meaning anion gap acidosis is present.

Calculated osms are 296 (2(140) + 28/2.8 + 108/18).

Osm gap is 1 (296–295), essentially normal, and rules out osmotically active ingestion.

When you add the change in anion gap (22–12 = 10) to his bicarbonate (15), you get 25, close enough to 24 that you can declare there are no other simultaneous metabolic processes.

31–1, D. Learning objective: *Interpret acid-base abnormalities in the context of clinical information to develop a reasonable differential diagnosis.* He has been taking large doses of aspirin for back pain. Aspirin causes a primary respiratory alkalosis by stimulating CNS breathing centers to hyperventilate, as well as an anion gap acidosis due to salicylic acid. His melena is likely from NSAID-induced gastritis. Other less likely explanations of his acid-base derangements would have to invoke two separate processes. Early sepsis could cause an anion gap acidosis with compensatory hyperventilation, although the pH should be less than 7.4, reflecting the primary acidosis.

31–2, A. Learning objective: *Identify the primary acid-base derangement.* Acidemia with a low bicarbonate gives her a primary metabolic acidosis.

31–2, B. Learning objective: *Identify the compensatory acid-base derangement.* Low pCO_2 from hyperventilating creates a compensatory respiratory alkalosis.

31–2, C. Learning objective: *Identify all coexisting acid-base derangements by calculating anion gap and osmolar gap, and comparing the change in anion gap to the change in bicarbonate (delta-delta).*

Anion gap is 32 (130 − (88 + 10))

Calculated osms are 310 (2(130) + 28/2.8 + 720/18)

Osm gap is 5 (315 − 310)

Using delta-delta, the rise in anion gap is 20 (32 − 12), and when you add this to the bicarbonate, you get 30 (20 + 10). Because this is greater than 24, a metabolic alkalosis is also present.

31–2, D. Learning objective: *Interpret acid-base abnormalities in the context of clinical information.* She has diabetic ketoacidosis (polyuria, polydypsea, and high glucose), causing an anion gap acidosis. She has some respiratory compensation, blowing off CO_2 to reduce her acidemia. Additionally, she is experiencing a coexisting metabolic alkalosis, probably from vomiting acidic stomach contents.

▶ ACUTE RENAL FAILURE ANSWERS

31–3, A. Learning objective: *Diagnose prerenal ARF.* Prerenal hypovolemia due to decreased PO intake and vomiting is most likely. This is supported by the BUN/Cr ratio of greater than 20 and a low urine output (oliguria less than or equal to 400 mL/24 hours). He may also have ATN from prolonged prerenal azotemia. The patient should be catheterized to rule-out concurrent bladder outlet obstruction, and then given IV normal saline. FeNa and urine sed-iment exam are indicated. Urine sediment should show hyaline casts, unless hypovolemia has caused ATN, in which case there may be granular and "muddy brown" casts.

31–3, B. Learning objective: *Calculate FeNa.* FeNa is 0.6, consis-tent with prerenal ARF.

31–3, C. Learning objective: *Anticipate and manage complications of acute renal failure.* He may develop volume overload, periph-eral and pulmonary edema, and even CHF. He is at risk for elec-trolyte imbalances and acidemia. He should have strict measurement of his input and output, along with daily weights, which are most accurate. Daily exam should include vital signs, mental status exam, jugular venous pressure, heart and lung exam, and extremity exam for edema. Labs should include CBC, chemistries, calcium, magnesium, and phosphorus. Obtain CXR and ECG, especially if K^+ is elevated. Re-establish urine output with normal saline resuscitation. Use diuretics only for volume overload. Dose all medications according to renal function. Adjust diet for renal failure (low sodium and potassium) and avoid medications containing potassium and magnesium (antacids).

31–4, A. Learning objective: *Recognize postrenal azotemia.* This elderly man has acute urinary retention from anticholinergic med-ication superimposed on likely benign prostatic hypertrophy or possibly prostate cancer. The suprapubic mass is his bladder.

31–4, B. Learning objective: *Look for postobstructive diuresis.* After catheter placement, high volume diuresis may cause elec-trolyte wasting. Monitor and replace output and electrolytes.

31–5, A. Learning objective: *Recognize interstitial nephritis.* Active urine sediment with protein and eosinophils (93% spe-cific for acute interstitial nephritis, AIN) indicates interstitial nephritis due to piperacillin. Patients with AIN have rash, fever, and peripheral eosinophilia approximately 30% of the time (rare with NSAID-induced AIN). Her single kidney with chronic catheterization means that obstruction should be considered; change the catheter and order ultrasound to evaluate for hydronephrosis. Consider urinary tract infection, although this in itself would be unlikely to elevate her creatinine.

31–5, B. Learning objective: *Manage acute interstitial nephritis.* Most cases resolve by stopping the presumed causative medica-tion. For persistent renal failure, prednisone may be necessary.

31–6, A. Learning objective: *Recognize a pulmonary-renal syn-drome.* He has renal failure with borderline anemia, history of sinusitis and ongoing lung disease, elevated blood pressure of uncertain duration, and TMP/SMX use. The differential for his azotemia includes Wegener's granulomatosis (sinus, lung, and renal involvement), elevation in creatinine due to TMP/SMX, or chronic renal impairment due to hypertension. Other diagnoses would be less likely although other causes of pulmonary and renal disease should be considered, e.g., SLE, Goodpasture's disease. Postrenal obstruction due to BPH is also possible in a middle-aged man.

31–6, B. Learning objective: *Order appropriate tests to investigate the cause of glomerulonephritis.* An ANA (SLE), c-ANCA (Wegener's), ESR, UA (for RBC casts), and CXR are a minimum work-up. Prostate exam and percussion of his bladder help rule-out postrenal obstruction, as does catheterization for a postvoid residual. The highest-yield diagnostic test for Wegener's granulomatosis is renal biopsy, but because he has sinus and lung disease, a trans-bronchial or sinus biopsy might be sufficient and less invasive.

31–6, C. Learning objective: *Recognize the urine sediment findings in acute glomerulonephritis.* Urine sediment might show cre-nated, dysmorphic red cells, evidence of red cells exposed to a high osmotic gradient in the tubules, and red cell casts from RBCs compacted in the tubules. Look at a fresh urine sample yourself because casts decompose quickly! In contrast, RBCs from the bladder will not be dysmorphic, nor will they form casts.

31–7, A. Learning objective: *Recognize nephrotic syndrome and list its causes.* This patient has nephrotic syndrome (renal failure with edema, 24-hour urine protein greater than 3.5 grams, and dyslipi-demia). The most likely causes of his nephrotic syndrome include his heroin use, HIV nephropathy, polyarteritis nodosa (related to hep-atitis B), ibuprofen use (although interstitial nephritis usually has less protein, less than 1.5 gm/24 hours), and renal disease, such as mem-branous nephropathy, or even minimal change disease, which is more common in children.

31–7, B. Learning objective: *Order appropriate tests to work-up nephrotic syndrome.* He should have an HIV test, a CBC, hepa-titis B and C serologies, p-ANCA, CXR, and probably a renal biopsy. ANA reflexive panel and ESR might be helpful.

31–7, C. Learning objective: *Recognize the urine abnormalities of nephrotic syndrome.* Oval fat bodies and Maltese-like crosses are found in the urine sediment in nephrotic syndrome. You might also see other clues to etiology (e.g., WBC casts and eosinophils in interstitial nephritis).

► ELECTROLYTE DISTURBANCES AND FLUID MANAGEMENT ANSWERS

31–8, A. Learning objective: *Prioritize hyperkalemia as a life-threatening problem.* Hyperkalemia is most life-threatening because of the potential for lethal arrhythmias. Hypertension is likely baseline and can be addressed over days to weeks as long as there is no end-organ damage. Dyspnea with elevated JVP, rales, and edema are signs of moderate fluid overload, and should be addressed with diuretics or hemodialysis over hours to days. Metabolic nongap acidosis is likely chronic due to renal failure.

31–8, B. Learning objective: *State the ECG findings of hyperkalemia.* Moderate hyperkalemia causes peaked T waves. More severe hyperkalemia widens the QRS, reflecting the increased time for ventricular depolarization. With severe hyperkalemia, ECG looks like a sine wave with peaked Ts and wide QRS indistinguishable from each other in an undulating wave.

31–8, C. Learning objective: *Identify interventions for acute hyperkalemia and state the mechanism of each.* To avoid cardiac arrhythmia, first give IV calcium gluconate to rapidly stabilize cardiac membranes. Next, give IV glucose (an amp of D50) and insulin (five to ten units) to carry potassium into the intracellular space. Be careful not to give so much insulin as to cause hypoglycemia. Alkalinize with IV bicarbonate for a transient intracellular potassium shift. Kayexalate can be initiated with the acute therapies but is too slow acting to reverse severe hyperkalemia. Furosemide helps over hours if the patient is making urine. Use dialysis for severe hyperkalemia, although it takes some time to set up. Administer calcium, glucose with insulin, and bicarbonate while waiting for dialysis to begin.

31–9, A. Learning objective: *Use the details of a clinical situation to generate a list of probable causes of hyponatremia.* Hydrochlorothiazide could be causing a hypovolemic or euvolemic hyponatremia. She is systemically ill with confusion, dyspnea, and cough, suggesting cardiac or pulmonary pathology. Cough and dyspnea could be heart failure, not unlikely in a woman with multiple risk factors for CHF (hypertension, smoking, and alcohol use). She also has risk factors for pneumonia and for lung tumor, either of which could lead to SIADH.

31–9, B. Learning objective: *Recognize the importance of volume status in the work-up of hyponatremia.* Evaluate fluid status to direct further inquiry. Orthostatic vital signs, dry mucous membranes, and poor skin turgor indicate decreased volume. Hypoxia, rales, jugular vein distention, or leg or sacral edema indicate fluid overload. The lack of either group of signs indicates euvolemia. Cachexia might make you suspicious of tumor. Focal signs of lung consolidation may make you think of pneumonia or tumor. Hoarse voice, dry skin, and coarse hair suggest hypothyroidism. Focal neurologic exam might make you worry about a CNS tumor.

31–9, C. Learning objective: *Design appropriate work-up for euvolemic hyponatremia.* Obtain CXR to look for pneumonia or tumor. Without lung findings to explain hyponatremia, evaluate further with a head CT and consider LP. TSH is also a reasonable consideration.

31-9, D. Learning objective: *State options for managment of SIADH.* She most likely has SIADH due to pneumonia, although we have not totally ruled out the possibility of a lung tumor. Treat with free water restriction to about 500–1500 mL/day. As an alternative, one may use IV normal saline along with free water restriction over the first day for more rapid response, especially if sodium is very low (less than 120). Patients seizing from low sodium can be given 3% hypertonic IV saline. Whatever the approach, raise sodium by no more than 1–2 mEq/hour in the first few hours, then by 8 mEq total over the first 24 hours. Follow sodium levels hourly initially until rate of rise is stable. If hyponatremia does not resolve with treatment of pneumonia, think about diuretic or perhaps an occult lung tumor as a contributing cause.

▶ HYPERTENSION ANSWERS

31-10, A. Learning objective: *Identify factors contributing to hypertension.* Oral contraceptives, NSAIDs, acute pain, and excessive alcohol use can all contribute to her hypertension.

31-10, B. Learning objective: *Design appropriate follow-up for patients in whom mild hypertension is found.* Recheck within the next two months or so, before she forgets to return.

31-10, C. Learning objective: *Counsel patients appropriately about lifestyle modifications to lower blood pressure.* With a single measurement under nonextenuating circumstances, her BP may well normalize, so she can continue birth control pills. NSAIDs are also appropriate for short-term management of pain and inflammation. You need to address her alcohol use. Regardless of whether it has increased her blood pressure, she is drinking enough to cause significant medical and social sequelae. Intervention in a young woman is more likely to succeed than in older, more chronic alcohol users. Use your CAGE questions for further screening.

31-11, A. Learning objective: *Recognize side effects of nifedipine and find alternative treatment for three reasons:* 1) unacceptable side-effects (constipation and lower extremity edema are common with calcium channel blockers); 2) increased mortality with short-acting calcium channel blockers; 3) compliance is made difficult. She has to take a pill three times a day, and poor compliance may be why her blood pressure is still elevated.

31-11, B. Learning objective: *Perform appropriate initial evaluation for hypertension in patients with unclear prior evaluation.* With a patient that is new to you, begin at the beginning. If she has not had diet and exercise counseling, review with her. Examine her for end-organ damage. Perform a careful eye and heart exam, and, at minimum, obtain a lab panel of electrolytes and renal function. Next, consider whether she could have secondary causes for her hypertension. On the one hand, her hypertension has been long-standing, so further testing is probably not indicated. On the other hand, her age alone puts her at risk for renal artery stenosis, so if more than two medications do not control her pressure, consider a renal artery duplex.

31–11, C. Learning objective: *Choose appropriate antihypertensive therapy in a patient with gout and bradycardia.* Whereas her lower extremity edema invites a low dose diuretic, the increase in uric acid may cause her gout to flare. A β-blocker may also be a poor choice in this patient because her pulse is bradycardic. Many elderly patients have bradycardia or borderline heart block from impaired electrical conduction in the heart as a consequence of degeneration/aging, not ischemia per se. In patients with a low pulse (less than 60), check an ECG before starting a β-blocker. A calcium channel blocker such as diltiazem or verapamil may delay conduction at the AV node and worsen heart block. An α-blocker is a cheap alternative, but orthostatic hypotension puts older patients at risk for falls. An ACEI may be the best choice— check renal function after a week of therapy.

31–12, A. Learning objective: *Identify features on history and exam that suggest reasons for hypertension.* Potential factors include family history, obesity, Cushing's disease (depression, obesity, diabetes, stretch marks, and low potassium), hyperaldosteronism, and sleep apnea (fatigue, falling asleep while driving, and obesity).

31–12, B. Learning objective: *Order appropriate tests for suspected secondary causes of hypertension in an obese patient with hypokalemia.* Perform serial work-up beginning with a 24-hour cortisol since she has several stigmata of Cushing's. Other tests to do in serial fashion include renal artery study (diabetes puts her at risk for vascular disease), aldosterone/renin ratio (low potassium also occurs with hyperaldosteronism), and sleep study looking for apnea.

31–12, C. Learning objective: *Begin treatment for hypertension with lifestyle modification.* Lifestyle modification is imperative in this patient. Weight loss and exercise will help not only her hypertension but also her diabetes. Just ten pounds can make a big change in medication requirements. This patient has stage 2 hypertension and so medications are indicated *while* she works on her lifestyle changes. Control other risk factors for coronary heart disease by checking cholesterol, treating diabetes, and starting estrogen replacement unless contraindicated.

> ▶ **NEUROLOGY ANSWERS**

32–1, A. Learning objective: *Recognize delirium and distinguish it from dementia.* This patient has waxing and waning mental status with inattention, classic for delirium. The cognitive deficits of dementia, in contrast, usually develop slowly over months to years. Attention remains intact until very late.

32–1, B. Learning objective: *List a differential diagnosis for delirium.* Differential includes infection (meningitis, pyelonephritis, cholangitis), electrolyte abnormality (hyponatremia, hypercalcemia most likely), seizures, stroke, myocardial infarction, and medication effect.

32–1, C. Learning objective: *Plan appropriate work-up for a patient with delirium.* Obtain CBC, chemistry panel, calcium, liver function tests, oxygen saturation, ECG, CXR. If a cause is not readily apparent, consider head CT and LP. Results show Na 140, Cl 110, HCO_3^- 27, Ca 14 (normal less than 10.5), normal LFTs, ECG (aside from a shortened QT interval), and CXR.

32–1, D. Learning objective: *Identify hypercalcemia as a cause of delirium. Recognize that a low anion gap in a patient with hypercalcemia suggests multiple myeloma.* Hypercalcemia explains the patient's dehydrated volume status and delirium. The low anion gap is a clue that perhaps multiple myeloma is the culprit.

32–1, E. Learning objective: *Design further tests to confirm the cause of hypercalcemia.* In this patient with the low anion gap a focused work-up for myeloma is appropriate to include serum and urine protein electrophoresis. If positive, check bone survey to look for the characteristic punched-out lesions. In other patients, in whom the diagnosis of myeloma is not suspected, it is best to start with an intact parathyroid hormone measurement as hyperparathyroidism is most common. If negative, review history and exam for signs of malignancy, update all overdue cancer screening, and pursue any other suggestive findings with further work-up for malignancy. Consider granulomatous disease such as TB and sarcoid—CXR is a good place to start for these. See chapter on calcium abnormalities for more suggestions.

32–2, A. Learning objective: *List a differential diagnosis for first-time seizure.* Differential includes new onset true epilepsy, cocaine, alcohol withdrawal, electrolyte disorder, especially hyponatremia or hypocalcemia, focal CNS infection (i.e., toxoplasmosis in the setting of advanced HIV infection), primary or metastatic brain tumor, or stroke but unlikely based on his age.

32–2, B. Learning objective: *Ask a pertinent history to reveal potential causes of seizure.* Ask about history of epilepsy, substance use including alcohol and cocaine, HIV risk factors, and signs of tumor (weight loss, headache).

32–2, C. Learning objective: *Design a work-up to rule-out structural and metabolic causes of first-time seizure.* Obtain CBC, chemistry panel, calcium, magnesium, toxicology screen, head CT scan, and LP. Testing reveals a mildly elevated WBC, slightly low calcium and magnesium, mild anion gap acidosis, negative toxicology screen, and normal head CT scan. LP reveals a mild pleocytosis. After all the tests, the patient's girlfriend reveals to you that he usually drinks very heavily but stopped abruptly two days ago.

32–2, D. Learning objective: *State appropriate treatment for alcohol withdrawal seizures.* With the further history, he likely is having an alcohol withdrawal seizure. Treatment is supportive with observation, seizure precautions (padded bed rails), hydration, thiamine, and electrolyte replacement as needed. Most alcohol withdrawal seizures are single seizures. If seizing recurs, an IV benzodiazepine such as lorazepam can be given. Do not give phenytoin for alcohol withdrawal seizures. Advise the patient to abstain from alcohol in the future.

▶ DEPRESSION ANSWERS

33–1, A. Learning objective: *Outline a differential diagnosis for an elderly woman with mild memory deficits.* Early Alzheimer's disease, multi-infarct dementia, electrolyte abnormalities, polypharmacy, vitamin B_{12} deficiency, alcohol abuse, pulmonary or genitourinary infections, thyroid disease, subdural hemorrhage, and depression might all be contributing factors in this woman. Recognize that absence of depressed mood does *not* exclude the diagnosis of depression.

33–1, B. Learning objective: *Devise questions for history in a woman in whom you suspect depression may be a possibility.* Ask about sleep pattern, anhedonia, depressed mood, suicidality, change in appetite, weight loss or gain, concentration, and excessive guilt. To further investigate nonpsychiatric causes, inquire about recent blood glucose recordings (has she had hypoglycemic episodes), balance or gait difficulties suggesting stroke or vitamin B_{12} deficiency, falls contributing to subdural hemorrhage, heat/cold intolerance, constipation, or other findings of thyroid disease. Because a family history makes some conditions more likely, ask patients about family history of depression, bipolar disorder, dementia, or stroke.

33–1, C. Learning objective: *Order appropriate labs when considering depression in an elderly patient.* Order TSH, vitamin B_{12} level, electrolytes, calcium, and consider a urinalysis if GU symptoms are present. If there are abnormalities on the neurological exam or a recent fall, consider a contrast CT scan.

33–1, D. Learning objective: *Identify a trial of SSRI as a reasonable course in an elderly patient with cognitive deficits, otherwise normal labs and exam, and findings consistent with depression.* In this patient, start an SSRI with cautions about side-effects and expected response within four weeks. If she does not improve, consider switching to a second agent. Retest memory when and if depressive symptoms improve.

33–2, A. Learning objective: *List criteria for depression.* This patient has at least five of these criteria: depressed mood, sleep disruption, agitation, trouble concentrating, decreased appetite, and suicidality.

33–2, B. Learning objective: *Clarify risk of suicide in a depressed patient.* Ask him about suicidal ideation and any specific plans. Find out whether he has access to guns, prescription medications, and so on.

33–2, C. Learning objective: *When patients are reluctant to take medications, explore the source of their resistance.* Ask this young man about his father's response to medications, because older treatments were often not well-tolerated and, at times, ineffective. Inquire further about manic-depressive symptoms in him and his father. Ask if he has been on medications previously and how he responded. Inquire as to his attitude about depression and medical therapy. Many patients consider depression a character flaw.

33–2, D. Learning objective: *Identify alternative methods of treating depression.* This young man needs intensive treatment for his depression, but it is his right to refuse medication. Offer him counseling as an option, particularly given his acute grief over his ended relationship. Provide him with several names and phone numbers of reliable therapists. Recommend that he abstain from all alcohol and substance abuse. He should exercise to a good sweat three to five times a week.

▶ ASTHMA ANSWERS

34–1, A. Learning objective: *In new or worsening asthma, ask about precipitants.* In her new house, are there carpets, wood stoves, pets (previously or currently)? Is she newly exposed to cigarette smoke? Has she changed jobs, now with an occupational exposure? Do her symptoms resolve when she travels back to her prior residence, suggesting allergies or exposures. Has she been sick recently with upper respiratory symptoms?

34–1, B. Learning objective: *Identify the indications, risks, and benefits of regular use of inhaled corticosteroids.* In light of her increase in symptom frequency, exacerbations, and nighttime symptoms, she is classified as having at least mild persistent asthma. Anti-inflammatory therapy is necessary, specifically an inhaled corticosteroid. Inhaled corticosteroids provide the most potent and consistently effective long-term control of asthma by inhibiting production of cytokines and other inflammatory mediators, thereby reversing airway inflammation and decreasing airway hyperresponsiveness.

34–1, C. Learning objective: *Outline the risks and benefits of inhaled corticosteroid therapy.* Inhaled steroids will decrease her symptoms and will prevent the remodeling that leads to irreversible pulmonary damage. Although the negative impact of low-dose inhaled steroids is not clear, long-term use of high-dose inhaled steroids can cause osteoporosis, immunosuppression, elevated intraocular pressure, altered bone homeostasis, and cataract formation. Minimize systemic absorption by mouth-rinsing after each administration and by use of spacer devices. For all patients, recommend preventive measures for osteoporosis and consider DXA screening (see osteoporosis chapter).

34–2, A. Learning objective: *Recognize signs of severe asthma exacerbation and outline an action plan.* This patient has a severe asthma exacerbation. Her ability to speak only in short sentences is an early sign of impending respiratory failure. Instruct her to take 60 mg of prednisone if she has some at home and to go to an ED immediately. She should not drive herself and an EMT should be called if necessary.

34–2, B. Learning objective: *Describe the evaluation and treatment for acute asthma exacerbation.* Check vital signs, give IV corticosteroids, and begin continuous albuterol via nebulizer. Follow serial vital signs, including pulsus paradoxus (significant decrease in systolic pressure with inspiration). Look for use of accessory muscles of respiration and paradoxical abdominal motion. Observe the expiratory to inspiratory (E/I) ratio, often increased with airway obstruction. Listen to the lungs for air movement, wheezing. Obtain ABG. Although URI is the most likely precipitant, consider a CXR to look for signs of pneumonia and an ECG to evaluate for cardiac ischemia. Sputum can be thick and greenish even in the absence of infection, but a sputum culture might be helpful. Watch for trends in vital signs and exam. With any sign of worsening, hospitalize immediately, preferably in an ICU.

34–2, C. Learning objective: *Recognize respiratory failure in severe asthma exacerbations.* Common signs of impending respiratory failure include presence of a worsening pulsus paradoxus, decrease in respiratory rate, use of accessory muscles that suggests fatigue, and prolongation of the expiratory phase leading to an increased E/I ratio. Wheezing is often a difficult sign to interpret because a patient who has severely compromised air movement may have NO wheezing or air movement. As she improves, diffuse wheezing may appear. Obtain an ABG and hospitalize for significant hypoxemia or hypercarbia. It is important to recognize early respiratory failure and intubate with mechanical ventilation in a controlled setting, not after the patient exhibits hemodynamic compromise.

> ► CHRONIC OBSTRUCTIVE PULMONARY DISEASE ANSWERS

34–3, A. Learning objective: *Distinguish COPD from asthma.* This patient almost certainly has COPD rather than asthma. Her consistent (rather than episodic) dyspnea on exertion, tobacco history, age of symptom onset, suggestion of bullous disease on CXR, and fixed obstructive defect on spirometry all favor the diagnosis of COPD.

34–3, B. Learning objective: *List the risk factors for COPD.* Although her COPD may be entirely the result of smoking, the basilar predominance of bullous changes on CXR and diagnosis prior to age 45 raise the possibility of α_1-antitrypsin deficiency, a rare genetic disorder. Low serum enzyme levels help to make the diagnosis. Intravenous injection of crushed Ritalin tablets is an even more rare cause of early onset, basilar-predominant emphysema.

34–3, C. Learning objective: *Devise a medication regimen appropriate for a patient with stable COPD.* The highest priority in this patient is weaning her off prednisone. Long-term oral steroids are not indicated for the treatment of COPD and have serious long-term side-effects. The patient is using a large amount of albuterol; the addition of a long-acting β_2-agonist and/or a scheduled anticholinergic inhaler is appropriate. Theophylline is an option if there is an inadequate response to first-line bronchodilators. If she's symptomatic despite the mentioned interventions, a trial of inhaled corticosteroid is reasonable. If her FEV_1 fails to improve, inhaled steroid should be discontinued as there is an increased risk of osteoporosis associated with chronic use. The patient may benefit from enzyme augmentation therapy if she has α_1-antitrypsin deficiency.

34–4, A. Learning objective: *Patients with COPD have airflow obstruction and hence his FEV₁/FVC should be less than 70%.* His FEV_1 at 25% of predicted is consistent with severe disease, and his lung volumes likely will include an increased total lung capacity (TLC) indicating hyperinflation and an elevated residual volume (RV) as a result of air trapping. Diffusing capacity for carbon monoxide (DLCO) is usually severely decreased in patients with severe emphysema, reflecting destruction of the lung parenchyma. A relatively preserved DLCO should prompt consideration of a large reversible component to airflow obstruction as seen in patients with asthma. The chronic, compensated CO_2 retention and hypoxemia seen on his ABG are consistent with his advanced disease.

34–4, B. Learning objective: *State the indications for supplemental oxygen in COPD patients.* Long-term oxygen therapy for greater than 15 hours per day reduces mortality in chronically hypoxemic patients with COPD and is indicated in this patient. LTOT is indicated for all patients with PaO_2 less than or equal to 55 mm Hg or with PaO_2 between 55 and 60 mm Hg in the presence of pulmonary hypertension, right heart failure, or polycythemia (HCT greater than 55%). The patient's exam is consistent with cor pulmonale and right heart failure. Intermittent supplemental oxygen may improve quality of life in patients that desaturate during exercise or sleep, but has not been shown to decrease mortality.

34–4, C. Learning objective: *Identify smoking as the most effective way to slow progression of COPD.* Smoking cessation is the most effective way to slow disease progression. This patient's prognosis is poor. The FEV_1 is the best predictor of mortality in patients with COPD. Individuals with an FEV_1 greater than 50% predicted have a life expectancy close to smokers without airflow obstruction. This patient, however, has an estimated five-year survival of only about 30%. Although the course of disease is highly variable among individuals with comparable degrees of airflow obstruction, this patient's hypoxemia and cor pulmonale place him at greater risk of mortality.

▶ PULMONARY EMBOLISM ANSWERS

34–5, A. Learning objective: *Describe the history and examination findings of PE, and list other disorders that can present similarly.* The patient's shortness of breath and asymmetric lower extremity edema suggest DVT and PE as the leading diagnosis. Asthma is possible, but she is not currently wheezing. Her cough could indicate pneumonia, although she is afebrile with a normal lung exam. Consider pneumothorax or angina, although she would most likely have chest pain.

34–5, B. Learning objective: *List this patient's risk factors for thrombus formation.* This patient has two important risk factors for PE: oral contraceptive use, causing a high estrogen state, and leg trauma, which could cause blood vessel intimal damage.

34–5, C. Learning objective: *Describe an appropriate work-up for a patient with suspected PE.* CXR and ECG will help rule-out pneumonia, pneumothorax, and MI, but cannot confirm a diagnosis of PE. CBC, PT, and PTT are necessary before starting heparin. If any risk factors are present for GI bleeding (heavy NSAID use, previous ulcer), perform a stool guaiac test. ABG will allow calculation of the A-a gradient. To evaluate for PE, a V/Q scan and lower extremity doppler ultrasound are indicated in this patient with normal cardiopulmonary reserve and physical exam findings of a DVT. In this case, V/Q scan was high probability and ultrasound revealed a large thrombus.

34–5, D. Learning objective: *Outline the therapy for PE using heparin and warfarin.* After H & P, the treating team correctly had a high clinical suspicion for PE and started IV heparin before the V/Q scan and ultrasound. IV heparin is dosed 80 units/kg bolus (5000–10000 U) followed by 18 U/kg/hr (approximately 1000 U/hr). The PTT is monitored frequently, initially every six hours, to maintain it between 60 and 80. After confirming the diagnosis, the heparin can be switched to LMWH. Patients can be taught to inject LMWH themselves subcutaneously. LMWH has the advantage over IV unfractionated heparin in that it does not require monitoring of the PTT. Thus patients can be treated at home with LMWH vs. in the hospital with IV heparin. Warfarin should be started on the first day heparin is given, at a dose of 5 mg per day. The PT and INR must be monitored closely—at least every other day initially—until the INR is at the target range of 2.0–3.0. The heparin can then be discontinued, and warfarin continued usually for six months.

34–6, A. Learning objective: *Generate a differential diagnosis for dyspnea in an acutely ill patient.* This patient's shortness of breath, productive cough, fever, and hypoxia suggest that he has pneumonia. He may have community-acquired pneumonia, postobstructive pneumonia due to the cancer, or aspiration pneumonia. He may also have worsening lung cancer, myocardial infarction, or PE.

34–6, B. Learning objective: *Recognize hypoxia and list potential causes.* The sudden hypoxia, elevated JVP, and loud P_2 are concerning for PE with right heart strain. Although he has pneumonia, he is clinically improved, and so worsening pneumonia would be unlikely to cause new hypoxia. This patient is at risk for PE due to his underlying cancer, age, and immobility. His hypoxia may also be due to cardiac disease (angina/MI or CHF) or pneumothorax. Anemia could contribute.

34–6, C. Learning objective: *Describe a diagnostic work-up for PE in a hospitalized patient with cardiopulmonary disease.* Helical CT will be more helpful than a V/Q scan due to the underlying pulmonary infiltrates. A V/Q would most likely be nondiagnostic. A lower extremity ultrasound would be helpful if positive for DVT. If the ultrasound were negative, it would still be possible that the entire DVT had embolized, and further testing would be needed. If ultrasound and helical CT were nondiagnostic, proceed to pulmonary angiogram given the high clinical suspicion in this case. Obtain CBC, PT, PTT before considering treatment for PE. ECG is indicated to rule-out MI.

34–6, D. Learning objective: *State the indications for thrombolytic therapy for PE.* This patient has hemodynamic compromise, with hypotension and signs of acute right heart failure most likely due to PE. Secure the ABCs, increase oxygen to 100%, and consider intubation. Give a normal saline bolus of 500 mL and consider dopamine to increase the blood pressure. In this case, ultrasound showed bilateral DVTs and helical CT showed a large PE. A life-threatening PE with hypotension or right heart failure warrants the consideration of thrombolysis with tPA.

▶ **GOUT ANSWERS**

35–1, A. Learning objective: *Choose appropriate therapy for acute gout with attention to risk factors.* This patient has an acute attack of gout. Decisions about treatment are complicated by his other medical problems. He should not receive NSAIDs because of his renal insufficiency. Colchicine is also more toxic in patients with renal insufficiency. Steroid treatment would likely markedly raise his blood sugars, which appear under poor control (Hgb_{alc} 10 + random glucose 350). Injecting his joint with steroids is the best option.

35–2, A. Learning objective: *Chose appropriate therapy for acute gout with attention to risk factors.* This patient presents with a gouty attack involving a major joint (knee). He has chronic renal insufficiency and hypertension complicating his treatment options. An NSAID is usually the first choice but should not be used in this patient because of his renal insufficiency. NSAIDs also could make his antihypertensive regimen less effective. Colchicine in full treatment doses is more toxic in patients with renal insufficiency and should be avoided. The best option would be a knee injection with corticosteroid, and 10–20 mg of triamcinolone would work well. Another option would be a five to seven day course of oral prednisone.

35–2, B. Learning objective: *Decide when to institute prophylactic medication to prevent gout attacks and decide on the best treatment options.* This patient has had three attacks in the past year. He would benefit from preventive treatment because he is extremely likely to have recurrences. The timing of starting therapy with urate-lowering medication is important. Therapy should not be started during an acute attack because it may prolong the acute attack. Low dose colchicine (.6 mg a day) can be used to bridge the gap between the acute attack and urate-lowering therapy. Allopurinol is the best option because probenecid is only effective in patients with normal renal function.

▶ **RHEUMATOID ARTHRITIS ANSWERS**

35–3, A. Learning objective: *Recognize early manifestations of rheumatoid arthritis and be aware of other disorders that might mimic RA.* Rheumatoid arthritis is the most likely diagnosis but patients with systemic lupus erythematosus may have similar presentation. Objective joint swelling rules-out fibromyalgia alone as the cause of her symptoms. Duration of symptoms rules-out viral disorders associated with arthritis such as parvovirus B19.

35–3, B. Learning objective: *Order appropriate labs in a patient newly diagnosed with rheumatoid arthritis.* A CBC is indicated because some patients may manifest anemia as part of rheumatoid arthritis. The sedimentation rate and CRP may be elevated. Normal studies do not exclude RA. Rheumatoid factor is indicated. This test is more for prognostic value than diagnosis, because many other disorders can have rheumatoid factor. High titers of rheumatoid factor are associated with a worse prognosis, in particular, worse joint disease and risk of extra-articular features. A high titer of ANA with a negative or slightly positive RF would point more to the diagnosis of SLE. X-rays of the hands in early rheumatoid arthritis are usually normal except for juxta-articular osteopenia. In more aggressive disease, marginal joint erosions may be present.

35–3, C. Learning objective: *Recognize the importance of early treatment of rheumatoid arthritis.* In a patient with active synovitis and positive rheumatoid factor, early treatment is important. Patients are usually initially placed on hydroxychloroquine 400 mg/day, followed immediately by methotrexate given once per week starting with a dose of 7.5 mg. An NSAID may give symptomatic relief.

35–4, A. Learning objective: *Recognize extra-articular manifestations of rheumatoid arthritis.* Patients with rheumatoid arthritis may develop extra-articular manifestations such as rheumatoid vasculitis; peripheral neuropathy often secondary to vasculitis; compression neuropathies, such as carpal tunnel syndrome; rheumatoid nodules, including pulmonary nodules; or Felty's syndrome, characterized by leukopenia and splenomegaly. This patient has a neuropathy secondary to rheumatoid vasculitis. Extra-articular manifestations including vasculitis are usually associated with high titers of rheumatoid factor. In the differential diagnosis of foot drop is a peroneal nerve compression caused by prolonged crossing of the legs or radiculopathy.

35–4, B. Learning objective: *Order appropriate tests for a new, significant neuropathy.* Nerve conduction test distinguishes a vasculitic neuropathy from a compression syndrome neuropathy. ESR is usually elevated in these patients, and rheumatoid factor is generally strongly positive.

35–4, C. Learning objective: *Choose appropriate treatment for this disorder.* Treat patients with neuropathy secondary to rheumatoid vasculitis with prednisone 60 mg/day and cyclophosphamide 1–2 mg/kg/day. Prednisone is gradually reduced. After three months of cyclophosphamide treatment, azathioprine can be substituted.

► SYSTEMIC LUPUS ERYTHEMATOSUS ANSWERS

35–5, A. Learning objective: *List the common causes of polyarticular symmetric inflammatory arthritis and recognize other features suggestive of lupus.* Possible causes of polyarticular symmetric joint inflammation include postviral arthritis, SLE, RA, and psoriatic or reactive arthritis. Other features of her presentation (oral ulcers, photosensitivity, pleuritis, spontaneous abortion) suggest lupus and are not characteristic of the other conditions on this list.

35–5, B. Learning objective: *Know and use diagnostic criteria for lupus.* This patient meets five criteria for lupus: oral ulcers, arthritis, photosensitivity, malar rash, and probable serositis (episodes of chest pain). If ANA is positive, lupus is a nearly certain diagnosis.

35–5, C. Learning objective: *Order appropriate labs to evaluate a patient with probable lupus.* Order ANA with autoantibody reflexive panel, CBC with differential, partial thromboplastin time (PTT), erythrocyte sedimentation rate (ESR), complement levels (C3, C4, and CH_{50}), RPR or VDRL, BUN, creatinine, and urinalysis. A positive ANA and anti–double-stranded DNA, in combination with her symptoms, make lupus highly likely. Low complement levels and elevated ESR suggest disease activity. Elevated BUN and creatinine, or active urine sediment, indicate renal involvement. Prolonged PTT or falsely positive VDRL or RPR suggests antiphospholipid antibody syndrome. CBC is important to detect thrombocytopenia, anemia, and leukopenia—all treatable complications of lupus. She has positive ANA and anti–double-stranded DNA, ESR of 50, and low complement level.

35–5, D. Learning objective: *Design appropriate therapy for mild lupus.* In choosing therapy, you must balance the risks and benefits of each medication. Because this patient has relatively mild disease (i.e., no serious or life-threatening organ involvement, such as rapidly progressing renal disease or psychosis), start with an NSAID and hydroxychloroquine (the least toxic medications). If she does not improve, consider adding low-dose steroids.

► VASCULITIS ANSWERS

35–6, A. Learning objective: *Recognize the presentation of giant cell arteritis.* The most likely diagnosis is giant cell arteritis, given the patient's age, morning shoulder stiffness and pain, likely temporal headache, and jaw claudication.

35–6, B. Learning objective: *Order appropriate diagnostic tests for temporal arteritis.* She needs an ESR to confirm the inflammatory nature of her symptoms and a temporal artery biopsy.

35–6, C. Learning objective: *Appropriately treat giant cell arteritis.* Prednisone in a dose of 40–60 mg/day is the usual therapy given in order to prevent blindness. People with jaw claudication are at increased risk of visual changes that can be permanent. Some physicians add low-dose aspirin to the regimen, at least initially.

35–7, A. Learning objective: *Recognize the presentation of small vessel vasculitis.* A patient with "rheumatoid arthritis" who does not really have RA but has polyarticular joint symptoms, along with palpable petechiae, should prompt one to consider hepatitis C infection. The use of IV drugs earlier in life is an important piece of history. Other causes of joint pain and petechiae could include lupus, hepatitis B, or endocarditis.

35–7, B. Learning objective: *Order appropriate diagnostic tests to look for hepatitis and endocarditis in patients with palpable purpura.* Liver function tests are not adequate in most cases. Serologies for hepatitis B and C with PCR confirm viral presence if hepatitis C is positive. A blood culture and a careful listen to the heart are helpful in endocarditis. Rheumatoid factor is commonly positive in hepatitis C patients as are cryoglobulins.

35–7, C. Learning objective: *Treat hepatitis C-associated vasculitis.* Treatment of hepatitis C is beyond the scope of this chapter, but for the associated small vessel vasculitis, such as the one presented, NSAIDs may be sufficient. If not, colchicine, low-dose prednisone, (less than 15 mg), hydroxychloroquine (400 mg/day), or dapsone may be effective in these patients.

▶ ALCOHOL ANSWERS

36–1, A. Learning objective: *State the common causes of abdominal pain associated with alcohol use.* Nausea, vomiting, low-grade fevers, and abdominal pain are likely caused by alcoholic hepatitis. Pancreatitis is also possible. Gastritis from alcohol use is less likely.

36–1, B. Learning objective: *Order appropriate tests for evaluating abdominal pain in a patient with history of alcohol abuse.* Order transaminases, bilirubin, amylase, alkaline phosphatase, and a CBC. If he has alcoholic hepatitis you would expect his AST to be two to three times greater than his ALT. Pancreatic amylase would be elevated if he has acute pancreatitis. A CBC identifies a low hematocrit (GI tract bleeding) and an elevated WBC (alcoholic hepatitis and pancreatitis). Consider a CXR to look for aspiration pneumonia.

36–1, C. Learning objective: *Understand common electrolyte disorders associated with heavy alcohol use.* Low magnesium, calcium, potassium, and phosphate levels are likely in the setting of chronic alcohol use.

36–2, A. Learning objective: *Recognize alcoholic ketoacidosis.* This patient has an anion gap acidosis in the setting of heavy alcohol use. Consider an ingestion of methanol or ethylene glycol in addition to alcoholic ketoacidosis in your differential. The lack of an osmolar gap makes those ingestions unlikely. Treat alcoholic ketoacidosis with fluid resuscitation containing glucose. Remember to check magnesium level, replace electrolytes, and give thiamine and multivitamin with folate.

36–2, B. Learning objective: *Treat alcohol withdrawal appropriately.* He should receive benzodiazepines in adequate doses possibly every two to four hours initially. He would probably also benefit from a β-blocker because he is tachycardic and hypertensive.

▶ DRUG USE ANSWERS

36–3, A. Learning objective: *Outline an appropriate drug history.* Questions about drug use should be integrated into the history-taking. Make sure your patient feels safe with you and sees you as nonjudgmental, respectful, and confidential. If she does not initially report injection drug use, ask her again, emphasizing that the information is essential in properly diagnosing and treating her arm infection.

36–3, B. Learning objective: *Describe the infectious complications of IV drug use.* This infection is probably cellulitis, an infection of the skin. Examine carefully for signs of abscess (area of fluctuance), septic arthritis (joint effusion and extreme pain on passive range of motion), osteomyelitis (changes on x-ray or bone scan), and/or endocarditis (high fever and sometimes a heart murmur).

36–3, C. Learning objective: *Treat IVDU-associated infections.* If this patient has cellulitis alone, has a fever lower than 38.5°C, and is able to tolerate food and medicine, prescribe oral dicloxacillin or cephalexin and arrange for a follow-up exam within a few days. Small abscesses may be drained in the office and treated the same way. Patients with large abscesses, septic arthritis, osteomyelitis, or endocarditis should be admitted for IV antibiotics and further evaluation. Patients with vomiting and dehydration likewise should be admitted. In either case, a drug-related infection is a situation in which your patient may be most motivated to start drug treatment. Consider counseling, screening, and vaccination for hepatitis A, B, and C, as well as HIV. Anticipate heroin withdrawal in daily users of this drug who are hospitalized.

36–4, A. Learning objective: *Describe opiate withdrawal.* You can expect that over a period of days this patient will develop some or all of these symptoms: dilated pupils, rhinorrhea, muscle cramps, bone and joint aches, abdominal cramps, nausea, vomiting, diarrhea, and piloerection. You would not expect him to have fever, tachycardia, or hypertension as a result of opiate withdrawal. These findings would require further evaluation.

36–4, B. Learning objective: *Devise an approach to a patient with chronic drug use.* You may be able to help this patient most by providing information and resources in a nonaccusatory, nonjudgmental way. Establishing trust over several visits and keeping appropriate boundaries with him will also help. Tapering the opiate dose slowly will minimize the withdrawal symptoms. Addressing the underlying addiction is essential.

▶ ABNORMAL PAP SMEARS ANSWERS

37–1, A. Learning objective: *Plan appropriate follow-up for a Pap smear showing ASCUS.* If HPV subtyping is available, and the result is positive for concerning HPV subtype, send directly for colposcopy. If the subtype is negative, or for all newly diagnosed ASCUS where subtyping is unavailable, follow-up with a repeat Pap smear in four to six months. If results are normal, she will need follow up Pap smears every four to six months until she has had three consecutive normals. If any subsequent Pap smear shows ASCUS or higher-grade changes, referral for colposcopy is required. The Pap test is a cytologic examination that only includes the cells on the surface of the cervix. These findings must be confirmed by tissue biopsy. Although this patient may consult a gynecologic oncologist if she wishes, her management requires colposcopy by a gynecologist to determine tissue diagnosis first.

37–1, B. Learning objective: *Describe the association of specific strains of HPV and cervical dysplasia.* HPV is strongly associated with cervical dysplasia. Certain strains of HPV, such as 16 and 18, have been associated with development of invasive cervical cancer. HPV DNA testing is not currently widely used in clinical practice. When available, HPV DNA testing is helpful primarily for identifying patients with newly diagnosed ASCUS whose test is positive, and who should therefore be referred directly for colposcopy, rather than returning for repeat Pap smear.

▶ ABNORMAL UTERINE BLEEDING ANSWERS

37–2, A. Learning objective: *Identify a clinical scenario suggestive of polycystic ovarian syndrome.* This patient's primary oligomenorrhea, hirsutism, obesity, and acanthosis nigricans are strongly suggestive of polycystic ovarian syndrome (PCOS). This is a poorly understood condition with heterogenous presentation. Despite the suggestive name, the anatomic finding of polycystic ovaries is variably present. There is a significant degree of controversy regarding the basic pathophysiologic mechanism of disease. Most experts agree that there is inappropriate feedback involving the ovarian-pituitary axis, leading to relative hyperandrogenism. An LH to FSH ratio of greater than 2:1 can be confirmatory, but its absence would not rule it out. It is not necessary to perform a pelvic ultrasound. A TSH and prolactin level should also be done to rule-out thyroid and pituitary disease.

37–2, B. Learning objective: *Recognize the association of insulin resistance and endometrial cancer in patients with PCOS.* Polycystic ovarian syndrome has been associated with insulin resistance and endometrial cancer. Exclude these by fasting glucose and endometrial monitoring by ultrasound or biopsy. Guidelines for frequency or mode of screening don't currently exist.

37–2, C. Learning objective: *Prescribe oral contraceptives to prevent unwanted pregnancy, regulate cycles, and prevent atypical endometrial changes.* Amenorrhea or oligomenorrhea can lead to endometrial hyperplasia and atypia. Patients with PCOS should receive oral contraceptive pills to help regulate endometrial shedding. This also protects against pregnancy, as infertility cannot be assumed. Patients who do not desire contraception may choose instead to use cyclic medroxyprogesterone to induce menstruation, every three months.

▶ BREAST HEALTH ANSWERS

37–3, A. Learning objective: *Design appropriate work-up for a breast lump.* Order diagnostic mammogram. Unless a clearly benign finding is noted, perform US and FNA.

37–3, B. Learning objective: *Plan follow-up when work-up for a breast lump is negative.* A negative "triple test"—physical exam without suspicious features, negative mammogram, and benign FNA—reduces, but does not eliminate, the possibility of cancer. Perform follow-up exams every three to six months for at least a year to assure stability.

37–3, C. Learning objective: *Recognize indications for referral of patients with abnormal breast findings.* Suspicious mammogram, US, or FNA should prompt early referral. Referral is also indicated if the mass enlarges over time.

37–4, A. Learning objective: *Identify the role of ultrasound in work-up of abnormal breast lesions.* US is useful, especially when mammogram is difficult to interpret due to high breast density. Alternately, FNA results may reveal a cyst or cytology consistent with a fibroadenoma.

37–4, B. Learning objective: *Appropriately manage a fibroadenoma.* Fibroadenomas are benign, disorganized breast tissue. Indications for removal are: size greater than 2 cm, rapid growth, and discomfort.

37–4, C. Learning objective: *Appropriately manage a simple breast cyst.* If US of the mass clearly demonstrates a simple cyst, no further follow-up is necessary. If the mass is bothersome to the patient or interferes with mammography or physical exam, aspirate under US guidance.

▶ MENOPAUSE ANSWERS

37–5, A. Learning objective: *Recognize that menopause is a clinical diagnosis.* No further testing is required.

37–5, B. Learning objective: *Design hormone replacement therapy for a perimenopausal woman.* A cyclic regimen might be preferred in women in the transition whose ovaries continue to produce some sex hormones at irregular intervals. It may be possible to regulate cycles by this regimen. Be sure to review risks and benefits before initiating HRT.

37–5, C. Learning objective: *Understand importance and method of evaluating out-of-phase or prolonged bleeding in a woman on HRT greater than six to 12 months.* Consider an endometrial biopsy or a pelvic ultrasound to evaluate the endometrial lining and rule-out hyperplasia, malignancy, or structural abnormality such as polyp or fibroid.

37–5, D. Learning objective: *Use progestin to stabilize endometrium.* If the endometrial biopsy and uterine ultrasound are normal, the next step is to increase progestin to foster transformation of the proliferating endometrium. Alternatively, very-low-dose birth control pills can be used to completely capture cycles and establish regular bleeding.

▶ OSTEOPOROSIS ANSWERS

37–6, A. Learning objective: *List osteoporosis risk factors.* This patient has several clear risk factors: weight less than 127 pounds, current smoking, and probable family history given her mother's posture—dowager's hump, or kyphosis, from chronic vertebral compression fractures. She does not exercise and most likely has low calcium intake because of her lactose intolerance.

37–6, B. Learning objective: *Be familiar with current NOF osteoporosis screening recommendations.* Screening recommendations vary, and the USPSTF is currently reviewing their screening recommendations. In the meantime, the NOF recommendations applied to this case are as follows: This patient is not older than age 65, when the NOF recommends all women should be screened for osteoporosis. She has several risk factors for osteoporosis and so should have been screened after age 50 some twelve years ago.

37–6, C. Learning objective: *State the best screening test for osteoporosis.* Dual-electron-X-ray absorptometry (DEXA) scan is the standardized test for osteoporosis. Other tests, such as urine metabolic markers of bone turnover or heel or wrist ultrasound, typically obtained at shopping malls, may indicate the possibility of osteoporosis, but are not reliable enough to direct treatment. Rather, their results may prompt the DEXA scan, which is the standardized measure of osteoporosis. Another option in this patient is to obtain a lateral CXR to screen for compression fractures. If present and no secondary cause is suspected (i.e., pathologic fracture of multiple myeloma), the fragility fracture makes the diagnosis of osteoporosis without a DEXA scan required.

37–6, D. Learning objective: *Identify nonpharmacologic measures for osteoporosis prevention.* The patient should stop smoking, which will decrease her risk for osteoporosis and potentially improve her reflux symptoms. She should begin weight-bearing exercise and start taking vitamin D and calcium daily.

37–7, A. Learning objective: *Interpret T-score result.* The T-score of –2.3 indicates 2.3 standard deviations below the average bone density of a 25-year-old white woman. This is consistent with osteopenia, which is defined as T-score between –1.0 and –2.5.

37–7, B. Learning objective: *Outline when to begin pharmacologic treatment in osteopenia.* Although this patient does not have osteoporosis, based on current NOF guidelines, treatment should be started because her T-score is less than –2.0. In fact, because of her risk factor of family history, therapy would be started for a T-score of only –1.5. These guidelines are under review and may become slightly more stringent. (Please see the NOF website at the end of the osteoporosis chapter for current recommendations.)

37–7, C. Learning objective: *Design pharmacologic treatment for osteoporosis in this patient with a history of deep venous thrombosis (DVT).* Because of this patient's history of DVT, hormone therapy is not appropriate. In her case, a bisphosphonate is an excellent choice. Alendronate at 70 mg a week is reasonable. As with all osteoporosis prevention and treatment, ascertain that the patient is getting adequate vitamin D, calcium, and weight-bearing exercise.

1. A 50-year-old healthy man has been recently diagnosed with hypertension. Other than his BP of 160/100, he has no concerning findings on physical exam. An ECG, urinalysis, basic chemistry panel, and lipid panel are normal. Despite a six-month course of nonpharmacologic management, his blood pressure remains elevated. Which class of antihypertensive medication would you choose for treatment based on existing evidence that it decreases morbidity and mortality from hypertension?

   A. Thiazide diuretics

   B. α-Blockers

   C. Calcium channel blockers

   D. Angiotensin receptor blockers

   E. Nitrates

2. A 70-year-old woman with hypertension reports shortness of breath, orthopnea, and paroxysmal nocturnal dyspnea. She reports no chest pain or syncope but has a cough producing frothy sputum. On exam HR is 104, BP 100/76, RR 26, and oxygen saturation is 92% on room air. Her JVP is 14 cm and she has bibasilar crackles, an S_3 and pitting edema to her knees bilaterally. Which of the following studies would you order next?

   A. Exercise treadmill test

   B. Cardiac catheterization

   C. Echocardiogram

   D. Coxsackie virus titers

   E. Persantine-thallium scan

3. A 59-year-old woman with COPD has been on prednisone 10 mg PO qd for two years. Seven days ago she developed a diarrheal illness that progressed to nausea and vomiting. She has not taken any medications for three days due to her nausea. Over the last twenty-four hours she has had two syncopal episodes as well as severe fatigue and weakness. Which of the following lab results would be most consistent with adrenal insufficiency?

   A. Random cortisol of 22 μg/dL

   B. Metabolic alkalosis

   C. Hyperglycemia

   D. Hypokalemia

   E. Hyponatremia

4. A 50-year-old alcoholic is found lying in an alley. He is brought to the ED. His alcohol level is three times the legal limit. Additional laboratory tests show a BUN of 71 and creatinine of 4.2, up from his baseline of 1.1. A urine dipstick shows 3+ blood but is otherwise negative. Urine microscopy shows no red or white blood cells but occasional renal tubular cells and muddy brown casts. The cause of his renal failure is most likely:

   A. Hepatitis B
   B. Hypotension
   C. Interstitial nephritis
   D. Rhabdomyolysis
   E. Urinary obstruction

5. A 33-year-old man is referred for a renal artery duplex as a part of a hypertension evaluation. The test comes back positive. The renal artery duplex is highly sensitive (92%) and specific (94%) for renal artery stenosis as a cause of hypertension. The incidence of renal artery stenosis in the population is 2%. Which of the following statements is accurate in interpreting the results of the test for the patient?

   A. The test rules in the diagnosis of renal artery stenosis because of its high sensitivity.
   B. The test rules out the diagnosis of renal artery stenosis because of its high specificity.
   C. The high sensitivity and specificity reliably predict the accuracy of the diagnosis.
   D. The low disease incidence results in a low positive predictive value for the test.
   E. The low disease incidence results in a low negative predictive value for the test.

6. A 42-year-old woman comes to clinic reporting that she has had three disabling headaches this month. She describes a regular pattern of unilateral throbbing with associated nausea and vomiting. The headache was so disabling that she has had to lie down. She is worried that she may have a brain tumor or stroke. What is the most likely cause of this headache?

   A. Subarachnoid hemorrhage
   B. Cluster headache
   C. Tension-type headache
   D. Migraine headache
   E. Brain tumor

7. A 36-year-old woman presents for evaluation of headache. She reports she has had headaches for the past 14 months, occurring at the occiput and sometimes behind her right eye. Medications: sertraline, OCP. Her physical exam, including neurologic exam, is normal. What testing would you recommend?

   A. ESR

   B. CT without contrast

   C. CT with contrast

   D. MRI

   E. No testing

8. A sexually active, athletic 23-year-old male comes to clinic with an exquisitely painful right knee. The patient reports that the knee has become progressively painful over the last day, and he notes swelling and warmth to the touch. Small amounts of knee flexion and extension cause extreme pain. What is the most appropriate initial diagnostic study?

   A. Knee films

   B. Arthrocentesis

   C. Uric acid

   D. CBC

   E. MRI

9. A 20-year-old college student presents to the student health service with sore throat, low-grade fever, and fatigue. Physical exam reveals bilateral lymphadenopathy of the neck, axilla, and groin. She has previously been in excellent health and reports no weight loss or night sweats. CBC and differential show many atypical lymphocytes. What is the most likely cause of this student's illness?

   A. Gonorrhea

   B. Human immunodeficiency virus

   C. Mononucleosis

   D. Hodgkin's disease

   E. Herpes simplex virus

10. A 34-year-old man with a long history of alcohol abuse presents to clinic with nausea and abdominal pain. He has been drinking heavily (beer and vodka) for the past three weeks but stopped yesterday because of severe pain and nausea. What abnormalities would you expect to see?

    A. Low phosphate, high magnesium, low bicarbonate, high amylase, high calcium

B. Low phosphate, low magnesium, low bicarbonate, high amylase, low calcium

C. High phosphate, high magnesium, high bicarbonate, high amylase, low calcium

D. Low phosphate, low magnesium, high bicarbonate, normal amylase, low calcium

E. High phosphate, low magnesium, low bicarbonate, high amylase, high calcium

11. A 72-year-old World War II veteran is hospitalized with congestive heart failure. He develops pain involving the great toe shortly after admission. The toe appears red and warm and is extremely painful to the touch. He informs you that this is probably a recurrence of his gout. Which medication would you choose in initially treating this patient?

    A. Indomethacin

    B. Prednisone

    C. Allopurinol

    D. Probenecid

    E. Do not treat without arthrocentesis

12. A 45-year-old man comes to clinic for a general physical exam. You note that he was diagnosed with ulcerative colitis at age 25. He reports that he has not had much problem with the colitis over the years. He denies melena, hematochezia, or change in stool pattern. The most appropriate recommendation for colorectal cancer screening in this patient is:

    A. Annual digital rectal exam

    B. Annual stool occult blood testing

    C. Flexible sigmoidoscopy

    D. Colonoscopy

    E. Delay screening until age 50

13. A 40-year-old woman has a WBC of 40,000 and a high serum leukocyte alkaline phosphatase score. What is the most appropriate next step in her work-up?

    A. Referral for possible bone marrow transplant

    B. Infection work-up

    C. Begin hydroxyurea

    D. Chromosome analysis

    E. Bone marrow biopsy

14. A 65-year-old man presents with hemoptysis, dyspnea, and cough. He recently quit smoking. CXR demonstrates a mediastinal mass. CT scan confirms the mass and an additional lesion is found in the liver. A biopsy of the mediastinal mass confirms a diagnosis of non–small-cell lung cancer. What is the most appropriate intervention at this point?

    A. Begin chemotherapy
    B. Referral for surgical resection
    C. Biopsy of the liver lesion
    D. Further staging including head CT and bone scan
    E. Referral for hospice services

15. An unstable patient is airlifted to your medical center. The referring physician notes that the patient had a metabolic acidosis. The osmolar gap was 15, and oxalate crystals were seen in the urine. The most likely cause of this patient's acidosis is:

    A. Uremia
    B. Aspirin ingestion
    C. Ketoacidosis
    D. Sepsis
    E. Ethylene glycol ingestion

16. A 43 year-old woman with a 23-year history of type 1 diabetes is seen in clinic with fatigue and postprandial nausea. Laboratory test results are as follows: Na 136, Cl 112, K 5.3, HCO_3 14, BUN 16, Cr 1.3, Glu 146, Hb_{alc} 6.8. What is the most likely cause for the patient's low HCO_3?

    A. Diabetic ketoacidosis
    B. Renal tubular acidosis
    C. Lactic acidosis
    D. Recurrent vomiting
    E. Aspirin ingestion

17. A 23-year-old man is noted to have sudden onset of nausea, vomiting, and headache. He appears lethargic and has difficulty answering questions. You consider the diagnosis of encephalitis. What is the most appropriate intervention at this point?

    A. Begin IV acyclovir
    B. Lumbar puncture
    C. Head CT
    D. EEG
    E. MRI

18. A 49-year-old man has worsening hypertension over the past six months. Home blood pressure readings have been 180-200/100-110. Three years ago, he had a normal blood pressure reading. His physical exam is unremarkable. Laboratory test results are reading as follows: Na 138, K 2.9, BUN 10, Cr 1.2, and Glu 90. A renal duplex scan is negative. What would be the next best step?

    A. No testing, treat essential hypertension

    B. Aldosterone/renin ratio

    C. 24-hour urine catecholamines

    D. TSH

    E. Abdominal CT scan

19. A 29-year-old alcoholic man presents with fever, headache, and mental status changes. His physical examination is significant for nuchal rigidity, a Kernig's sign, and disorientation on mental status examination. Laboratory tests reveal HCT 36, MCV 104, and WBC 23,000. What organism is the most likely cause of his symptoms?

    A. *Streptococcus pneumoniae*

    B. *Neisseria meningitidis*

    C. *Haemophilus influenzae*

    D. *Listeria monocytogenes*

    E. Coxsackie virus

20. A 65-year-old smoker has an HDL cholesterol of 30 and an LDL cholesterol of 170. You advise him that his cholesterol is too high and suggest which of the following?

    A. A goal LDL of 160

    B. Step 1 Diet with the goal of lowering his cholesterol to 130

    C. Mild to moderate consumption of alcohol to raise his HDL cholesterol

    D. A goal LDL cholesterol of 100

    E. Repeat cholesterol screening every five years

21. A 64-year-old man comes to your clinic for follow-up after being hospitalized eight weeks ago for a "small heart attack." He has stopped smoking, started walking 2 miles daily, watches his diet carefully, and "feels terrific." He is taking atenolol 25 mg and an aspirin daily. He asks you if he should do anything else. A complete fasting lipid panel was obtained: Total cholesterol is 198, triglycerides 95, LDL 132, and HDL 30. Which of the following treatments would you recommend?

A. Continue diet and exercise therapy for another six months.
B. Simvastatin 20 mg qd
C. Niacin 2–3 gm per day in divided doses
D. Gemfibrozil 600 mg bid
E. Cholestyramine 4 gm bid with meals

22. A 72-year-old man with a history of hypertension and hyperlipidemia presents with four hours of substernal chest pressure radiating to his left arm. He also reports nausea and
sweatiness. On examination, his BP is 100/74, HR is 98, and
RR is 22. He is pale and diaphoretic and has a II/VI systolic
murmur and clear lungs. An ECG shows normal sinus rhythm
with 3-mm ST elevations in leads V2-V4 compared to an ECG
two months ago that was normal. His CXR shows no infiltrates
or cardiomegaly. The next most appropriate course of action
would be:

A. Obtain an echocardiogram to evaluate his murmur.
B. Give aspirin and thrombolytics if there are no
contraindications.
C. Give aspirin, start heparin, and a β-blocker, and rule-out
for a myocardial infarction.
D. Give aspirin, and start heparin and a calcium channel
blocker for unstable angina.
E. Order a ventilation/perfusion scan to evaluate for a
pulmonary embolus.

23. A 70-year-old woman with a history of advanced osteoarthritis of her knees and hips presents with chest pressure, which
occurs with emotional distress and exertion. The chest pressure does not radiate, and she has no associated dyspnea.
ECG shows left bundle branch block. What diagnostic test
would be most helpful?

A. Exercise treadmill test
B. Exercise treadmill with thallium
C. Echocardiogram
D. Dipyridamole (Persantine) thallium
E. Exercise echocardiogram

24. A 44-year-old alcoholic man reports sharp epigastric pain radiating to his back. He has had similar pains in his epigastrium
for years that are exacerbated by alcohol use. The patient's
current symptoms started after a seven-day binge and have
been increasing over the last three weeks. The symptoms have
markedly intensified in the past 24 hours. Initially the pain was

improved by eating but it is now constant. He states that he has also been having loose stools, which are now black in color. Which of the following abdominal x-ray findings would be most worrisome given his likely diagnosis?

A. Subdiaphragmatic "free" air

B. Multiple pancreatic calcifications

C. Dilated small bowel with air-fluid levels

D. Markedly dilated colon

E. Pneumatosis intestinalis (air in the bowel wall)

25. A 50-year-old woman with a history of heavy alcohol use presents to her primary care physician with new onset abdominal swelling. She denies any pain or fever. On physical exam her BP is 96/70, HR is 110, and she has evidence of shifting dullness in the abdomen. The most appropriate way to evaluate the cause of her ascites is:

A. Abdominal CT scan

B. Abdominal ultrasound

C. Pelvic ultrasound

D. Paracentesis

E. Colonoscopy

26. A 45-year-old man with long-standing cirrhosis due to hepatitis B comes to clinic to establish care. He denies any weight loss, abdominal swelling, or pain. Which of the following tumor markers would be the best screen for hepatocellular carcinoma?

A. β-HCG

B. CEA

C. α-Fetoprotein

D. CA 125

E. BrCA-1

27. A 69-year-old man with a history of COPD is hospitalized in an intensive care unit with respiratory failure. He is on a ventilator for five days. On the sixth day, he becomes febrile and a blood culture reveals *Pseudomonas aeruginosa*. Which antibiotic has the best pseudomonal coverage?

A. Trimethoprim-sulfamethoxazole

B. Ceftriaxone

C. Ampicillin/sulbactam

D. Ceftazidime

E. Vancomycin

28. A 72-year-old man presents for evaluation of his fatigue. He states that he drinks one fifth of whiskey each day and has a poor diet. Laboratory tests show a hematocrit of 28 with an MCV of 109. Which of the following would you expect to see on his peripheral blood smear?

    A. Schistocytes

    B. Tear Drops

    C. Döhle bodies

    D. Hypersegmented neutrophils

    E. Spherocytes

29. A 40-year-old woman reports a cough for the last eight months. She does not smoke or take any medications, and she reports no fever or hemoptysis. Over the last year, she has gained 20 pounds because her new job does not allow time for exercise. Her cough tends to be worse after dinner and when she is trying to go to sleep at night. She recently stopped drinking alcohol and thinks that the cough improved some after stopping. Which of the following is the most appropriate initial therapy based on her history?

    A. Azithromycin

    B. Diphenhydramine

    C. Nasal steroid spray

    D. Albuterol metered-dose inhaler

    E. Omeprazole

30. A 32-year-old woman complains of cough for one week associated with a runny nose, pressure in her ears, fever to 38°C, and muscle aches. Her ear pressure, fever, and myalgias have resolved, but her cough is keeping her awake at night. Guaifenesin cough syrup has not helped. On examination, vital signs are normal and ears and lungs are normal. Throat shows cobblestoning. The best treatment is:

    A. Azithromycin for five days

    B. Amoxicillin for five days

    C. Albuterol MDI as needed

    D. Codeine cough syrup

    E. Fexofenadine as needed

31. A 23-year-old woman with a history of allergies presents in March with a cough worse with exercise that has bothered her all winter. She has not had a recent URI and is otherwise well. Examination shows a healthy, thin woman with normal vital signs, normal HEENT and lung exam, and skin exam shows a red, scaling rash on her fingers and the back of one

hand, which she attributes to her job as a housecleaner. The best thing to do first is:

A. Order a CXR.
B. Start ranitidine at bedtime.
C. Order PFTs with methacholine challenge test.
D. Start albuterol 30 minutes before exercise.
E. Start nasal steroids and diphenhydramine.

32. A 33-year-old woman reports intermittent loose stools for the past year. Her symptoms are associated with crampy abdominal pain and a bloating sensation. Defecation seems to relieve the discomfort. She has not noticed any blood in her stool. When her symptoms are flaring, she sometimes needs to have five to seven bowel movements a day to control the discomfort. Between episodes, however, she is often constipated. The most likely cause of this patient's diarrhea is:

A. Inflammatory bowel disease
B. Irritable bowel syndrome
C. *Giardia lamblia* infection
D. Lactose intolerance
E. Celiac sprue

33. A 72-year-old woman reports two weeks of episodic dizziness. She describes the room "spinning in circles" when she gets in and out of bed or if she looks up toward the ceiling. The episodes typically last less than 2 minutes. She denies any hearing problems or tinnitus. On examination, a Hallpike-Dix maneuver produces rotary nystagmus. The most likely cause of this patient's symptoms is:

A. Benign positional vertigo
B. Acute labyrinthitis
C. Meniere's syndrome
D. Brain stem ischemia
E. Acoustic neuroma

34. A 58-year-old man with a history of a myocardial infarction presents with lightheadedness and palpitations. He takes aspirin and a β-blocker and occasionally needs a sublingual nitroglycerin tablet for exertional chest pain. His rhythm strip is shown below:

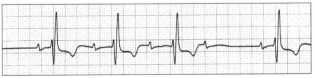

This rhythm is best described as:

A. First-degree AV nodal block
B. Second-degree AV nodal block, Mobitz type I (Wenckebach)

602

Practice Test

C. Second-degree AV nodal block, Mobitz type II

D. Third-degree nodal block

E. Junctional rhythm

35. A 30-year-old man presents with chest pain. He describes the pain as crushing substernal chest pressure radiating to his left arm. It started one hour after eating lunch and is associated with nausea and sweatiness. On examination, he is pale and diaphoretic but has normal vital signs and a normal heart and lung examination. An ECG during the exam is normal, but his pain improves ten minutes after taking a sublingual nitroglycerin tablet. The most likely cause of this patient's chest pain is:

A. Myocardial infarction

B. Pulmonary embolus

C. Esophageal spasm

D. Aortic dissection

E. Pericarditis

36. A 59-year-old Peruvian woman reports nausea and achy epigastric pain for the last two months. She does not drink alcohol or take any medications and has not had any vomiting or diarrhea. *H. pylori* serology is positive. Which of the following causes of dyspepsia will respond to *H. pylori* eradication?

A. Gastroesophageal reflux disease

B. Irritable bowel syndrome

C. Chronic pancreatitis

D. Diabetic gastroparesis

E. Peptic ulcer disease

37. A 31-year-old construction worker reports that she feels tired all the time. She has trouble getting through the workday and worries that she may have a serious illness. Her fatigue has worsened since she was recently promoted to foreman, a job that involves longer work hours and a higher stress level. Which of the following symptoms are concerning for a physical rather than a psychological cause of her fatigue?

A. Symptoms relieved by sleep

B. Symptoms increased during periods of stress

C. Symptoms better later in the day

D. Symptoms for the last ten months

E. Symptoms that began at the time her father died

38. A 50-year-old woman with long-standing alcohol abuse and cirrhosis presents with hematemesis. Her BP is 120/80, her HR is 95, and she has spider telangiectasias, palmar erythema, and splenomegaly. Her hematocrit is 28. An EGD shows bleeding esophageal varices that are successfully banded. She improves over the next several days in the hospital and is able to be discharged home. In addition to abstinence from alcohol, what is the best prophylaxis against a repeat variceal bleed?

   A. Omeprazole
   B. Lisinopril
   C. Perphenazine
   D. Nadolol
   E. Cisapride

39. A 31-year-old woman presents with pain and swelling in her wrists and hands. She also has pain in the ball of her foot. She has a history of pneumococcal pneumonia with sepsis one year ago and two prior spontaneous abortions in the past four years. On examination, she has spongy, tender swelling in the wrists and MCP and MTP joints. Laboratory test results are as follows: HCT 33, platelets 114,000, BUN 20, Cr 1.2, and urinalysis 2+ protein with 10–30 red cells/high power field. Which lab test is the most likely to confirm a diagnosis?

   A. ANA
   B. Rheumatoid factor
   C. ESR
   D. c-ANCA
   E. Total complement (CH50)

40. A 40-year-old man presents to establish health care. He has no chronic diseases and has had no preventive health screening. Review of systems reveals no concerning symptoms, and his physical examination is normal. Which of the following screening tests would be most appropriate to do in this patient?

   A. Prostate specific antigen
   B. *Helicobacter pylori* serologies
   C. Total cholesterol
   D. Fecal occult blood test
   E. Flexible sigmoidoscopy

41. A 50-year-old man reports pain in his lower back since lifting a heavy crate. He rested and took ibuprofen without relief. He

has restricted his activity and is worried that he may not be able to ski this winter because of his pain. Which of the following would be most concerning for a dangerous cause of this patient's low back pain?

A. New onset of marked constipation

B. No improvement after two weeks of ibuprofen

C. No relief with weekly chiropractic intervention

D. Pain in the lower back with straight leg raise

E. Worsened symptoms after seven days of bed rest

42. A 43-year-old female injection drug user presents with fever, right upper quadrant pain, and diarrhea. She has been sharing needles but has no history of hepatitis or HIV. On examination, she is jaundiced and has tenderness in her right upper quadrant. Her AST is 468, her ALT is 650, and serologies are consistent with hepatitis B infection. Which of the following statements about hepatitis B virus is most correct?

A. Approximately 80% of patients with hepatitis B develop chronic infection.

B. HB_eAg indicates increased infectivity.

C. HB_cIgM indicates chronic infection.

D. HBV requires coinfection with hepatitis D virus to replicate.

E. HBV infection does not respond to alpha-interferon treatment.

43. A 20-year-old man with C3 HIV disease (CD_4 count 29/viral load 23,000) returns to clinic for discussion of therapy options. He has previously taken AZT, then ddI monotherapy. He is interested in treatment and has not missed previous clinic visits. What therapy do you recommend?

A. Lamivudine (3TC) + zidovudine (AZT)

B. Stavudine (D4T) + lamivudine (3TC)

C. Indinavir + zidovudine (AZT) + didanosine (DDI)

D. Nelfinavir + stavudine (D4T) + lamivudine (3TC)

E. Zidovudine (AZT) + stavudine (D4T) + zalcitabine (ddC)

44. A 32-year-old HIV-positive patient reports difficult and painful swallowing for three days. Her CD_4 count was 100 last month, but she has done well other than occasional oral thrush. She takes trimethoprim/sulfamethoxazole, D4T, 3TC, and nelfinavir. Her examination is remarkable for a temperature of 38.5°C and oral thrush. The most likely cause of this patient's symptoms is:

A. Hairy leukoplakia

B. CMV esophagitis

C. HSV esophagitis

D. Candidal esophagitis

E. D4T related esophageal ulcerations

45. A 25-year-old woman presents with four days of dysuria and frequency. She has had no fevers or flank pain. She has one sexual partner with no new partners in the past 12 months. Physical examination is unremarkable. What test(s) should be ordered?

    A. Urinalysis

    B. Urinalysis and urine culture

    C. Urinalysis, urine culture, and chlamydia culture

    D. Urinalysis, urine culture, gonorrhea culture, and chlamydia culture

    E. Urine culture

46. A 37-year-old man with C3 HIV disease and a history of injection drug use presents with fever, weight loss, and nonproductive cough. He has adenopathy in the axilla and neck. His CXR shows bilateral hilar and paratracheal adenopathy. No infiltrates are present. What is the most likely cause?

    A. *Pneumocystis carinii*

    B. Sarcoidosis

    C. *Mycobacterium tuberculosis*

    D. Endocarditis

    E. Persistent generalized lymphadenopathy

47. A 41-year-old man with a long history of recurrent sinusitis reports a new episode of nasal discharge, cough, and fatigue. On physical examination, he has crusted blood in the nares and a tender right maxillary sinus with opacification on transillumination. CXR reveals bilateral nodules. Laboratory test results are as follows: HCT 33, WBC 10,000, BUN 33, Cr 2.6, and urinalysis shows 2+ protein, 0–3 WBCs, and 30–50 RBCs. What test is the most likely to explain his sinus disease and laboratory findings?

    A. ANA

    B. Anticardiolipin antibody

    C. ESR

    D. c-ANCA

    E. CEA

48. A 27-year-old elementary school teacher is seen for evaluation of fever and cough. She has had a nonproductive cough for the past five days, myalgias, sore throat, and fevers (T_{max} 101.8°F). On examination, she has rhonchi and wheezes in the right lower lobe. Laboratory test results are as follows: WBC 10.8, HCT 37, and CXR shows a subsegmental right lower lobe infiltrate. What is the most likely organism?

    A. *Haemophilus influenzae*

    B. Influenza A

    C. Mixed anaerobes

    D. *Mycoplasma pneumoniae*

    E. *Streptococcus pneumoniae*

49. A 79-year-old woman presents with fever, nausea, vomiting, jaundice, and right upper quadrant pain. Laboratory test results are as follows: bilirubin 2.5, alkaline phosphatase 360, and WBC 23,000. Ultrasound shows gallstones and dilated common bile duct. What is the most appropriate course of action?

    A. Consult surgery for urgent cholecystectomy

    B. Treat with IV azithromycin

    C. Treat with IV cefazolin

    D. Treat with IV ampicillin

    E. Consult a gastroenterologist for emergent ERCP

50. A 33-year-old injection drug user presents with a three-day history of cough, fever, and pleuritic chest pain. Cardiac examination reveals a grade II/VI systolic murmur, normal skin examination, and bilateral rhonchi on chest auscultation. CXR shows bilateral, patchy peripheral infiltrates. What test is most important for making a diagnosis?

    A. Three sets of blood cultures

    B. Chest CT scan

    C. Sputum Gram stain

    D. Echocardiogram

    E. Sputum culture

51. A 33-year-old woman presents with fatigue and weight gain. She reports a family history of hypothyroidism. Which set of clinical features would be most consistent with hypothyroidism?

    A. Macroglossia, tachypnea, increased CPK, amenorrhea

    B. Amenorrhea, bradycardia, increased cholesterol, cool skin

    C. Macroglossia, tachycardia, increased cholesterol, menorrhagia

D. Menorrhagia, increased CPK, increased cholesterol, carpal tunnel syndrome

E. Amenorrhea, decreased cholesterol, bradycardia, macroglossia

52. A 47-year-old obese man presents for annual examination. He reports a family history of type 2 diabetes. A screening fasting blood glucose is 200. He begins a diet, loses 10 pounds over three months, and a repeat fasting blood glucose is 160 with an Hb_{alc} of 7.8. Cholesterol is 220 with triglycerides of 400 and HDL 30. What is the best initial therapy for this patient?

A. Insulin

B. Metformin

C. Metformin + sulfonylurea

D. Rosiglitazone

E. Sulfonylurea + troglitazone

53. A 45-year-old woman with type I diabetes for 18 years presents as a new patient for evaluation. Her physical examination is remarkable for nonproliferative diabetic retinopathy and a BP of 146/92. Laboratory test results are as follows: Hgb_{alc} 7.0, BUN 12, Cr 0.8, and urinalysis shows trace protein. What would you recommend for this patient?

A. Follow blood pressure, no treatment at this time

B. Begin hydrochlorothiazide

C. Begin ACE inhibitor

D. Begin calcium channel blocker

E. Begin β-blocker

54. A 34-year-old pregnant woman from Cambodia who is in her second trimester presents with increasing dyspnea on exertion. She has also coughed up occasional bloody sputum. On examination, she has a low-pitched diastolic murmur heard best at the apex. What is the most likely diagnosis?

A. Bacterial pneumonia

B. Primary pulmonary hypertension

C. Aortic regurgitation

D. Aortic stenosis

E. Mitral stenosis

55. A 25-year-old man with HIV infection and a CD_4 count of 100 presents with fever, headache, and mild photophobia. Funduscopic examination reveals normal optic discs, and the patient has a nonfocal neurologic examination. Diagnostic evaluation should begin with which of the following?

A. Lumbar puncture

B. Head CT scan

C. Monitor clinical symptoms

D. Begin IV acyclovir

E. Begin IV amphotericin

56. A 54-year-old man presents to the hospital with a six-month history of fever, night sweats, and weight loss. CT scan reveals evidence of multiple tumors confined above the diaphragm. Biopsy reveals low-grade lymphoma. What is the correct stage of this patient's non-Hodgkin's lymphoma?

A. I

B. IB

C. II

D. IIB

E. IIIB

57. A 55-year-old man with type 2 diabetes reports progressive lower-extremity pain over the last three months. The pain is bilateral and varies from being a burning pain to an uncomfortable tingling sensation. It started in his feet and has progressed to involve both ankles. The pain is most bothersome at night. On examination, an ankle/brachial index is 1.1, and he has decreased vibration and proprioception in his feet. What is the most likely cause of this patient's leg pain?

A. Peripheral vascular disease

B. Venous obstruction

C. Nocturnal cramps

D. Multiple myeloma

E. Diabetic peripheral neuropathy

58. A 30-year-old female smoker reports three days of left lower extremity swelling. She denies any trauma to the leg and states that in the last day it has started aching as well. She has also developed a low-grade temperature but denies chills, sweats, or rash. Which of the following would increase her risk of deep venous thrombosis the most?

A. Corticosteroid therapy

B. History of asthma

C. History of myocardial infarction

D. History of nephrotic syndrome

E. Laparoscopic cholecystectomy

59. A 31-year-old man undergoes HIV testing because his partner is newly HIV positive; he is found to be HIV positive by ELISA and by Western blot. He has no symptoms, and his examination is normal. Which of the following statements is correct regarding the initial management of this patient?

    A. Start azithromycin prophylaxis against *Mycobacterium avium* if his CD-count is less than 50.

    B. Start trimethoprim-sulfamethoxazole prophylaxis against *Pneumocystis* if his CD_4 count is less than 500.

    C. Check an HIV viral load only when the patient becomes symptomatic.

    D. Start AZT monotherapy if his CD_4 count is less than 200

    E. Check a p24 antigen to verify the ELISA and Western blot results.

60. A 73-year-old woman is seen for evaluation of urinary incontinence. She reports she is unable to make it to the bathroom in time to urinate. She has frequent (three to four) episodes of incontinence each day. She does not have problems with incontinence when coughing or sneezing. Her only other medical problem is long-standing hypertension that is treated with an ACE inhibitor. What would you recommend?

    A. Pelvic muscle exercises

    B. An α-blocker (doxazosin)

    C. Bladder muscle relaxant (oxybutynin)

    D. Hydrochlorothiazide

    E. Stop ACE inhibitor.

61. A 26-year-old female with asthma presents with increasing symptoms. She reports that she has had to increase use of her β-agonist inhaler from once a week six months ago to once or twice a day. She started using a corticosteroid inhaler one month ago and has not noticed much improvement. Her medical history includes migraine headaches of recent onset and depression. Medications: albuterol two puffs prn, beclomethasone inhaler four puffs twice a day, ibuprofen 400mg tid, sertraline 50mg qd. What would you recommend?

    A. Increase potency of inhaled steroid to fluticasone

    B. Scheduled albuterol use instead of prn

    C. Add a leukotriene inhibitor

    D. Allergy testing

    E. Stop ibuprofen

PRACTICE **TEST** ANSWERS

1. **A** (31—Hypertension)
2. **C** (24—Congestive heart failure)
3. **E** (26—Adrenal disorders)
4. **D** (31—Acute renal failure)
5. **D** (6—How to interpret sensitivity and specificity)
6. **D** (17—Headache)
7. **E** (17—Headache)
8. **B** (19—Joint pain)
9. **C** (22—Lymphadenopathy)
10. **B** (36—Alcohol)
11. **B** (35—Gout)
12. **D** (29—Colon Cancer)
13. **B** (29—Leukemia)
14. **D** (29—Lung Cancer)
15. **E** (31—Acid Base Disturbances)
16. **B** (31—Acid Base Disturbances)
17. **A** (30—Encephalitis)
18. **B** (31—Hypertension)
19. **A** (30—Meningitis)
20. **B** (26—Hyperlipidemia)
21. **B** (26—Hyperlipidemia)
22. **B** (24—Ischemic heart disease)
23. **D** (24—Ischemic heart disease)
24. **A** (6—How to read an abdominal film)
25. **D** (6—How to perform basic procedures and body fluid analysis)
26. **C** (6—How to interpret abnormal laboratory tests)
27. **D** (6—How to use antibiotics)
28. **D** (8—Anemia)
29. **E** (10—Cough)
30. **C** (10—Cough)
31. **D** (10—Cough)
32. **B** (11—Diarrhea)
33. **A** (12—Dizziness and syncope)
34. **B** (24—Common cardiac arrhythmias)

35. **C** (9—Chest pain)
36. **E** (13—Dyspepsia)
37. **A** (15—Fatigue)
38. **D** (16—Gastrointestinal bleeding)
39. **A** (35—Systemic lupus erythematosus)
40. **C** (18—Healthy patients)
41. **A** (20—Low back pain)
42. **B** (27—Liver disease)
43. **D** (30—HIV infection primary care)
44. **D** (30—HIV infection complications)
45. **A** (30—Urinary tract infections)
46. **C** (30—Tuberculosis)
47. **D** (35—Vasculitis)
48. **D** (30—Pneumonia)
49. **E** (27—Biliary tract disease)
50. **A** (30—Endocarditis)
51. **D** (26—Thyroid Disease)
52. **B** (26—Diabetes)
53. **C** (26—Diabetes)
54. **E** (24—Valvular heart disease)
55. **B** (30—Meningitis)
56. **D** (29—Non-Hodgkin's lymphoma)
57. **E** (21—Lower extremity pain)
58. **D** (21—Lower extremity swelling)
59. **A** (30—HIV infection primary care)
60. **C** (28—Geriatrics)
61. **E** (34—Asthma)

Appendix I

Important Drug Side Effects

Symptom	Associated Medications
Constipation	Antihistamines Calcium Calcium channel blockers (non-dihydropyridines > dihydropyridines*) Iron Narcotics Tricyclic antidepressants
Diarrhea	Antibiotics β-blockers Colchicine Digoxin Magnesium-containing antacids Metformin Milk of magnesia SSRIs
Edema	Calcium channel blockers, dihydropyridines Estrogen NSAIDs Pioglitazone Progesterone Rosiglitazone Testosterone
Urinary Retention	Calcium channel blockers Sedating antihistamines (diphenhydramine, chlorpheniramine) Tricyclic antidepressants
Confusion	Antidepressants Benzodiazepines H_2 blockers Narcotics NSAIDs (rare) Quinolones Oxybutinin Sedating antihistamines (diphenhydramine, chlorpheniramine)

*Non-dihydropyridines = diltiazem, verapamil
Dihydropyridines = amlodipine, felodipine, nifedipine

Appendix II

Common Drug-related Changes in Electrolytes and Glucose

Bicarbonate

Decreased	Nucleoside reverse transcriptase inhibitor
	Metformin
Increased	Corticosteroids
	Diuretics (especially thiazides)

Calcium

Increased	Thiazide diuretics

Glucose

Increased	Niacin, protease inhibitors, corticosteroids, megestrol

Magnesium

Decreased	Diuretics, amphotericin B, cisplatin

Potassium

Decreased	Diuretics, both thiazide and loop
	Carbiplatinum/cisplatinum
	Corticosteroids, especially fludrocortisone
	Gentamicin, tobramycin
Increased	ACE inhibitors
	Cyclosporine
	NSAIDs
	Potassium-sparing diuretics
	TMP/SMX

Sodium

Decreased	ACE inhibitors
	Antidepressants (SSRI > TCAs)
	Carbamazepine, valproic acid
	Chlorpropamide
	Cyclophosphamide
	Neuroleptics
	Thiazide diuretics
Increased	Lithium (via nephrogenic DI)

Index

Note: Page numbers followed by f refer to figures; those followed by t refer to tables, and those followed by b refer to boxed material.

630